Injury & Trauma Sourcebook

Learning Disabilities Sourcebook,
2nd Edition

Leukemia Sourcebook

Liver Disorders Sourcebook

Lung Disorders Sourcebook

Medical Tests Sourcebook, 2nd Edition

Men's Health Concerns Sourcebook,
2nd Edition

Mental Health Disorders Sourcebook,
3rd Edition

Mental Retardation Sourcebook

Movement Disorders Sourcebook

Muscular Dystrophy Sourcebook

Obesity Sourcebook

Osteoporosis Sourcebook

Pain Sourcebook, 2nd Edition

Pediatric Cancer Sourcebook

Physical & Mental Issues in Aging
Sourcebook

Podiatry Sourcebook, 2nd Edition

Pregnancy & Birth Sourcebook,
2nd Edition

Prostate Cancer Sourcebook

Prostate & Urological Disorders
Sourcebook

Rehabilitation Sourcebook

Respiratory Diseases & Disorders
Sourcebook

Sexually Transmitted Diseases
Sourcebook, 3rd Edition

Sleep Disorders Sourcebook,
2nd Edition

Smoking Concerns Sourcebook

Sports Injuries Sourcebook, 3rd Edition

Stress-Related Disorders Sourcebook

Stroke Sourcebook

Substance Abuse Sourcebook

Surgery Sourcebook

Thyroid Disorders Sourcebook

Transplantation Sourcebook

Traveler's Health Sourcebook

Urinary Tract & Kidney Diseases &
Disorders Sourcebook, 2nd Edition

Vegetarian Sourcebook

Women's Health Concerns Sourcebook,
2nd Edition

Workplace Health & Safety Sourcebook

Worldwide Health Sourcebook

Teen Health Series

Abuse & Violence Information
for Teens

Alcohol Information for Teens

Allergy Information for Teens

Asthma Information for Teens

Body Information for Teens

Cancer Information for Teens

Complementary & Alternative
Medicine Information for
Teens

Diabetes Information for Teens

Diet Information for Teens,
2nd Edition

Drug Information for Teens,
2nd Edition

Eating Disorders Information
for Teens

Fitness Information for Teens

Learning Disabilities Information
for Teens

Mental Health Information for
Teens, 2nd Edition

Pegnancy Information for Teens

Sexual Health Information for
Teens

Skin Health Information for
Teens

Sports Injuries Information
for Teens

Suicide Information for Teens

Tobacco Information for Teens

Endocrine and Metabolic Disorders SOURCEBOOK

Second Edition

Health Reference Series

Second Edition

Endocrine and Metabolic Disorders SOURCEBOOK

Basic Consumer Health Information about Hormonal and Metabolic Disorders that Affect the Body's Growth, Development, and Functioning, Including Disorders of the Pancreas, Ovaries and Testes, and Pituitary, Thyroid, Parathyroid, and Adrenal Glands, with Facts about Growth Disorders, Addison Disease, Cushing Syndrome, Conn Syndrome, Diabetic Disorders, Multiple Endocrine Neoplasia, Inborn Errors of Metabolism, and More

Along with Information about Endocrine Functioning, Diagnostic and Screening Tests, a Glossary of Related Terms, and Directories of Additional Resources

Edited by
Joyce Brennfleck Shannon

Omnigraphics

P.O. Box 31-1640 • Detroit, MI 48231-1640

Bibliographic Note

Because this page cannot legibly accommodate all the copyright notices, the Bibliographic Note portion of the Preface constitutes an extension of the copyright notice.

Edited by Joyce Brennfleck Shannon

Health Reference Series

Karen Bellenir, *Managing Editor*
David A. Cooke, M.D., *Medical Consultant*
Elizabeth Collins, *Research and Permissions Coordinator*
Cherry Stockdale, *Permissions Assistant*
EdIndex, Services for Publishers, *Indexers*

* * *

Omnigraphics, Inc.

Matthew P. Barbour, *Senior Vice President*
Kay Gill, *Vice President—Directories*
Kevin Hayes, *Operations Manager*
David P. Bianco, *Marketing Director*

* * *

Peter E. Ruffner, *Publisher*

Frederick G. Ruffner, Jr., *Chairman*

Copyright © 2007 Omnigraphics, Inc.

ISBN 978-0-7808-0952-9

Library of Congress Cataloging-in-Publication Data

Endocrine and metabolic disorders sourcebook : basic consumer health information about hormonal and metabolic disorders that affect the body's growth, development, and functioning, including disorders of the pancreas, ovaries and testes, and pituitary, thyroid, parathyroid, and adrenal glands, with facts about growth disorders, Addison disease, Cushing syndrome, Conn syndrome, diabetic disorders, multiple endocrine neoplasia, inborn errors of metabolism, and more; along with information about endocrine functioning, diagnostic and screening tests, a glossary of related terms, and directories of additional resources / edited by Joyce Brennfleck Shannon. -- 2nd ed.
  p. cm. -- (Health reference series)
  Includes bibliographical references and index.
  Summary: "Provides basic consumer health information about diagnosis and treatment of endocrine system and metabolic function disorders. Includes index, glossary of related terms, and other resources"--Provided by publisher.
  ISBN 978-0-7808-0952-9 (hardcover : alk. paper) 1. Endocrine glands--Diseases-- Popular works. 2. Metabolism--Disorders--Popular works. I. Shannon, Joyce Brennfleck.
  RC648.E418 2007
  616.4--dc22
                                                                          2007018894

This book is printed on acid-free paper meeting the ANSI Z39.48 Standard. The infinity symbol that appears above indicates that the paper in this book meets that standard.

Printed in the United States

Table of Contents

Visit www.healthreferenceseries.com to view *A Contents Guide to the Health Reference Series*, a listing of more than 13,000 topics and the volumes in which they are covered.

Part II: The Pituitary Gland and Growth Disorders

Part III: Thyroid and Parathyroid Gland Disorders

Part IV: Adrenal Gland Disorders

Part V: Pancreatic and Diabetic Disorders

Part VI: Disorders of the Ovaries and Testes

Part VII: Other Disorders of Endocrine and Metabolic Functioning

Part VIII: Additional Help and Information

Preface

About This Book

The endocrine system includes the pituitary, adrenal, and thyroid glands, the pancreas, and the ovaries and testes. These glands secrete hormones that regulate metabolism, the process that supplies the body's cells with energy. Abnormal levels of hormones, whether too high or too low, disrupt normal functioning and compromise health. Sometimes the symptoms of dysfunction appear so gradually they are hardly noticed. Hypothyroidism, for example, can remain undetected for years. Other disruptions, such as diabetic shock, can appear suddenly, progress quickly, and be life threatening.

Endocrine and Metabolic Disorders Sourcebook, Second Edition provides updated information about the endocrine system and its role in the regulation of human growth, organ function, and metabolic control. Readers will learn about growth disorders, hypothyroidism, diabetic disorders, Addison disease, Cushing syndrome, pheochromocytoma, multiple endocrine neoplasia type 1, inborn errors of metabolism, and other disorders, including facts about symptoms, diagnosis, and treatment. A glossary and directories of resources provide additional help and information.

Readers seeking more information about some of the topics in this book may wish to consult these additional volumes in Omnigraphics' *Health Reference Series*:

- Thyroid and parathyroid disorders: *Thyroid Disorders Sourcebook, First Edition*

- Diabetic and pancreatic disorders: *Diabetes Sourcebook, Third Edition*

- Ovarian disorders: *Women's Health Concerns, Second Edition*

- Disorders of the testes: *Men's Health Concerns Sourcebook, First Edition*

- Hereditary disorders and syndromes: *Genetic Disorders Sourcebook, First Edition*

How to Use This Book

This book is divided into parts and chapters. Parts focus on broad areas of interest. Chapters are devoted to single topics within a part.

Part I: Endocrine Functioning and Metabolism describes the endocrine system, the various endocrine glands and their hormones, and the processes of metabolism and energy balance. Chemicals that disrupt the endocrine process are discussed. Individual chapters explain prenatal tests, newborn screening, and genetic counseling.

Part II: The Pituitary Gland and Growth Disorders discusses growth disorders in children and adults. It explains the evaluation process and the use of growth hormone therapy. It also describes pituitary tumors, prolactinomas, and other diseases related to the pituitary gland, including acromegaly, Cushing disease, and diabetes insipidus.

Part III: Thyroid and Parathyroid Gland Disorders offers facts about proper thyroid functioning and common dysfunctions, including thyroiditis, Hashimoto thyroiditis, hypothyroidism, hyperthyroidism, Graves disease, and thyroid nodules. It also describes disorders of the parathyroid glands and discusses related cancers.

Part IV: Adrenal Gland Disorders provides facts about diseases of adrenal insufficiency, including Addison disease, Conn syndrome, Cushing syndrome, and pheochromocytoma, along with information about adrenal gland cancer and congenital adrenal conditions. The management of adrenal insufficiency and the use of laparoscopic techniques for adrenal gland removal are also described.

Part V: Pancreatic and Diabetic Disorders provides information about pancreas function tests and the management of pancreatitis, insulin resistance, diabetes mellitus, and hypoglycemia. Facts about pancreatic and islet cell cancer and Zollinger-Ellison syndrome are also included.

Part VI: Disorders of the Ovaries and Testes describes disorders that result when sex gland hormone production is not balanced. These include hypogonadism, gynecomastia, menstrual problems, polycystic ovarian syndrome, premature ovarian failure, and precocious puberty.

Part VII: Other Disorders of Endocrine and Metabolic Functioning presents information about inherited enzyme deficiencies and other syndromes and diseases that result from, or impact, hormonal and metabolic processes.

Part VIII: Additional Help and Information includes a glossary of related terms, a guide to resources for children with special needs, and a directory of organizations able to provide more information about endocrine and metabolic disorders.

Bibliographic Note

This volume contains documents and excerpts from publications issued by the following U.S. government agencies: National Cancer Institute (NCI); NCI Surveillance Epidemiology and End Results (SEER); National Human Genome Research Institute; National Institute of Child Health and Human Development (NICHD); National Institute of Diabetes and Digestive and Kidney Diseases (NIDDK); National Institute of Environmental and Health Sciences (NIEHS); National Institute of Neurological Disorders and Stroke (NINDS); National Institute on Aging (NIA); National Institutes of Health (NIH) Clinical Center; National Library of Medicine; and National Women's Health Information Center (NWHIC).

In addition, this volume contains copyrighted documents from the following organizations: A.D.A.M, Inc.; American Academy of Family Physicians; American Academy of Otolaryngology–Head and Neck Surgery; American Association for Clinical Chemistry; American Association of Clinical Endocrinologists; American Heart Association; American Liver Foundation; American Thyroid Association; BSCS; Children's Hospital and Regional Medical Center; Cleveland Clinic; Hormone Foundation; Magic Foundation; Muscular Dystrophy Association–USA; National Adrenal Diseases Foundation; National Marrow Donor Program; National Newborn Screening and Genetics Resource Center; National Organization for Rare Disorders (NORD); National Urea Cycle Disorders Foundation; Nemours Foundation; Society of American Gastrointestinal Endoscopic Surgeons (SAGES); Thyroid Foundation of America; and Washington State Department of Health–Newborn Screening Program.

Full citation information is provided on the first page of each chapter or section. Every effort has been made to secure all necessary rights to reprint the copyrighted material. If any omissions have been made, please contact Omnigraphics to make corrections for future editions.

Acknowledgements

In addition to the listed organizations, agencies, and individuals who have contributed to this *Sourcebook*, special thanks go to managing editor Karen Bellenir, research and permissions coordinator Liz Collins, and document engineer Bruce Bellenir for their help and support.

About the Health Reference Series

The *Health Reference Series* is designed to provide basic medical information for patients, families, caregivers, and the general public. Each volume takes a particular topic and provides comprehensive coverage. This is especially important for people who may be dealing with a newly diagnosed disease or a chronic disorder in themselves or in a family member. People looking for preventive guidance, information about disease warning signs, medical statistics, and risk factors for health problems will also find answers to their questions in the *Health Reference Series*. The *Series*, however, is not intended to serve as a tool for diagnosing illness, in prescribing treatments, or as a substitute for the physician/patient relationship. All people concerned about medical symptoms or the possibility of disease are encouraged to seek professional care from an appropriate health care provider.

A Note about Spelling and Style

Health Reference Series editors use *Stedman's Medical Dictionary* as an authority for questions related to the spelling of medical terms and the *Chicago Manual of Style* for questions related to grammatical structures, punctuation, and other editorial concerns. Consistent adherence is not always possible, however, because the individual volumes within the *Series* include many documents from a wide variety of different producers and copyright holders, and the editor's primary goal is to present material from each source as accurately as is possible following the terms specified by each document's producer. This sometimes means that information in different chapters or sections may follow other guidelines and alternate spelling authorities. For example, occasionally a copyright holder may require that eponymous terms be shown in possessive forms (Crohn's disease *vs.* Crohn disease) or that British spelling norms be retained (leukaemia *vs.* leukemia).

Locating Information within the Health Reference Series

The *Health Reference Series* contains a wealth of information about a wide variety of medical topics. Ensuring easy access to all the fact sheets, research reports, in-depth discussions, and other material contained within the individual books of the *Series* remains one of our highest priorities. As the *Series* continues to grow in size and scope, however, locating the precise information needed by a reader may become more challenging.

A Contents Guide to the Health Reference Series was developed to direct readers to the specific volumes that address their concerns. It presents an extensive list of diseases, treatments, and other topics of general interest compiled from the Tables of Contents and major index headings. To access *A Contents Guide to the Health Reference Series*, visit www.healthreferenceseries.com.

Medical Consultant

Medical consultation services are provided to the *Health Reference Series* editors by David A. Cooke, M.D. Dr. Cooke is a graduate of Brandeis University, and he received his M.D. degree from the University of Michigan. He completed residency training at the University of Wisconsin Hospital and Clinics. He is board-certified in Internal Medicine. Dr. Cooke currently works as part of the University of Michigan Health System and practices in Brighton, MI. In his free time, he enjoys writing, science fiction, and spending time with his family.

Our Advisory Board

We would like to thank the following board members for providing guidance to the development of this *Series*:

- Dr. Lynda Baker,
  Associate Professor of Library and Information Science,
  Wayne State University, Detroit, MI

- Nancy Bulgarelli,
  William Beaumont Hospital Library, Royal Oak, MI

- Karen Imarisio,
  Bloomfield Township Public Library, Bloomfield Township, MI

- Karen Morgan,
  Mardigian Library, University of Michigan-Dearborn,
  Dearborn, MI

- Rosemary Orlando,
  St. Clair Shores Public Library, St. Clair Shores, MI

Health Reference Series *Update Policy*

The inaugural book in the *Health Reference Series* was the first edition of *Cancer Sourcebook* published in 1989. Since then, the *Series* has been enthusiastically received by librarians and in the medical community. In order to maintain the standard of providing high-quality health information for the layperson the editorial staff at Omnigraphics felt it was necessary to implement a policy of updating volumes when warranted.

Medical researchers have been making tremendous strides, and it is the purpose of the *Health Reference Series* to stay current with the most recent advances. Each decision to update a volume is made on an individual basis. Some of the considerations include how much new information is available and the feedback we receive from people who use the books. If there is a topic you would like to see added to the update list, or an area of medical concern you feel has not been adequately addressed, please write to:

Editor
Health Reference Series
Omnigraphics, Inc.
615 Griswold Street
Detroit, MI 48226
E-mail: editorial@omnigraphics.com

Part One

Endocrine Functioning and Metabolism

Chapter 1

Introduction to the Endocrine System

The endocrine system, along with the nervous system, functions in the regulation of body activities. The nervous system acts through electrical impulses and neurotransmitters to cause muscle contraction and glandular secretion. The effect is of short duration, measured in seconds, and localized. The endocrine system acts through chemical messengers called hormones that influence growth, development, and metabolic activities. The action of the endocrine system is measured in minutes, hours, or weeks, and is more generalized than the action of the nervous system.

There are two major categories of glands in the body—exocrine and endocrine.

- **Exocrine glands** have ducts that carry their secretory product to a surface. These glands include the sweat, sebaceous and mammary glands, and the glands that secrete digestive enzymes.

- **Endocrine glands** do not have ducts to carry their product to a surface. They are called ductless glands. The word endocrine is derived from the Greek terms *endo*, meaning within, and *krine*, meaning to separate or secrete. The secretory products of endocrine glands are called hormones and are secreted directly into

This chapter includes "Introduction to the Endocrine System," and "Endocrine Glands and Their Hormones," from National Cancer Institute–Surveillance Epidemiology and End Results (NCI-SEER), 2000. The text was reviewed in February 2007 by Dr. David A. Cooke, M.D., Diplomate, American Board of Internal Medicine.

the blood. Hormones are then carried throughout the body where they influence only those cells that have receptor sites for that hormone.

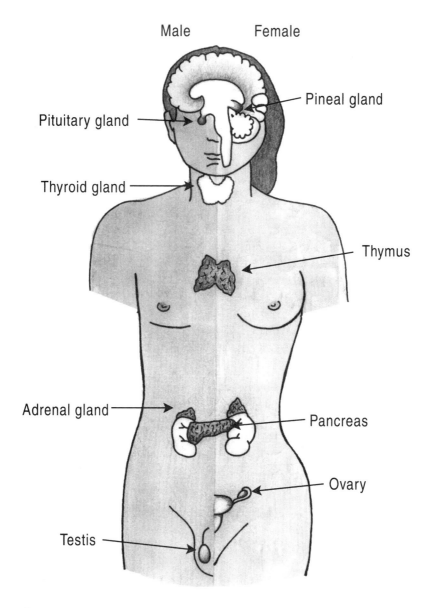

Figure 1.1. *Endocrine Organs of the Human Body (Source: NCI–SEER, redrawn for Omnigraphics by Alison DeKleine, 2007.)*

Endocrine Glands and Their Hormones

The endocrine system is made up of the endocrine glands that secrete hormones. Although there are eight major endocrine glands scattered throughout the body, they are still considered to be one system because they have similar functions, similar mechanisms of influence, and many important interrelationships.

Some glands also have non-endocrine regions that have functions other than hormone secretion. For example, the pancreas has a major exocrine portion that secretes digestive enzymes and an endocrine portion that secretes hormones. The ovaries and testes secrete hormones and also produce the ova and sperm. Some organs, such as the stomach, intestines, and heart, produce hormones, but their primary function is not hormone secretion.

Pituitary Gland

The pituitary gland or hypophysis is a small gland about one centimeter in diameter or the size of a pea. It is nearly surrounded by bone as it rests in the sella turcica, a depression in the sphenoid bone. The gland is connected to the hypothalamus of the brain by a slender stalk called the infundibulum.

There are two distinct regions in the gland: the anterior lobe (adenohypophysis) and the posterior lobe (neurohypophysis). The activity of the adenohypophysis is controlled by releasing hormones from the hypothalamus. The neurohypophysis is controlled by nerve stimulation.

Hormones of the Anterior Lobe (Adenohypophysis)

Growth hormone is a protein that stimulates the growth of bones, muscles, and other organs, by promoting protein synthesis. This hormone drastically affects the appearance of an individual because it influences height. If there is too little growth hormone in a child, that person may become a pituitary dwarf of normal proportions but small stature. An excess of the hormone in a child results in an exaggerated bone growth, and the individual becomes exceptionally tall or a giant.

Thyroid-stimulating hormone, or thyrotropin, causes the glandular cells of the thyroid to secrete thyroid hormone. When there is a hypersecretion of thyroid-stimulating hormone, the thyroid gland enlarges and secretes too much thyroid hormone.

Adrenocorticotropic hormone reacts with receptor sites in the cortex of the adrenal gland to stimulate the secretion of cortical hormones, particularly cortisol.

Gonadotropic hormones react with receptor sites in the gonads, or ovaries and testes, to regulate the development, growth, and function of these organs.

Prolactin hormone promotes the development of glandular tissue in the female breast during pregnancy and stimulates milk production after the birth of the infant.

Hormones of the Posterior Lobe (Neurohypophysis)

Antidiuretic hormone promotes the reabsorption of water by the kidney tubules resulting in less water being lost as urine. This mechanism conserves water for the body. Insufficient amounts of antidiuretic hormone cause excessive water loss in the urine.

Oxytocin causes contraction of the smooth muscle in the wall of the uterus. It also stimulates the ejection of milk from the lactating breast.

Pineal Gland

The pineal gland, also called pineal body or epiphysis cerebri, is a small cone-shaped structure that extends posteriorly from the third ventricle of the brain. The pineal gland consists of portions of neurons, neuroglial cells, and specialized secretory cells called pinealocytes. The pinealocytes synthesize the hormone melatonin and secrete it directly into the cerebrospinal fluid which takes it into the blood. Melatonin affects reproductive development and daily physiologic cycles.

Thyroid Gland

The thyroid gland is a very vascular organ that is located in the neck. It consists of two lobes, one on each side of the trachea, just below the larynx, or voice box. The two lobes are connected by a narrow band of tissue called the isthmus. Internally, the gland consists of follicles which produce thyroxine and triiodothyronine hormones. These hormones contain iodine.

About 95 percent of the active thyroid hormone is thyroxine, and most of the remaining five percent is triiodothyronine. Both of these require iodine for their synthesis. Thyroid hormone secretion is regulated by a negative feedback mechanism that involves the amount of circulating hormone, hypothalamus, and adenohypophysis.

If there is an iodine deficiency, the thyroid cannot make sufficient hormone. This stimulates the anterior pituitary to secrete thyroid-stimulating hormone which causes the thyroid gland to increase in size in a vain attempt to produce more hormones. But, it cannot produce more hormones because it does not have the necessary raw material, iodine. This type of thyroid enlargement is called simple goiter or iodine deficiency goiter.

Calcitonin is secreted by the parafollicular cells of the thyroid gland. This hormone opposes the action of the parathyroid glands by reducing the calcium level in the blood. If blood calcium becomes too high, calcitonin is secreted until calcium ion levels decrease to normal.

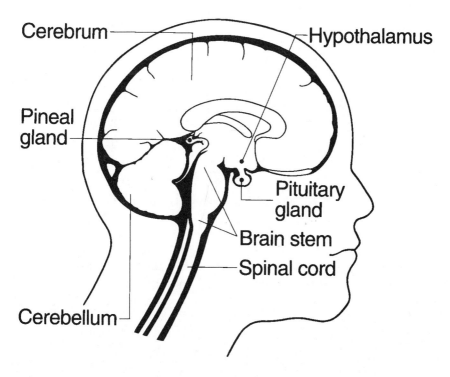

Figure 1.2. Pituitary and Pineal Glands (Source: National Cancer Institute, 2001)

Parathyroid Gland

Four small masses of epithelial tissue are embedded in the connective tissue capsule on the posterior surface of the thyroid glands. These are parathyroid glands, and they secrete parathyroid hormone or parathormone. Parathyroid hormone is the most important regulator of blood calcium levels. The hormone is secreted in response to low blood calcium levels, and its effect is to increase those levels.

Hypoparathyroidism, or insufficient secretion of parathyroid hormone, leads to increased nerve excitability. The low blood calcium levels trigger spontaneous and continuous nerve impulses which then stimulate muscle contraction.

Adrenal Gland

The adrenal, or suprarenal, gland is paired with one gland located near the upper portion of each kidney. Each gland is divided into an outer cortex and an inner medulla. The cortex and medulla of the adrenal gland, like the anterior and posterior lobes of the pituitary, develop from different embryonic tissues and secrete different hormones. The adrenal cortex is essential to life, but the medulla may be removed with no life-threatening effects.

The hypothalamus of the brain influences both portions of the adrenal gland but by different mechanisms. The adrenal cortex is regulated by negative feedback involving the hypothalamus and adrenocorticotropic hormone; the medulla is regulated by nerve impulses from the hypothalamus.

Hormones of the Adrenal Cortex

The adrenal cortex consists of three different regions with each region producing a different group or type of hormones. Chemically, all the cortical hormones are steroid.

Mineralocorticoids are secreted by the outermost region of the adrenal cortex. The principal mineralocorticoid is aldosterone which acts to conserve sodium ions and water in the body. Glucocorticoids are secreted by the middle region of the adrenal cortex. The principal glucocorticoid is cortisol which increases blood glucose levels.

The third group of steroids secreted by the adrenal cortex is the gonad corticoids, or sex hormones. These are secreted by the innermost region. Male hormones called androgens, and female hormones called estrogens are secreted in minimal amounts in both sexes by the adrenal cortex, but their effect is usually masked by the hormones from the testes and ovaries. In females, the masculinization effect of androgen secretion may become evident after menopause when estrogen levels from the ovaries decrease.

Hormones of the Adrenal Medulla

The adrenal medulla develops from neural tissue and secretes two hormones, epinephrine and norepinephrine. These two hormones are secreted in response to stimulation by sympathetic nerve, particularly during stressful situations. A lack of hormones from the adrenal medulla produces no significant effects. Hypersecretion, usually from a tumor, causes prolonged or continual sympathetic responses.

Pancreas

The pancreas is a long, soft organ that lies transversely along the posterior abdominal wall, posterior to the stomach, and extends from the region of the duodenum to the spleen. This gland has an exocrine portion that secretes digestive enzymes that are carried through a duct to the duodenum. The endocrine portion consists of the pancreatic islets which secrete glucagons and insulin.

Alpha cells in the pancreatic islets secrete the hormone glucagons in response to a low concentration of glucose in the blood. Beta cells in the pancreatic islets secrete the hormone insulin in response to a high concentration of glucose in the blood.

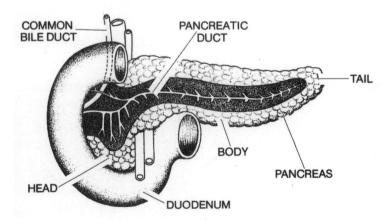

Figure 1.3. Anatomy of the Pancreas (Source: National Cancer Institute)

Gonads: Primary Reproductive Organs

The gonads, the primary reproductive organs, are the testes in the male and the ovaries in the female. These organs are responsible for producing the sperm and ova, but they also secrete hormones and are considered to be endocrine glands.

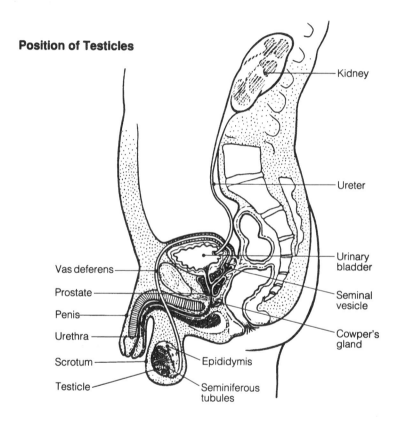

Position of Testicles

Kidney

Ureter

Vas deferens

Prostate

Penis

Urethra

Scrotum

Testicle

Epididymis

Seminiferous tubules

Urinary bladder

Seminal vesicle

Cowper's gland

Figure 1.4. Male Reproductive Anatomy (Source: National Cancer Institute)

Testes

Male sex hormones, as a group, are called androgens. The principal androgen is testosterone which is secreted by the testes. A small amount is also produced by the adrenal cortex. Production of testosterone begins during fetal development, continues for a short time after birth, nearly ceases during childhood, and then resumes at puberty. This steroid hormone is responsible for:

- growth and development of the male reproductive structures;
- increased skeletal and muscular growth;
- enlargement of the larynx accompanied by voice changes;
- growth and distribution of body hair; and
- increased male sexual drive.

Testosterone secretion is regulated by a negative feedback system that involves releasing hormones from the hypothalamus and gonadotropins from the anterior pituitary.

Ovaries

Two groups of female sex hormones are produced in the ovaries, the estrogens and progesterone. These steroid hormones contribute to the development and function of the female reproductive organs and sex characteristics. At the onset of puberty, estrogen promotes:

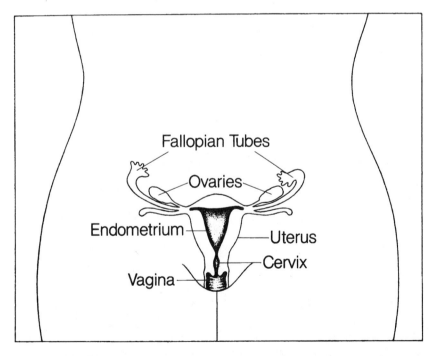

Figure 1.5. *Female Reproductive Anatomy (Source: National Cancer Institute)*

- development of the breasts;
- distribution of fat evidenced in the hips, legs, and breast; and
- maturation of reproductive organs such as the uterus and vagina.

Progesterone causes the uterine lining to thicken in preparation for pregnancy. Together, progesterone and estrogens are responsible for the changes that occur in the uterus during the female menstrual cycle.

Other Endocrine Glands

In addition to the major endocrine glands, other organs have some hormonal activity as part of their function. These include the thymus, stomach, small intestines, heart, and placenta.

The thymus gland produces thymosin which plays an important role in the development of the body's immune system.

The lining of the stomach, the gastric mucosa, produces a hormone called gastrin in response to the presence of food in the stomach. This hormone stimulates the production of hydrochloric acid and the enzyme pepsin which are used in the digestion of food.

The mucosa of the small intestine secretes the hormones secretin and cholecystokinin. Secreting stimulates the pancreas to produce a bicarbonate-rich fluid that neutralizes the stomach acid. Cholecystokinin stimulates contraction of the gallbladder which releases bile. It also stimulates the pancreas to secrete digestive enzyme.

The heart also acts as an endocrine organ in addition to its major role of pumping blood. Special cells in the wall of the upper chambers of the heart, called atria, produce a hormone called atrial natriuretic hormone, or atriopeptin.

The placenta develops in the pregnant female as a source of nourishment and gas exchange for the developing fetus. It also serves as a temporary endocrine gland. One of the hormones it secretes is human chorionic gonadotropin which signals the mother's ovaries to secrete hormones to maintain the uterine lining, so that it does not degenerate and slough off in menstruation.

Chapter 2

Endocrine Gland Hormones

Chapter Contents

Section 2.1

Hormone Characteristics and Functions

"Characteristics of Hormones," from National Cancer Institute–Surveillance Epidemiology and End Results (NCI-SEER), 2000. Updated in February 2007 by Dr. David A. Cooke, M.D., Diplomate, American Board of Internal Medicine.

Chemical Nature of Hormones

Chemically, hormones may be classified as either proteins or steroids. All of the hormones in the human body, except the sex hormones and those from the adrenal cortex, are proteins or protein derivatives.

Mechanism of Hormone

Action hormones are carried by the blood throughout the entire body, yet they affect only certain cells. The specific cells that respond to a given hormone have receptor sites for that hormone. This is sort of a lock and key mechanism. If the key fits the lock, then the door will open. If a hormone fits the receptor site, then there will be an effect. If a hormone and a receptor site do not match, then there is no reaction. All the cells that have receptor sites for a given hormone make up the target tissue for that hormone. In some cases, the target tissue is localized in a single gland or organ. In other cases, the target tissue is diffuse and scattered throughout the body so that many areas are affected. Hormones bring about their characteristic effects on target cells by modifying cellular activity.

Most **protein hormones** react with receptors on the surface of the cell, and the sequence of events that results in hormone action is relatively rapid. Steroid hormones typically react with receptor sites inside a cell. Because this method of action actually involves synthesis of proteins, it is relatively slow.

Control of Hormone Action

Hormones are very potent substances, which means that very small amounts of a hormone may have profound effects on metabolic processes.

Because of their potency, hormone secretion must be regulated within very narrow limits in order to maintain homeostasis in the body.

Many hormones are controlled by some form of a negative feedback mechanism. In this type of system, a gland is sensitive to the concentration of a substance that it regulates. A negative feedback system causes a reversal of increases and decreases in body conditions in order to maintain a state of stability or homeostasis. Some endocrine glands secrete hormones in response to other hormones. The hormones that cause secretion of other hormones are called tropic hormones. A hormone from gland A causes gland B to secrete its hormone. A third method of regulating hormone secretion is by direct nervous stimulation. A nerve stimulus causes gland A to secrete its hormone.

Section 2.2

Hormones Regulate the Digestive Process

Excerpts from "Your Digestive System and How It Works," National Institute of Diabetes and Digestive and Kidney Diseases (NIDDK), NIH Publication No. 04–2681, May 2004.

The digestive system is a series of hollow organs joined in a long, twisting tube from the mouth to the anus. Inside this tube is a lining called mucosa. In the mouth, stomach, and small intestine, the mucosa contains tiny glands that produce juices to help digest food.

Two solid organs, the liver and the pancreas, produce digestive juices that reach the intestine through small tubes. In addition, parts of other organ systems (for instance, nerves and blood) play a major role in the digestive system.

Why is digestion important?

When we eat such things as bread, meat, and vegetables, they are not in a form that the body can use as nourishment. Our food and drink must be changed into smaller molecules of nutrients before they can be absorbed into the blood and carried to cells throughout the body. Digestion is the process by which food and drink are broken down into their smallest parts so that the body can use them to build and nourish cells and to provide energy.

How is food digested?

Digestion involves the mixing of food, its movement through the digestive tract, and the chemical breakdown of the large molecules of food into smaller molecules. Digestion begins in the mouth, when

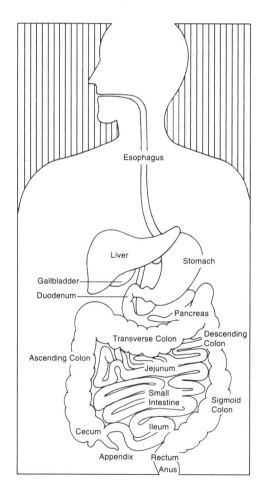

Figure 2.1. The Digestive System

we chew and swallow, and is completed in the small intestine. The chemical process varies somewhat for different kinds of food.

Production of Digestive Juices

The glands that act first are in the mouth—the salivary glands. Saliva produced by these glands contains an enzyme that begins to digest the starch from food into smaller molecules.

The next set of digestive glands is in the stomach lining. They produce stomach acid and an enzyme that digests protein. One of the unsolved puzzles of the digestive system is why the acid juice of the stomach does not dissolve the tissue of the stomach itself. In most people, the stomach mucosa is able to resist the juice, although food and other tissues of the body cannot.

After the stomach empties the food and juice mixture into the small intestine, the juices of two other digestive organs mix with the food to continue the process of digestion. One of these organs is the pancreas. It produces a juice that contains a wide array of enzymes to break down the carbohydrate, fat, and protein in food. Other enzymes that are active in the process come from glands in the wall of the intestine or even a part of that wall.

The liver produces yet another digestive juice—bile. The bile is stored between meals in the gallbladder. At mealtime, it is squeezed out of the gallbladder into the bile ducts to reach the intestine and mix with the fat in our food. The bile acids dissolve the fat into the watery contents of the intestine, much like detergents that dissolve grease from a frying pan. After the fat is dissolved, it is digested by enzymes from the pancreas and the lining of the intestine.

Control and Regulation of the Digestive System

Hormone Regulators

A fascinating feature of the digestive system is that it contains its own regulators. The major hormones that control the functions of the digestive system are produced and released by cells in the mucosa of the stomach and small intestine. These hormones are released into the blood of the digestive tract, travel back to the heart and through the arteries, and return to the digestive system where they stimulate digestive juices and cause organ movement.

The hormones that control digestion are gastrin, secretin, and cholecystokinin (CCK):

- **Gastrin** causes the stomach to produce an acid for dissolving and digesting some foods. It is also necessary for the normal growth of the lining of the stomach, small intestine, and colon.

- **Secretin** causes the pancreas to send out a digestive juice that is rich in bicarbonate. It stimulates the stomach to produce pepsin, an enzyme that digests protein, and it also stimulates the liver to produce bile.

- **CCK** causes the pancreas to grow and to produce the enzymes of pancreatic juice, and it causes the gallbladder to empty.

Additional hormones in the digestive system regulate appetite:

- **Ghrelin** is produced in the stomach and upper intestine in the absence of food in the digestive system and stimulates appetite.

- **Peptide YY** is produced in the GI tract in response to a meal in the system and inhibits appetite. Both of these hormones work on the brain to help regulate the intake of food for energy.

Nerve Regulators

Two types of nerves help to control the action of the digestive system. Extrinsic (outside) nerves come to the digestive organs from the unconscious part of the brain or from the spinal cord. They release a chemical called acetylcholine and another called adrenaline. Acetylcholine causes the muscle of the digestive organs to squeeze with more force and increase the push of food and juice through the digestive tract. Acetylcholine also causes the stomach and pancreas to produce more digestive juice. Adrenaline relaxes the muscle of the stomach and intestine and decreases the flow of blood to these organs.

Even more important, though, are the intrinsic (inside) nerves which make up a very dense network embedded in the walls of the esophagus, stomach, small intestine, and colon. The intrinsic nerves are triggered to act when the walls of the hollow organs are stretched by food. They release many different substances that speed up or delay the movement of food and the production of juices by the digestive organs.

Section 2.3

Can Hormones Prevent Aging?

"Pills, Patches, and Shots: Can Hormones Prevent Aging?"
National Institute on Aging (NIA), updated December 29, 2005.

We could not survive without hormones. They are among the most common and vital chemical messengers in the body. From head to toe, each moment of life, they signal cells to perform tasks that range from the ordinary to the extraordinary. Among their many roles, hormones help regulate body temperature, blood pressure, and blood sugar levels. In childhood, they help us grow up. In the teen years, they are the driving force behind puberty. But what influence, if any, the natural decline in some hormones has on the aging process in middle and late life is unclear. Although a few proponents are convinced that hormone supplements can favorably alter the aging process and have advocated their widespread use, the scientific evidence supporting this premise is, for the most part, sketchy.

For more than a decade, the National Institute on Aging (NIA), a component of the Federal Government's National Institutes of Health, has supported and conducted studies of replenishing hormones to find out if they may help reduce frailty and improve function in older people. These studies have focused on hormones known to decline as we grow older:

- dehydroepiandrosterone (DHEA),
- growth hormone,
- melatonin,
- testosterone, and
- menopausal hormones, such as estrogen and progesterone.

The results from these NIA-sponsored studies and other research projects likely will improve our understanding of the pros and cons of hormone supplementation. Until the results of these studies are compiled, analyzed, and a consensus among scientists is reached, recommendations to use supplemental hormones and hormone-like molecules to influence the aging process and health problems associated with aging should be viewed with skepticism. It is not yet known, for instance, how much is too much or too little, and when or whether hormone supplements should be taken at all.

What Is a Hormone?

Hormones are powerful chemicals that help keep our bodies working normally. The term hormone is derived from the Greek word, *hormo*, which means to set in motion. And that is precisely what hormones do in the body. They stimulate, regulate, and control the function of various tissues and organs. Made by specialized groups of cells within structures called glands, hormones are involved in almost every biological process including sexual reproduction, growth, metabolism, and immune function. These glands, including, the pituitary, thyroid, adrenals, ovaries and testes, release various hormones into the body as needed.

Levels of some hormones like parathyroid hormone which helps regulate calcium levels in the blood and bone, actually increase as a normal part of aging and may be involved in bone loss leading to osteoporosis. But the levels of a number of other hormones, such as testosterone in men and estrogen in women, tend to decrease over time. In other cases, the body may fail to make enough of a hormone due to diseases and disorders that can develop at any age. When this occurs, hormone supplements—pills, shots, topical gels, and medicated skin patches—may be prescribed.

Unproven claims that taking hormone supplements can make people feel young again, or that they can slow or prevent aging, have been hot news items for several years. The reality is that no one has yet shown that supplements of these hormones prevent frailty or add years to people's lives. And while some supplements provide health benefits for people with genuine deficiencies of certain hormones, they also can cause harmful side effects. In any case, people who have diagnosed hormone deficiencies should take them only under a doctor's supervision. Remember: More is not necessarily better. The right balance of hormones helps us stay healthy, but the wrong amount might be damaging.

Heed the Warnings

The NIA recognizes that some hormone-like products are available over the counter and can be used without consulting a physician. The

Institute discourages individuals from self-medicating with these products for a number of reasons. First, these products are marketed as dietary supplements, and therefore, are not regulated by the Food and Drug Administration (FDA) in the same way as drugs. This is an important distinction because the requirements for marketing a dietary supplement are very different from those that apply to hormones marketed as drugs. Unlike drug manufacturers, a firm selling dietary supplements does not need FDA approval of its products and does not need to prove that its products are safe and effective before marketing. Also, there is no specific guarantee that the substance in the container is authentic, or that the indicated dosage is accurate. Because of these differing standards, hormone-like substances that are sold as dietary supplements may not be as thoroughly studied as drug products, and therefore, the potential consequences of their use are not well-understood or defined. In addition, these over-the-counter products may interfere with other medications you are taking.

Therefore, the NIA does not recommend taking any supplement, including DHEA and melatonin, that is touted as an anti-aging remedy because no supplement has been proven to serve this purpose. The influence of these supplements on a person's health is unknown, particularly when taken over a long period of time. Talk to your doctor if you are interested in any form of hormone supplementation.

How Hormones Work

Most hormones exist in very low concentrations in the bloodstream. Each hormone molecule travels through the blood until it reaches a cell with a receptor that it matches. Then, the hormone molecule latches onto the receptor and sends a signal into the cell. These signals may instruct the cell to multiply, to make proteins or enzymes, or to perform other vital tasks. Some hormones can even stimulate a cell to release other hormones. However, no single hormone affects all cells in the same way. One hormone, for example, may stimulate a cell to perform one task, while the same hormone can have an entirely different influence over another cell. The response of some cells to hormonal stimulation also may change throughout life.

Hormone supplements, particularly if taken without medical supervision, may adversely affect this complex system. These supplements, for instance, may not behave exactly the same way as our own naturally produced hormones have because the body may process them differently. In addition, natural hormone production is not constant, so circulating blood levels may vary significantly over a 24-hour period. Hormone supplements cannot replicate these fluctuations. As a result, high doses of supplements, whether pills, shots, gels, or skin patches, may result in excessive and unhealthy amounts of hormones in the blood. Hormone supplements also may compound any negative effects caused by hormones naturally produced by the body.

Finally, most of the processes in the body are tightly controlled and regulated. Too much stimulation can elicit natural responses to inhibit a hormone's action. The body's system of checks and balances is complicated, and the notion that hormone supplements can improve function may be an oversimplification.

Dehydroepiandrosterone (DHEA)

Dehydroepiandrosterone or DHEA is made from cholesterol by the adrenal glands which sit on top of each kidney. Production of this substance peaks in the mid-20s and gradually declines with age in most people. What this drop means or how it affects the aging process, if at all, is unclear. In fact, scientists are somewhat mystified by DHEA and have not fully sorted out what it does in the body. However, researchers do know that the body converts DHEA into two hormones that are known to affect us in many ways: estrogen and testosterone.

Supplements of DHEA can be bought without a prescription and are sold as anti-aging remedies. Some proponents of these products claim that DHEA supplements improve energy, strength, and immunity. DHEA is also said to increase muscle and decrease fat. Right now, there is no consistent evidence that DHEA supplements do any of these things in people, and there is little scientific evidence to support the use of DHEA as a rejuvenating hormone. Although the long-term (over one year) effects of DHEA supplements have not been studied, there are early signs that these supplements, even when taken briefly, may have several detrimental effects on the body including liver damage.

In addition, some people's bodies make more estrogen and testosterone from DHEA than others. There is no way to predict who will make more and who will make less. Researchers are concerned that DHEA supplements may cause high levels of estrogen or testosterone in some people. This is important because testosterone may play a role in prostate cancer, and higher levels of estrogen are associated with an increased risk of breast cancer. It is not yet known for certain if supplements of estrogen and testosterone, or supplements of DHEA, also increase the risk of developing these types of cancer. In women, high testosterone levels can cause acne and growth of facial hair.

Overall, the studies that have been done so far do not provide a clear picture of the risks and benefits of DHEA. For example, some studies in older people show that DHEA helps build muscle and reduce fat, but other studies do not. Researchers are working to find more definite answers about the effects of DHEA on aging, muscles, and the immune system. In the meantime, people who are thinking about taking supplements of this hormone should understand that its effects are not fully known. Some of these unknown effects might turn out to be harmful.

Growth Hormone

Human growth hormone (hGH) is made by the pituitary gland, a pea-sized structure located at the base of the brain, and is important for normal development and maintenance of tissues and organs. It is especially important for normal growth in children.

Studies have shown that injections of supplemental hGH are helpful to certain people. Sometimes children are unusually short because their bodies do not make enough hGH. When they receive injections of this hormone, their growth improves. Young adults who have no pituitary gland (because of surgery for a pituitary tumor, for example) cannot make the hormone and they become obese. When they are given hGH, they lose weight.

Like some other hormones, blood levels of hGH often decrease as people age, but this may not necessarily be bad. At least one epidemiological study, for instance, suggests that people who have high levels of hGH are more apt to die at younger ages than those with lower levels of the hormone. Studies of animals with genetic disorders that suppress growth hormone production and secretion also suggest that reduced growth hormone secretion may prolong survival in some species.

Although there is no conclusive evidence that hGH can prevent aging, some people spend a great deal of money on supplements. These supplements are claimed, by some, to increase muscle, decrease fat, and to boost an individual's stamina and sense of well being. Shots— the only proven way of getting the body to make use of supplemental hGH—can cost more than $15,000 a year. They are available only by prescription and should be given by a doctor. In any case, people in search of the fountain of youth may have a hard time finding a doctor who will give them shots of hGH because so little is known about the long-term risks and benefits of this controversial treatment. Some dietary supplements, known as human growth hormone releasers, are marketed as a low-cost alternative to hGH shots. But claims that these over-the-counter products retard the aging process are unsubstantiated. While some studies have shown that supplemental hGH does increase muscle mass, it seems to have little impact on muscle strength or function. Scientists are continuing to study hGH, but they are watching their study participants very carefully because side effects can be serious in older adults. These include diabetes and pooling of fluid in the skin and other tissues which may lead to high blood pressure and heart failure. Joint pain and carpal tunnel syndrome also may occur. A recent report that treatment of children with human pituitary growth hormone increases the risk of subsequent cancer is a cause for concern. Further studies on this issue are needed. Whether older people treated with hGH for extended periods have an increased risk of cancer is unknown.

For now, there is no convincing evidence hGH supplements will improve the health of those who do not suffer a profound deficiency of this hormone.

Melatonin

This hormone is made by the pineal gland, a structure in the brain. Contrary to the claims of some, secretion of melatonin does not necessarily decrease with age. Instead, a number of factors, including light and many common medications, can affect melatonin secretion in people of any age.

Melatonin supplements can be bought without a prescription. Some people claim that melatonin is an anti-aging remedy, a sleep remedy, and an antioxidant (antioxidants protect against free radicals, naturally occurring oxygen-related molecules that cause damage to the body). Early test tube studies suggested that, in large doses, melatonin might be effective against free radicals. However, cells produce antioxidants naturally, and in test tube experiments, cells reduce the amount they make when they are exposed to additional antioxidants. Claims that melatonin can slow or reverse aging are very far from proven. Studies of melatonin have been much too limited to support these claims and have focused on animals, not people. Research on sleep shows that melatonin does play a role in our daily sleep-wake cycle, and that supplements, in amounts ranging from 0.1 to 0.5 milligrams, can improve sleep in some cases. If melatonin is taken at the wrong time, though, it can disrupt the sleep-wake cycle. Other side effects may include confusion, drowsiness, and headache the next morning. Animal studies suggest that melatonin may cause some blood vessels to constrict, a condition that could be dangerous for people with high blood pressure or other cardiovascular problems.

These side effects are important to keep in mind since the dose of melatonin usually sold in stores—3 milligrams—can result in amounts in the blood from 10 to 40 times higher than normal. What long-term effects such high concentrations of melatonin may have on the body are still unknown. Until researchers find out more, caution is advised.

Testosterone

Ask an average man about testosterone, and he might tell you that this hormone helps transform a boy into a man. Or, he might tell that you that it has something to do with sex drive. Or, if he has read news stories in recent years, he might mention male menopause, a condition supposedly caused by diminishing testosterone levels in aging men. In reality, there is scant evidence that this controversial condition, also known as andropause, exists.

Testosterone is indeed a vital sex hormone that plays an important role in puberty. In men, testosterone not only regulates sex drive (libido), it also helps regulate bone mass, fat distribution, muscle mass and strength, and the production of red blood cells and sperm. But contrary to what some people believe, testosterone is not exclusively a male hormone. Women produce small amounts of it in their bodies as well. In men, testosterone is produced in the testes, the reproductive glands that also produce sperm. The amount of testosterone produced in the testes is regulated by the hypothalamus and the pituitary gland.

As men age, their testes often produce somewhat less testosterone than they did during adolescence and early adulthood when production of this hormone peaks. It is important to keep in mind that the range of normal testosterone production is large. It is unclear how much of a decline or how low a level of testosterone is needed to cause adverse effects. The likelihood that an aging man will ever experience a major shut down of hormone production similar to a woman's menopause, is very remote.

In fact, many of the changes that take place in older men often are incorrectly blamed on decreasing testosterone levels. Some men who have erectile difficulty (impotence), for instance, may be tempted to blame this problem on lowered testosterone. However, in many cases, erectile difficulties are due to circulatory problems, not low testosterone.

Still, some men may be helped by testosterone supplementation. These FDA approved products are prescribed for men whose bodies make very little or no testosterone—for example, men whose pituitary glands have been damaged or destroyed by trauma, infections or tumors, or whose testes have been damaged. For these few men who have extreme deficiencies, testosterone therapy in the form of patches, injections, or topical gels may offer substantial benefit. Testosterone products may help a man with exceptionally low testosterone levels maintain strong muscles and bones and increase sex drive. However, what effects testosterone replacement may have in healthy older men without these extreme deficiencies requires more research.

The NIA is investigating the role of testosterone therapy in delaying or preventing frailty. Results from preliminary studies involving small groups of men have been inconclusive, and it remains unclear to what degree supplementation of this hormone can sharpen memory or help men maintain stout muscles, sturdy bones, and robust sexual activity.

Many other questions remain about the use of this hormone in late life. It is unclear, for example, whether men who are at the lower end of the normal range of testosterone production would benefit from supplementation. Some investigators are also concerned about the long-term harmful effects that supplemental testosterone might have on the aging body. It is not yet known, for instance, if testosterone therapy increases the risk of prostate cancer, the second leading cause of cancer death among men. In addition to potentially promoting new prostate cancers, testosterone also may promote the growth of those that have already developed. Studies also suggest that supplementation might trigger excessive red blood cell production in some men. This side effect can thicken blood and increase a man's risk of stroke.

The bottom line: Although some older men who have tried testosterone therapy report feeling more energetic or younger, testosterone supplementation remains a scientifically unproven method for preventing or relieving any physical and psychological changes that men with normal testosterone levels may experience as they get older. Until more scientifically rigorous studies are conducted, the question of whether the benefits of testosterone replacement outweigh any of its potential negative effects will remain unanswered.

Estrogen and Progesterone

Estrogen and progesterone are hormones produced in a woman's ovaries before menopause. They play an important part in the menstrual cycle and pregnancy, but estrogen also helps maintain bone strength and might prevent heart disease and protect memory before menopause. For more than 60 years, estrogen has been used by millions of women to control the hot flashes and vaginal dryness that frequently occur with menopause. It is also used to prevent or treat osteoporosis, the loss of bone strength that often occurs after menopause. However, over time experts realized that estrogen could cause a thickening of the lining of the uterus (endometrium) and an increased risk of endometrial cancer. Doctors then began giving progestin, a synthetic form of progesterone, to protect the lining of the uterus. Using estrogen alone (in a woman whose uterus has been removed) or with a progestin (in women with a uterus) to treat the symptoms of menopause is called menopausal hormone therapy (MHT), formerly known as hormone replacement therapy.

Unlike other hormones described in this section, many large, reliable long-term studies of estrogen and its effects on the body have been conducted. These studies suggested that using estrogen after menopause could provide many important benefits.

But estrogen also is a good example of why it is important to wait until researchers have discovered both the benefits and risks of a hormone before it becomes widely used. While some women are helped by estrogen during and after menopause, others are placed at higher risk for certain diseases if they take it.

Early studies suggested menopausal hormone therapy could lower the risk for heart disease (the number one killer of women in the United States) in postmenopausal women. But results from the *Women's Health Initiative* (WHI), an important study of menopausal hormone therapy funded by the National Institutes of Health, now suggest that using estrogen with or without a progestin after menopause does not protect postmenopausal women (ages 50 and older) from heart disease and may even increase their risk. In 2002, WHI scientists reported that using estrogen plus progestin actually elevates some women's chance of developing heart disease, stroke, blood clots, and breast cancer. But they also found health benefits—not as many hip fractures and fewer cases of colorectal cancer. In 2004, the same scientists reported that using estrogen alone increased a woman's risk of stroke and blood clots, but protected women from hip fractures.

Some studies suggest that estrogen may protect against Alzheimer disease, but this has not yet been proven. In fact, in 2003, researchers in a WHI substudy, the *WHI Memory Study* (WHIMS) reported that women age 65 and older taking a combination of estrogen plus progestin were at twice the risk of developing dementia as women not taking any hormones. Again in 2004, these WHIMS scientists reported that using estrogen alone could increase the risk of developing dementia in women age 65 and older compared to women not taking any hormones. As a result of these studies, experts have concluded that the health risks of using menopausal hormone therapy may be greater than the health benefits. These risks may differ between women who have menopausal symptoms and those who do not. Nevertheless, the FDA has stated that women who want to use menopausal hormone therapy to control the symptoms of menopause should do so at the lowest effective dose for the shortest time needed.

But the question of these greater risks is still an important public health issue. Even small increases, when millions of women are using menopausal hormone therapy, could mean many more cases of heart disease, stroke, blood clots, and breast cancer.

So the decision whether to take estrogen is now far more complex and difficult than ever before. Questions about menopausal hormone therapy remain: Would using a different estrogen and/or progestin or another dose change the risks? Would the results be different if the hormones were given as a patch or cream, rather than a pill? Would taking the progestin less often be as effective and safe? Does starting menopausal hormone therapy around the time of menopause compared to beginning years later change the risks? Can we predict which women will benefit or be harmed by using menopausal hormone therapy? As answers to these and other questions are found, women and their doctors should frequently review the pros and cons of menopausal hormone therapy in order to make an informed choice based on a realistic assessment of personal risks and benefits.

Many Questions, Few Answers

The NIA sponsors research that will reveal more about the risks and benefits of hormone therapies and supplements. One goal is to determine whether DHEA, melatonin, and other hormonal supplements improve the health of older people, have no effect, or are actually harmful.

It is important to remember that these studies may not yield immediate or final answers, especially in the cases of DHEA, melatonin, and hGH, since research on these supplements is fairly new. Some of these studies, for example, may simply provide researchers with more information about what kinds of questions they should ask in their next studies. Research is a step-by-step process, and larger studies may be needed to give more definitive answers.

Until more is known about DHEA, melatonin, and hGH, consumers should view them with a good deal of caution and doubt. Despite what advertisements or stories in the media may claim, hormone supplements have not been proven to prevent aging. Some harmful side effects already have been discovered and additional research may uncover others.

More is known about estrogen, progesterone, and testosterone, and people with genuine deficiencies of these hormones should consult with their doctors about supplements. Meanwhile, people who choose to take any hormone supplement without a doctor's supervision should be aware that these supplements appear to have few clear benefits for healthy individuals, and no proven influence on the aging process.

Chapter 3

Metabolism: A Collection of Chemical Reactions

Every time you swallow a bite of sandwich or slurp a smoothie, your body works hard to process the nutrients you've eaten. Long after the dishes are cleared and the food is digested, the nutrients you've taken in become the building blocks and fuel needed by your body. Your body gets the energy it needs from food through a process called metabolism.

What Is Metabolism and What Does It Do?

Metabolism (pronounced: muh-tah-buh-lih-zum) is a collection of chemical reactions that takes place in the body's cells. Metabolism converts the fuel in the food we eat into the energy needed to power everything we do, from moving to thinking to growing. Specific proteins in the body control the chemical reactions of metabolism, and each chemical reaction is coordinated with other body functions. In fact, thousands of metabolic reactions happen at the same time—all regulated by the body—to keep our cells healthy and working.

Metabolism is a constant process that begins when we're conceived and ends when we die. It is a vital process for all life forms—not just humans. If metabolism stops, living things die.

This information was provided by TeensHealth, one of the largest resources online for medically reviewed health information written for parents, kids, and teens. For more articles like this one, visit www.TeensHealth.org, or www .KidsHealth .org. © 2004 The Nemours Foundation.

Here's an example of how the process of metabolism works in humans—and it begins with plants. First, a green plant takes in energy from sunlight. The plant uses this energy and a molecule called chlorophyll (which gives plants their green color) to build sugars from water and carbon dioxide. This process is called photosynthesis, and you probably learned about it in biology class.

When people and animals eat the plants (or, if they're carnivores, they eat animals that have eaten the plants), they take in this energy (in the form of sugar), along with other vital cell-building chemicals. The body's next step is to break the sugar down so that the energy released can be distributed to, and used as fuel by, the body's cells.

After food is eaten, molecules in the digestive system called enzymes break proteins down into amino acids, fats into fatty acids, and carbohydrates into simple sugars (such as glucose). In addition to sugar, both amino acids and fatty acids can be used as energy sources by the body when needed. These compounds are absorbed into the blood, which transports them to the cells. After they enter the cells, other enzymes act to speed up or regulate the chemical reactions involved with "metabolizing" these compounds. During these processes, the energy from these compounds can be released for use by the body or stored in body tissues, especially the liver, muscles, and body fat.

In this way, the process of metabolism is really a balancing act involving two kinds of activities that go on at the same time—the building up of body tissues and energy stores and the breaking down of body tissues and energy stores to generate more fuel for body functions:

- Anabolism (pronounced: uh-nah-buh-lih-zum), or constructive metabolism, is all about building and storing: It supports the growth of new cells, the maintenance of body tissues, and the storage of energy for use in the future. During anabolism, small molecules are changed into larger, more complex molecules of carbohydrate, protein, and fat.

- Catabolism (pronounced: kuh-tah-buh-lih-zum), or destructive metabolism, is the process that produces the energy required for all activity in the cells. In this process, cells break down large molecules (mostly carbohydrates and fats) to release energy. This energy release provides fuel for anabolism, heats the body, and enables the muscles to contract and the body to move. As complex chemical units are broken down into more simple substances, the waste products released in the process of catabolism are removed from the body through the skin, kidneys, lungs, and intestines.

Several of the hormones of the endocrine system are involved in controlling the rate and direction of metabolism. Thyroxine (pronounced: thigh-rahk-sun), a hormone produced and released by the thyroid (pronounced: thigh-royd) gland, plays a key role in determining how fast or slow the chemical reactions of metabolism proceed in a person's body.

Another gland, the pancreas (pronounced: pan-kree-us) secretes (gives off) hormones that help determine whether the body's main metabolic activity at a particular time will be anabolic or catabolic. For example, after eating a meal, usually more anabolic activity occurs because eating increases the level of glucose—the body's most important fuel—in the blood. The pancreas senses this increased level of glucose and releases the hormone insulin (pronounced: in-suh-lin), which signals cells to increase their anabolic activities.

Metabolism is a complicated chemical process, so it's not surprising that many people think of it in its simplest sense: as something that influences how easily our bodies gain or lose weight. That's where calories come in. A calorie is a unit that measures how much energy a particular food provides to the body. A chocolate bar has more calories than an apple, so it provides the body with more energy—and sometimes that can be too much of a good thing. Just as a car stores gas in the gas tank until it is needed to fuel the engine, the body stores calories—primarily as fat. If you overfill a car's gas tank, it spills over onto the pavement. Likewise, if a person eats too many calories, they "spill over" in the form of excess fat on the body.

The number of calories a person burns in a day is affected by how much that person exercises, the amount of fat and muscle in his or her body, and the person's basal metabolic rate. The basal metabolic rate, or BMR, is a measure of the rate at which a person's body "burns" energy, in the form of calories, while at rest. The BMR can play a role in a person's tendency to gain weight. For example, a person with a low BMR (who therefore burns fewer calories while at rest or sleeping) will tend to gain more pounds of body fat over time, compared with a similar-sized person with an average BMR who eats the same amount of food and gets the same amount of exercise.

What factors influence a person's BMR? To a certain extent, a person's basal metabolic rate is inherited—passed on through the genes the person gets from his or her parents. Sometimes health problems can affect a person's BMR. But people can actually change their BMR in certain ways. For example, exercising more will not only cause a person to burn more calories directly from the extra activity itself, but becoming more physically fit will increase BMR as well. BMR is also influenced by body composition—people with more muscle and less fat generally have higher BMRs.

Things That Can Go Wrong with Metabolism

Most of the time your metabolism works effectively without you giving any thought to it. But sometimes a person's metabolism can cause major mayhem in the form of a metabolic disorder. In a broad sense, a metabolic disorder is any disease that is caused by an abnormal chemical reaction in the body's cells. Most disorders of metabolism involve either abnormal levels of enzymes of hormones or problems with the functioning of those enzymes or hormones. When the metabolism of body chemicals is blocked or defective, it can cause a buildup of toxic substances in the body or a deficiency of substances needed for normal body function, either of which can lead to serious symptoms.

Some metabolic diseases and conditions include:

Hyperthyroidism (pronounced: hi-per-thigh-roy-dih-zum). Hyperthyroidism is caused by an overactive thyroid gland. The thyroid releases too much of the hormone thyroxine, which increases the person's basal metabolic rate (BMR). It causes symptoms such as weight loss, increased heart rate and blood pressure, protruding eyes, and a swelling in the neck from an enlarged thyroid (goiter). The disease may be controlled with medications or through surgery or radiation treatments.

Hypothyroidism (pronounced: hi-po-thigh-roy-dih-zum). Hypothyroidism is caused by a nonexistent or underactive thyroid gland, and it results from a developmental problem or a destructive disease of the thyroid. The thyroid releases too little of the hormone thyroxine, so a person's basal metabolic rate (BMR) is low. Not getting treatment for hypothyroidism can lead to brain and growth problems. Hypothyroidism slows body processes and causes fatigue, slow heart rate, excessive weight gain, and constipation. Teens with this condition can be treated with oral thyroid hormone to achieve normal levels in the body.

Inborn errors of metabolism. Some metabolic diseases are inherited. These conditions are called inborn errors of metabolism. When babies are born, they're tested for many of these metabolic diseases. Inborn errors of metabolism can sometimes lead to serious problems if they're not controlled with diet or medication from an early age. Examples of inborn errors of metabolism include galactosemia (babies born with this inborn error of metabolism do not have enough of the enzyme that breaks down the sugar in milk called galactose) and phenylketonuria (this problem is due to a defect in the enzyme that breaks down the amino acid phenylalanine, which is needed for normal growth and protein production). Teens may need to follow a certain diet or take medications to control metabolic problems they've had since birth.

Type 1 diabetes mellitus (pronounced: dye-uh-bee-teez meh-luh-tus). Type 1 diabetes occurs when the pancreas doesn't produce and secrete enough insulin. Symptoms of this disease include excessive thirst and urination, hunger, and weight loss. Over the long term, the disease can cause kidney problems, pain due to nerve damage, blindness, and heart and blood vessel disease. Teens with type 1 diabetes need to receive regular injections of insulin and control blood sugar levels to reduce the risk of developing problems from diabetes.

Type 2 diabetes. Type 2 diabetes happens when the body can't respond normally to insulin. The symptoms of this disorder are similar to those of type 1 diabetes. Many children and teens who develop type 2 diabetes are overweight, and this is thought to play a role in their decreased responsiveness to insulin. Some teens can be treated successfully with dietary changes, exercise, and oral medication, but insulin injections are necessary in other cases. Controlling blood sugar levels reduces the risk of developing the same kinds of long-term health problems that occur with type 1 diabetes.

Chapter 4

Energy Balance: Calorie Intake, Physical Activity, and Basal Metabolic Rate

Important Concepts Related to Energy Intake and Energy Output

The Energy Balance Equation

The energy balance equation includes terms that refer to energy intake and energy output. For some individuals, the equation must also include terms for the energy required for growth and for energy that is stored.

Energy In (Ein): Energy is available from the foods we eat; this energy input is represented by Energy In, or Ein. Although foods contain a number of nutrients, energy is provided by proteins, carbohydrates, and fats. Vitamins and minerals in foods, although essential for normal metabolic functions, do not contribute calories to our diets. Each gram of protein or carbohydrate we consume contributes four calories of energy. In contrast, fat provides nine calories per gram. Interestingly, alcohol has seven calories per gram. Alcohol-containing products have calories and few nutrients; their consumption may upset both energy balance and nutritional status.

A food calorie is the equivalent of 1,000 calories, or 1 kilocalorie. The food calorie is sometimes represented by Calorie, with a capital

C. In keeping with the usual format in nutrition studies, this chapter uses "calorie" to mean the food calorie. A food calorie (1 kilocalorie) is defined as the amount of energy required to raise the temperature of a liter of water one degree centigrade at sea level.

A balanced diet provides 45 to 65 percent of total daily calories as carbohydrate, most of which should be from complex carbohydrates such as starches; 10 to 35 percent of daily calories from protein; and no more than 30 percent of calories from fat. The needs of athletes and other more physically active people may differ in both energy and nutrient intakes depending on the intensity and duration of their physical activities. People with special needs due to illness or medications should consult a physician and a registered dietitian to create an appropriate plan to meet nutritional demands.

Energy Out (Eout): Total energy expenditure is represented by Energy Out, or Eout. Eout has three major components which added together provide an accurate measure of an individual's daily caloric requirement: the basal metabolic rate (BMR), the energy used for physical activity, and the thermic effect of food.

The BMR represents the energy used to carry out the basic metabolic needs of the body. Energy must be provided for maintaining a heartbeat, breathing, regulating body temperature, and carrying out other activities that we take for granted. Most of our daily energy expenditure, about 60 to 70 percent, is represented by our BMR. The BMR can be estimated as follows: for adult males, multiply the body weight (in pounds) by 10, and add double the body weight to this value (for a 160-pound male, BMR = 1,600 + (2 × 160) = 1,920 calories/day); for adult females, multiply the body weight by 10, and add the body weight to this value (for a 110-pound female, BMR = 1,100 + 110 = 1,210 calories/day).

BMR calculations, as in the examples given, are average estimations. A person's actual BMR changes over time. This depends on a number of factors, including several that distinguish groups of people.

- Age—Younger people have higher than average BMR. As children grow, their body composition (percent body fat and muscle mass) changes. As they continue to age, BMR decreases as the percent muscle mass decreases.

- Growth—Children and pregnant women have higher-than-average BMR.

- Height—Tall, thin people have higher than average BMR.

- Body composition—People with higher-than-average, or increased, muscle mass have higher-than-average BMR.

Other factors that cause variation within individuals include:

- Fever—Fever increases your BMR.

- Stress—Physical stress, such as recovering from an illness, increases your BMR; mental or emotional stress may lead to lethargy or depression and decrease your BMR.

- Inside or outside temperature—Both heat and cold raise your BMR.

- Fasting—Fasting lowers your BMR.

Physical activity amounts to about 20 to 30 percent of the body's total energy output. Energy expended during physical activity varies with the level and duration of the activity. It is also affected by the age, gender, height, and weight of the individual performing the activity. Examples of the calories used by different individuals for walking and running are presented in Table 4.1. The values in the table include the calories for BMR.

The "thermic effect of food" refers to the energy required to digest food. This term indicates what is usually obvious: we must expend some energy to make materials available in the body that will be used

Table 4.1. Energy Expended during Physical Activity

Individual	Calories Used Per Hour		
	Walking for pleasure (2.5–3.0 mph)	Walking for exercise (3.5–4.0 mph)	Running (5.0 mph)
12-year-old girl, 4'11", 92 pounds	187	203	426
12-year-old boy, 4'11", 89 pounds	188	204	430
30-year-old woman, 5'4", 133 pounds	204	221	465
30-year-old man, 5'10", 155 pounds	251	273	574

Compiled by BSCS staff using various health education resources.

for the production of much larger amounts of energy. The thermic effect of food can be estimated as approximately ten percent of total calories consumed. Because it makes a relatively small contribution to energy expended, the thermic effect of food is not included as part of Eout in this chapter.

As an alternative to adding the three terms previously discussed, daily caloric requirements (Eout) can also be estimated as follows:

- for less-active individuals: weight (in pounds) × 14 = estimated calories per day;

- for moderately active individuals (3 to 4 aerobic sessions per week): weight (in pounds) × 17 = estimated calories per day; and

- for active individuals (5 to 7 aerobic sessions per week): weight (in pounds) × 20 = estimated calories per day.

Using the Energy Balance Equation

The equation for energy balance is Ein = Eout. This means that caloric intake equals caloric output. It is the desirable condition for adults who are at a healthy weight. One way to understand the concept of energy balance is to use a two-pan balance analogy. On one pan of the balance are weights representing Ein (foods which contain carbohydrate, protein, fat, and alcohol). On the other pan are weights representing energy expenditures (Eout) as metabolic activities and physical activities (and the thermic effect of food). If adults consume more calories than are used for metabolic and physical activities, then Ein is greater than Eout, and the extra energy is stored as body fat. They are in a state of positive energy balance. The pan scale would tip to the Ein side. If adults lose weight (for example, with dieting), they are in a state of negative energy balance. In this case, Ein is less than Eout, and the pan scale would tip to the Eout side.

Healthy children and adolescents (until they stop growing) are in a state of positive energy balance. The extra calories are used primarily to increase the amount of important body tissues such as bone, muscle, blood, and body organs. Some of the extra calories may also be stored as body fat, which can be used at a later time as a source of energy. Thus, food components (protein, fat, and carbohydrate) taken into the body have the following fates: they can be used to fuel metabolic activities and physical activities; they can be incorporated into growing body tissues; and they can be stored as fat. If food intake contributes to all three of these fates, then Ein = Eout + energy for growth + energy that is stored, and the body is in positive energy balance. If

Ein is less than Eout + Egrowth for children or adolescents the body will be in negative energy balance and will not be able to grow properly.

Extra Ein is an important consideration during periods of growth. The amount of energy (calories) required for growth during most of a child's life accounts for about one to two percent of the youngster's daily energy intake. However, during infancy and adolescence, growth does have a significant impact on energy requirements. The appetites of healthy youngsters, at any age, are usually reliable guides to the amount of food they should eat. Presented with a well-balanced diet, healthy children will eat all they need. Importantly, attempts to force low-calorie diets on children and adolescents may interfere with normal growth processes. Furthermore, such diets alone have not been very successful in achieving long-term weight control. An important consideration is that growing children and adolescents are not in energy balance until they stop growing. Rather, they are in positive energy balance, taking in more energy than is expended in physical activities and in maintaining the BMR. That extra energy is used for growth.

In summary, there are two important concepts of energy balance for adolescents. First, to allow for normal body growth, more food energy must be consumed than can be accounted for solely on the basis of energy required for metabolic and physical activities. Second, insufficient energy intake may affect cellular metabolic activities, body weight, growth, tissue formation, and health.

Body Fat Composition

Understanding the relationship between energy requirements and desirable body weights should take into account, not only the total weight, but also the composition of the weight. This is important because muscle mass and body fat make different demands on daily energy requirements, and can have different long-term health consequences. Considerable variation among individuals in resting metabolic rates is due in part to variation in body composition, or more specifically, to the ratio of muscle to fat tissue in the body. Muscle tissue is more effective than fat at burning calories, expending more than three times as much energy as under resting conditions. Therefore, the ratio of muscle to fat tissue is an important determinant of the total daily energy requirement.

Significant changes in the ratio of muscle tissue to fat tissue occur during adolescence. In females, body fat increases from a mean of 17 percent of body weight to 25 percent of body weight during adolescence. Males, in contrast, experience a decline in body fat, from a mean of 18 percent of body weight to 11 percent of body weight during this period. In addition, the pattern of body fat distribution changes during adolescence: in both genders, body fat redistributes from peripheral sites to central sites (gluteal region in females, abdomen in males). These normal changes during adolescence are due primarily to genetic and physiologic factors. Nevertheless, energy balance still plays an important role in influencing the direction and magnitude of these changes. Because of changes in body composition with growth, weight is a less reliable measure of body composition for children and adolescents than for adults. Consequently, it is important to emphasize to students that great variation exists in body shapes and sizes among healthy individuals. Conditions of overweight and obesity should be diagnosed only by qualified health professionals and should not be based on appearance.

Body composition is a much better predictor of one's level of health and risk of disease than is weight. Muscle mass or a measure of body fat is used to assess body composition. Professionals estimate body-fat content using tools and techniques such as circumference measurements (of abdomen, hips); a height and hip-girth chart; ultrasound measurements; electrical impedance measurements; the caliper measurement method; and the water-weighing measurement method.

Body Mass Index (BMI)

BMI expresses the relationship between an individual's weight in kilograms (or pounds divided by 2.2) and height in meters (or inches divided by 39.4). For adults, the formula is BMI = weight divided by height^2. For children over two years old and adolescents, the formula is BMI = (weight in pounds divided by height in inches^2) × 703. BMI is a helpful indicator of obesity and underweight and has two primary uses. It can be used to screen and monitor a population for risks to health or for nutritional disorders. Alternatively, BMI, along with other necessary information, can be used to assess risks to health for an individual.

What does a BMI value mean? Scientists and health officials have arrived at classifications for adults, based on the effect that body weight has on disease and death as shown in Table 4.2.

Average BMI values rise throughout adolescence, and the changes are similar for both genders. Typical ranges for BMI during adolescence are 16 to 22 at age 12, rising to 18 to 25 at age 17. Students

Table 4.2. Body Mass Index Classification

Body Mass Index (BMI)	Classification
BMI less than 18.5	underweight
BMI between 18.5 and 24.9	healthy range
BMI between 25 and 29.9	overweight
BMI equal to or over 30.0	obese

need to appreciate these age-related trends in order to interpret correctly the BMI as an assessment tool for their own weight status. Students should also understand that the similar range of BMI for females and males during adolescence conceals significant gender differences in body composition. Adolescent females tend to have a higher ratio of fat to fat-free tissue than do males of comparable BMI. Students should understand that these gender-related differences in body composition are normal and that small gains in fat tissue and weight in girls are a normal part of physiological preparation for reproduction.

Factors Affecting Energy Intake

Portion size: Nutritionists caution that effective weight management places equal importance on both the kind and the amount of food consumed. However, in a recent survey by the American Institute for Cancer Research, 78 percent of those responding believed that the kind of food they eat is more important for managing weight than how much they eat. In part, this is attributed to advertising and emphasis on low-fat and fat-free foods. Trends in the food industry have also contributed to increased consumption. Competition has resulted in serving larger portion sizes. Fast-food restaurants have "super-sized" and "value" meals, while other restaurants have replaced the former industry standard 10-inch plate with a 12-inch plate. Interestingly, information from the U.S. Department of Agriculture shows that while the percentage of fat in the American diet dropped from 40 percent to 33 percent over the past 20 years, total daily caloric intake increased about eight percent, from 1,854 calories to 2,002 calories.

In many ways, these trends are not surprising. Our lack of concern about portion size may result from our general lack of understanding about what actually constitutes a serving of food. Even though today's food labels offer more complete nutrition information than they did in the past, the information is not always easy to translate into practical terms. For instance, to calculate our energy intake in calories, we must multiply the calories per serving given on the label by the number of servings we eat. But what is a serving? Serving size may not reflect what a person actually eats. Indeed, food consumption varies widely across the population, especially as a function of age. How many of us consume one ounce of dry cereal at breakfast? What is one ounce of dry cereal? How much is three ounces of meat? What is a medium apple as opposed to a small or a large apple? And a food-label serving size is not necessarily the same as a Food Guide Pyramid serving size. However, a label serving and a Food Guide Pyramid serving are each a standardized amount that reflects a certain nutritional content. No matter how confusing serving size might be, or how inconvenient it might be to determine the number of servings consumed, it should be apparent that no understanding of energy intake can be achieved without attention to the actual amounts of foods consumed. Consider the examples in Table 4.3 which provides a practical and simple means of estimating how much of various foods we consume.

Hunger and appetite: The input side of the energy balance equation, Ein, is controlled in large part through the opposing sensations of hunger and satiety. Hunger is a physiological state modulated by internal factors. It is often associated with the question, Is there anything to eat? Key to understanding the physiological control of body weight is understanding how eating behavior (food intake) and metabolism are coordinated. This area is complex, and a detailed understanding of the mechanisms is lacking. Early models of the control of food intake held that hunger was a simple response to stomach contractions or to temporary low concentrations of glucose, amino acids, or fatty acids circulating in the blood. In the past decade, however, this simplistic view has been refined into a more comprehensive model involving the nervous and endocrine systems.

Factors that may lead to decreased food intake include:

- increased blood glucose concentration;

- increased production of certain hormones (such as insulin, glucagon, gastrointestinal hormones, and pituitary hormones), certain peptides and proteins (such as those released during illness), or molecules involved in the function of the nervous system (such as serotonin);

- increased body temperature;

- stress (such as from illness or from emotional or mental causes);

- conditioned responses (such as taking small portions and eating slowly); and

- sensory mechanisms (such as mechanoreceptors in the stomach that sense stretching and chemoreceptors in the stomach that are sensitive to glucose and amino acids).

Factors that may lead to increased food intake include:

- sensory mechanisms (such as those relating to the pleasant smell and taste of food),

- stress (such as from emotional or mental causes),

- conditioned responses (such as learning to clean the plate or eat rapidly),

- pituitary hormones (such as growth hormone and prolactin), and

- brain peptides (such as the endogenous opiates and neuropeptide Y).

Although we do not yet understand all of the factors regulating food intake, it is clear that regulation is complex and involves the coordinated interaction of many signals.

Appetite is a learned condition influenced by both external and internal cues. It is often associated with the question, What do I want to eat? Appetite seems better related to energy need when we are regularly physically active. When physical activity is low, appetite may increase out of boredom or a need to do something. Eating also may be a means of achieving immediate satisfaction or gratification.

An important molecule that regulates energy balance through its effects on metabolism and appetite is leptin, a protein produced by fat cells. Leptin is able to reduce food intake, inhibit the synthesis and release of neuropeptide Y (a peptide that increases appetite), increase body temperature, increase metabolic rate, and reduce blood concentrations of glucose and insulin. The overall result is lower body weight and lower percentage of body fat.

How does integration of all the signals relating to hunger and appetite occur? Experiments have shown that specific regions of the brain integrate various inputs to control food intake. It is thought that the most important region for control of hunger and satiety is the hypothalamus. This structure lies deep in the center of the brain, and it regulates biologically-based motives such as hunger, thirst, and sex drive. The hypothalamus receives smell, taste, and visual inputs, and it senses changes in blood glucose concentration. One area of the hypothalamus contains the satiety center which tells us when to stop eating. A second area contains the hunger center. Other areas of the brain are involved in the regulation of hunger and satiety as well. Additionally, the brain stem regulates the mechanical events of eating, such as saliva production, chewing, and swallowing.

Genetics. Food intake and body weight, like all physiological variables, are influenced by genes. The genetics of feeding behavior has been studied in rodents, in which single gene mutations that result in increased feeding and obesity have been identified. Functional analysis of the ways the mutated products of these genes contribute to overeating began only recently.

Progress has been made in understanding the genetic relationship between two defective gene products in the mouse. These are the OB protein (also called leptin) which is the product of the recessive OB

Table 4.3. Estimating Amounts of Common Foods

Food	Amount	Estimated size
Apple, orange, pear, peach	1 medium	1 tennis ball
Cooked beans or peas	½ cup	1 cupcake wrapper
Cooked cereal	½ cup	1 cupcake wrapper
Cooked or raw vegetables	½ cup	½ baseball
Cut or mixed fruit	½ cup	½ baseball
Dry cereal	1 cup	2 cupcake wrappers
Meat, fish, or poultry	2 to 3 ounces	1 deck of cards
Natural cheese	1½ ounces	3 dominoes
Pasta	½ cup	1 cupcake wrapper
Peanut butter	2 tablespoons	1 golf or table tennis ball
Potato	1 medium	Size of standard computer mouse
Processed cheese	1½ ounces	2 9-volt batteries
Raw, leafy vegetables	1 cup	4 outer romaine or iceberg lettuce leaves
Rice	½ cup	1 cupcake wrapper

gene, and OB-R protein (leptin receptor) which is the product of the recessive DB gene. The initial observation was that a protein secreted by fat tissue of normal lean mice was absent in obese mice with two recessive OB genes. When leptin became available in recombinant form and was injected into obese mice with two recessive OB genes, they ate less and their metabolic heat production increased, followed by weight loss. Because of a mutation in the OB gene, mice with two recessive OB genes fail to produce leptin. Lacking leptin, which inhibits food intake, the mutants tend toward obesity.

Leptin may exert its inhibitory effect on food intake indirectly, by inhibiting production in the brain of the powerful eating stimulant neuropeptide Y and/or by increasing production of an appetite-suppressing brain peptide. In the recessive DB strain of obese mice, on the other hand, it is the receptor for leptin, OB-R, that is defective. In this case, a mutation in the receptor gene results in a receptor that has greatly reduced binding affinity for leptin in the brain. Such mutants fail to respond to injected leptin.

The first single-gene defect associated with human obesity was described only recently and involved leptin deficiency in both a child and an adult. However, most obese humans have high circulating concentrations of leptin and normal leptin receptors, so any defect in the leptin signaling pathway likely resides beyond the receptor and leads to a state of leptin resistance. Also, children with Prader-Willi syndrome, a genetic disorder caused by deletion of a small piece of chromosome 15 donated by the father, have a voracious appetite and insatiable hunger. They tend to become obese early in life. It is believed that genes for appetite regulation are contained on the missing piece of chromosome 15.

In general, the genetics of human food intake and obesity are not yet well understood. However, clear genetic effects do exist. Scientific studies have evaluated the contributions of genetic factors and the family environment to BMI. These studies have taken two different approaches. Some have compared adoptees with both their biological parents and their adoptive parents, while others have studied BMI in identical and fraternal twins. Scientists have concluded from these studies that BMI is under substantial genetic control. Additionally, one research study concluded that human obesity may be influenced by behaviors that themselves are regulated genetically. Nonetheless, some studies have indicated a large contribution of separate individual environmental influences on BMI.

The relative importance of genetics and environment to BMI is not clearly defined. What is clear, however, is that despite the popular attribution of overweight to glandular problems, known endocrine disorders are actually a rare cause of obesity.

Strategies for Achieving and Maintaining a Healthy Body Weight and Size

Attention to energy balance over time is required for promoting health and maintaining a stable body weight. For overweight people, steps must be taken to stop the weight gain and reduce weight to a healthy level, and then to maintain that healthy weight. Accomplishing these goals requires an understanding of energy balance—that is, of the general concepts of energy in and energy out. Individuals have direct control over both their food (calorie) intake and their physical activity level. By gaining knowledge of the caloric content of various foods and the caloric costs of various activities, individuals can evaluate their current E_{in} and E_{out} regimens and devise plans to achieve energy balance. People are generally surprised to learn just how small a contribution sedentary activities, such as watching television or playing video games, make to daily calorie expenditures. On the other hand, any type of physical activity, from running or playing sports to walking or household work, increases the number of calories the body uses.

As emphasized by the National Institute of Diabetes and Digestive and Kidney Disorders (NIDDK), the key to successful weight control and improved overall health is making physical activity a part of daily routine. Interestingly, behavioral research suggests that attempts to change the activity patterns of overweight students may be more effective when students are reinforced for choosing ways to limit their inactivity than when they are reinforced directly for activity.

How much physical activity is necessary?

The Dietary Guidelines for Americans recommends 30 minutes of physical activity a day for adults and 60 minutes a day for children and adolescents. A new report from the National Academy of Sciences recommends a goal of one hour per day total exercise for adults. The report indicates that energy expenditure is cumulative, including both low intensity activities, such as stair climbing and house cleaning, and more vigorous exercise, such as swimming and cycling. Sixty minutes of moderate physical activity most days of the week is recommended for children, adolescents, and teenagers up to age 18. Substantial health benefits may still be gained by accumulating at least 30 minutes of moderate-to-intense physical activity a day, at least five times a week. However, care should be taken not to exercise more frequently and more intensely than is required for good health or to compete well.

Developing appropriate strategies for achieving and maintaining a healthy body size and weight can be challenging for some individuals, and it may require more than one approach to the problem. Education may be necessary for an understanding of energy balance and basic nutrition principles. Counseling with an appropriate professional may be essential, for instance, for helping individuals find suitable physical activities and motivating factors. Counseling with a registered dietitian or other qualified professional may also be necessary for developing meals and daily food plans. Medical or psychological therapy may be necessary for dealing with issues of under-eating or overeating. Additionally, physical activity classes and programs should be available and accessible.

Chapter 5

What Is an Endocrinologist?

What is the endocrine system?

The endocrine system is a complex group of glands. Glands are organs that make hormones. These are substances that help to control activities in your body. Hormones control reproduction, metabolism (food burning and waste elimination), growth, and development. Hormones also control the way you respond to your surroundings, and they help to provide the proper amount of energy and nutrition your body needs to function. The endocrine glands include the thyroid, parathyroid, pancreas, ovaries, testes, adrenal, pituitary and hypothalamus.

What is an endocrinologist?

An endocrinologist is a specially trained doctor. Endocrinologists diagnose diseases that affect your glands. They know how to treat conditions that are often complex and involve many systems within your body. Your primary care doctor refers you to an endocrinologist when you have a problem with your endocrine system.

What do endocrinologists do?

Endocrinologists are trained to diagnose and treat hormone problems by helping to restore the normal balance of hormones in your system. Endocrinologists conduct basic research to learn the way glands work and clinical research to learn the best methods to treat patients. Endocrinologists develop new drugs and treatments for hormone problems. They take care of many conditions including:

- diabetes,
- thyroid diseases,
- metabolic disorders,
- over or under production of hormones,
- menopause,
- osteoporosis,
- hypertension,
- cholesterol (lipid) disorders,
- infertility,
- lack of growth (short stature), and
- cancers of the endocrine glands.

What type of medical training do endocrinologists receive?

Endocrinologists finish four years of medical school and then spend three or four years in an internship and residency program. These specialty programs cover internal medicine, pediatrics, or obstetrics and gynecology. They spend two or three more years learning how to diagnose and treat hormone conditions. Overall, an endocrinologist's training will take more than ten years.

What are the most common endocrine diseases and disorders?

Endocrine diseases and disorders can be grouped into several different areas. Some endocrinologists focus on one or two areas, such as diabetes, pediatric disorders, thyroid, or reproductive and menstrual disorders. Others work in all areas of endocrinology. Descriptions of the major areas of endocrinology follow.

Diabetes: Patients with diabetes have too much sugar in their blood. Recent studies have found that controlling blood sugar helps prevent serious problems that can be caused by diabetes. These can include problems with the eyes, kidneys, and nerves, which can lead to blindness, dialysis, or amputation. Endocrinologists treat diabetes with diet and medications, including insulin. They also work closely with patients to control blood sugar and monitor them so they can prevent health problems.

Thyroid: Patients with thyroid disorders often have problems with their energy levels. They may also have problems with muscle strength, emotions, weight control, and tolerating heat or cold. Endocrinologists treat patients with too much or too little thyroid hormone. They help patients reach a hormone balance by replacing or blocking thyroid hormone. Endocrinologists also receive special training to manage patients with thyroid growths, thyroid cancer, or enlarged thyroid glands.

Bone: Osteomalacia (rickets), which causes bones to soften, and osteoporosis are bone diseases that endocrinologists diagnose and treat. Osteoporosis is a disease that weakens your skeleton. Certain hormones act to protect bone tissue. When hormone levels are abnormal, bones can lose calcium and weaken. Menopause, loss of testicle function, and aging may put you at risk for bone fractures. Endocrinologists treat other disorders that can affect bones, such as too much parathyroid hormone and long-term use of steroids like prednisone.

Reproduction and Infertility: About one in ten American couples are infertile. Endocrine research has helped thousands of couples to have children. Endocrinologists diagnose and treat hormone imbalances that can cause infertility, and also assess and treat patients with reproductive problems. They work with patients who need hormone replacement. Problems that they treat include menopause symptoms, irregular periods, endometriosis, polycystic ovary syndrome (PCOS), premenstrual syndrome, and impotence.

Obesity and Overweight: Endocrinologists treat patients who are overweight or obese, sometimes because of metabolic and hormonal problems. When someone is obese they have too much body fat. Thyroid, adrenal, ovarian, and pituitary disorders can cause obesity. Endocrinologists also identify factors linked with obesity, such as insulin resistance and genetic problems.

Pituitary Gland: The pituitary is often called the master gland of the body because it controls other glands. The pituitary makes several important hormones. Over- or under-production of pituitary hormones can lead to infertility, menstrual disorders, growth disorders (acromegaly or short stature) and too much cortisol production (Cushing syndrome). Endocrinologists control these conditions with medications and refer patients who need surgery.

Growth: Children and adults can have effects from not making enough growth hormone. Pediatric endocrinologists treat children who suffer from endocrine problems that cause short stature and other growth disorders. Adults with growth hormone deficiency can experience emotional distress and fatigue. Safe and effective growth hormone replacement therapy is available for people whose growth hormone is abnormal.

Hypertension: Hypertension is high blood pressure, and it is a risk factor for heart disease. Up to 10% of people have hypertension because of too much aldosterone, a hormone produced in the adrenal glands. About half of these cases are caused by growths that can be removed with surgery. Conditions such as the metabolic syndrome, or a rare adrenal growth called a pheochromocytoma, may cause hypertension. These conditions also can be treated successfully.

Lipid Disorders: Patients with lipid disorders have trouble maintaining normal levels of body fats. One of the most common lipid disorders is hyperlipidemia—high levels of total cholesterol, low-density lipoprotein cholesterol (known as bad cholesterol), and/or triglycerides in the blood. High levels of these fats are linked to heart (coronary) disease, strokes, and peripheral vascular disease (problems with circulation in the legs). Endocrinologists are trained to detect factors that may be related to lipid disorders, such as hypothyroidism, drug use (such as steroids), or genetic or metabolic conditions. Lipid disorders can be found in several conditions that require special management, including the metabolic syndrome, polycystic ovary syndrome (PCOS), and obesity. Special diets, exercise, and medications, may be prescribed to manage hyperlipidemia and other lipid disorders.

Additional Information

Hormone Foundation
8401 Connecticut Ave., Suite 900
Chevy Chase, MD 20815-5817
Toll-Free: 800-HORMONE (467-6663)
Fax: 301-941-0259
Website: http://www.hormone.org
E-mail: hormone@endo-society.org

The Hormone Foundation's website offers a physician referral service to assist readers who wish to find an endocrinologist.

Chapter 6

Endocrine Disruptors

Over the past decade, a growing body of evidence suggests that numerous chemicals, both natural and man-made, may interfere with the endocrine system and produce adverse effects in humans, wildlife, fish, or birds. Scientists often refer to these chemicals as endocrine disruptors. These chemicals are found in many of the everyday products we use including some plastic bottles, metal food cans, detergents, flame retardants, food, toys, cosmetics, and pesticides. Although limited scientific information is available on the potential adverse human health effects, concern arises because endocrine disrupting chemicals, while present in the environment at very low levels, have been shown to have adverse effects in wildlife species, as well as in laboratory animals.

The difficulty of assessing public health effects is increased by the fact that people are typically exposed to multiple endocrine disruptors simultaneously. The National Institute of Environmental Health Sciences (NIEHS) and the National Toxicology Program (NTP) support research to understand how these chemicals work and to understand the effects that they may have in various animal and human populations with the long-term goals of developing prevention and intervention strategies to reduce any adverse effects.

What are endocrine disruptors?

Endocrine disruptors are naturally occurring compounds or manmade chemicals that may interfere with the production or activity of

National Institute of Environmental Health Sciences (NIEHS), June 2006.

hormones of the endocrine system leading to adverse health effects. Many of these chemicals have been linked with developmental, reproductive, neural, immune, and other problems, in wildlife and laboratory animals. Some scientists think these chemicals also are adversely affecting human health in similar ways resulting in declined fertility and increased incidences or progression of some diseases including endometriosis and cancers. These chemicals have also been referred to as endocrine modulators, environmental hormones, and endocrine active compounds. Environmental chemicals with estrogenic activity are probably the most studied; however, chemicals with anti-estrogen, androgen, anti-androgen, progesterone, or thyroid-like activity have also been identified.

What is the endocrine system? Why is it important?

The endocrine system is one of the body's main communication networks and is responsible for controlling and coordinating numerous body functions. Hormones are first produced by the endocrine tissues, such as the ovaries, testes, pituitary, thyroid and pancreas, and then secreted into the blood to act as the body's chemical messengers, where they direct communication and coordination among other tissues throughout the body. For example, hormones work with the nervous system, reproductive system, kidneys, gut, liver, and fat to help maintain and control:

- body energy levels;
- reproduction;
- growth and development;
- internal balance of body systems, called homeostasis; and
- responses to surroundings, stress, and injury.

Endocrine disrupting chemicals may interfere with the body's own hormone signals because of their structure and activity.

How do endocrine disruptors work?

From animal studies, researchers have learned much about the mechanisms through which endocrine disruptors influence the endocrine system and alter hormonal functions.

Endocrine disruptors can:

- Mimic or partly mimic naturally occurring hormones in the body like estrogens (the female sex hormone) and androgens (the male sex hormone) and thyroid hormones, potentially producing over-stimulation.

- Bind to a receptor within a cell and block the endogenous hormone from binding. The normal signal then fails to occur and the body fails to respond properly. Examples of chemicals that block or antagonize hormones are antiestrogens or anti-androgens.

- Interfere or block the way natural hormones or their receptors are made or controlled, for example, by blocking their metabolism in the liver.

Examples of Endocrine Disruptors

A wide and varied range of substances are thought to cause endocrine disruption. Chemicals that are known endocrine disruptors include diethylstilbestrol (the drug DES), dioxin and dioxin-like compounds, polychlorinated biphenyl (PCB), dichlorodiphenyltrichloroethane (DDT), and some other pesticides. Some chemicals, particularly pesticides and plasticizers, such as bisphenol A are suspected endocrine disruptors based on animal studies.

Bisphenol A (BPA) is a manmade chemical that can leach out of plastic products when heated. BPA is used in the manufacture of polycarbonate plastics, often used for food and beverage containers and epoxy resins found in dental sealants. Some endocrine disruptors occur among a group of chemicals referred to as phthalates, a class of chemicals that soften and increase the flexibility of polyvinyl chloride plastics. An example of a phthalate is a compound called di(2-ethylhexyl) phthalate (DEHP). DEHP is a high production volume chemical used in the manufacture of a wide variety of consumer products, such as building products, car products, clothing, food packaging, some children's products, and some polyvinyl chloride medical devices. An independent panel of experts assembled by the National Toxicology Program (NTP) found that DEHP may pose a risk to human development, especially for critically ill male infants.[1]

Phytoestrogens are naturally occurring substances in plants that have hormone-like activity. Examples of phytoestrogens are genistein and daidzein which can be found in soy-derived products. To specifically evaluate the effects that chemicals have on human reproduction, the National Toxicology Program (NTP) developed the Center for the Evaluation of Risks to Human Reproduction (CERHR). This center has evaluated the endocrine disruptor effects of seven phthalates and the phytoestrogen genistein found in soy infant formulas.[2]

Human Exposure to Endocrine Disruptors

People may be exposed to endocrine disruptors through the food and beverages they consume, medicine they take, and cosmetics they use. So, exposures may be through the diet, air, and skin. Some environmental endocrine disrupting chemicals, such as DDT, are highly persistent and slow to degrade in the environment making them potentially hazardous over an extended period of time.

Research on Endocrine Disruptors

The NIEHS has been a pioneer in conducting research on the health effects of endocrine disruptors for more than three decades starting with the endocrine disrupting effects of the pharmaceutical diethylstilbestrol (DES). From the 1940s to the 1970s, DES was used to treat women with high-risk pregnancies with the mistaken belief that it prevented miscarriage. In 1972, prenatal exposure to DES was linked with the development of a rare form of vaginal cancer in the DES-daughters, and with numerous non-cancerous changes in both sons and daughters. NIEHS researchers developed animal models of DES exposure that successfully replicated and predicted human health problems and have been useful in studying the mechanisms involved in DES toxic effects.[3] NIEHS researchers also showed the effects of DES and other endocrine disruptors involved the estrogen receptor protein mechanism.[4] Researchers are playing a lead role in uncovering the mechanisms of action of endocrine disruptors.

Today, scientists are:

- developing new models and tools to better understand how endocrine disruptors work;

- developing high throughput assays to determine which chemicals have endocrine disrupting activity;

- examining the long-term effects of exposure to various endocrine disrupting compounds during development, and on disease and dysfunction later in life;

- conducting epidemiological studies in human populations;

- developing new assessment and biomarkers to determine exposure and toxicity levels, especially how mixtures of chemicals impact individuals; and

• developing intervention and prevention strategies.

Prenatal and Developmental Exposure

Research shows that endocrine disruptors may pose the greatest risk during prenatal and early postnatal development when organ and neural systems are developing. In animals, adverse consequences, such as subfertility, premature reproductive senescence, and cancer are linked to early exposure, but they may not be apparent until much later in life.[5]

Researchers supported by NIEHS at the University of Cincinnati and the University of Illinois found that animals exposed to low doses of the natural human estrogen estradiol, or the environmental estrogen bisphenol A (BPA), during fetal development, and estradiol as adults were more likely to develop a precursor of prostate cancer than those who were not exposed. This suggests that exposure to environmental and natural estrogens during fetal development could affect the way prostate genes behave, and may lead to higher rates of prostate disease during aging.[6]

Exposures at Low Levels

In 2000, an independent panel of experts convened by the NIEHS and the National Toxicology Program (NTP) found that there was credible evidence that some hormone-like chemicals can affect test animal's bodily functions at very low levels—well below the no effect levels determined by traditional testing.[7] Although, there is little evidence to prove that low-dose exposures are causing adverse human health effects, there is a large body of research in experimental animals and wildlife suggesting that endocrine disruptors may cause:

• reductions in male fertility and declines in the numbers of males born;

• abnormalities in male reproductive organs;

• female reproductive diseases including fertility problems, early puberty, and early reproductive senescence; and

• increases in mammary, ovarian, and prostate cancers.

There are data showing that exposure to bisphenol A as well as other endocrine disrupting chemicals with estrogenic activity may have effects on obesity and diabetes. These data, while preliminary and only in animals, indicate the potential for endocrine disrupting agents to have effects on other endocrine systems not yet fully examined.

Transgenerational Effects

There is some evidence that endocrine disruptors may not only impact the individual directly exposed, but also future generations. Research from NIEHS investigators has shown that the adverse effects of DES in mice can be passed to subsequent generations even though they were not directly exposed. The increased susceptibility for tumors was seen in both the granddaughters and grandsons of mice who were developmentally exposed to DES.[8] Mechanisms involved in the transmission of disease were shown to involve epigenetic events.[9] Research funded by the NIEHS also found that endocrine disruptors may affect not just the offspring of mothers exposed during pregnancy, but future offspring as well. The researchers found that two endocrine disrupting chemicals caused fertility defects in male rats that were passed down to nearly every male in subsequent generations. This study suggests that the two compounds may have caused changes in the developing male germ cells, and that endocrine disruptors may be able to reprogram or change the expression of genes without mutating DNA.[10] The role of environmental endocrine disrupting chemicals in the transmission of disease from one generation to another is of great research interest to the NIEHS.

References

1. NTP Brief on the Potential Human Reproductive and Developmental Effects of Di(2-ethylhexyl) Phthalate (DEHP). Draft, May 2006.

2. CERHR website.

3. *Endocrinology* 147 (6) Supplement S11-S17, 2006.

4. *Developmental Biology*. 2001. 238:224-238.

5. *Environmental Health Perspectives* 103:83-87, 1995. *Endocrinology* 147 (6) Supplement S11-S17, 2006.

6. *Cancer Research*. 2006 June 1;66(11):5624-32.

7. National Toxicology Program's Report of the Endocrine Disruptors Low-Dose Peer Review, 2001.

8. *Carcinogenesis.* 2000 July 21;(7):1355-63. *Carcinogenesis* 19; 1655-1663.

9. *Cancer Research* 2000 60-235-237.

10. *Science* 3 June 20. Vol. 308. no. 5727, pp. 1466-1469.

Additional Information

National Institute of Environmental Health Sciences (NIEHS)
P.O. Box 12233
Research Triangle Park, NC 27709
Phone: 919-541-3345
TTY: 919-541-0731
Website: http://www.niehs.nih.gov
E-mail: webcenter@niehs.nih.gov

Chapter 7

Diagnostic Tests and Procedures for Endocrine and Metabolic Disorders

Neurological Diagnostic Tests and Procedures

Diagnostic tests and procedures are vital tools that help physicians confirm or rule out the presence of a neurological disorder or other medical condition. Researchers and physicians use a variety of diagnostic imaging techniques and chemical and metabolic analyses to detect, manage, and treat neurological disease. Some procedures are performed in specialized settings, conducted to determine the presence of a particular disorder or abnormality. Many tests that were previously conducted in a hospital are now performed in a physician's office, or at an outpatient testing facility, with little if any risk to the patient. Depending on the type of procedure, results are either immediate or may take several hours to process.

This chapter includes: Excerpts from "Neurological Diagnostic Tests and Procedures," National Institute of Neurological Disorders and Stroke (NINDS), NIH Publication No. 05–5380, updated December 18, 2006; and, "ERCP (Endoscopic Retrograde Cholangiopancreatography)," National Institute of Diabetes and Digestive and Kidney Diseases (NIDDK), NIH Publication No 05–4336, November 2004. Also, reprinted with permission, "Skin Biopsy for Diagnosis of Metabolic Diseases," and "Muscle Biopsy for Diagnosis of Metabolic Diseases," © 2006 The Cleveland Clinic Foundation, 9500 Euclid Avenue, Cleveland, OH 44195, www.clevelandclinic.org. Additional information is available from the Cleveland Clinic Health Information Center, 216-444-3771, toll-free 800-223-2273 extension 43771, or at http://www.clevelandclinic.org/health.

Common Screening Tests

Laboratory screening tests of blood, urine, or other substances are used to help diagnose disease, better understand the disease process, and monitor levels of therapeutic drugs. Certain tests, ordered by the physician as part of a regular check-up, provide general information, while others are used to identify specific health concerns. For example, blood and blood product tests can detect brain or spinal cord infection, bone marrow disease, hemorrhage, blood vessel damage, toxins that affect the nervous system, and the presence of antibodies that signal the presence of an autoimmune disease. Blood tests are also used to monitor levels of therapeutic drugs used to treat epilepsy and other neurological disorders. Genetic testing of deoxyribonucleic acid (DNA) extracted from white cells in the blood can help diagnose Huntington disease and other congenital diseases. Analysis of the fluid that surrounds the brain and spinal cord can detect meningitis, acute and chronic inflammation, rare infections, and some cases of multiple sclerosis. Chemical and metabolic testing of the blood can indicate protein disorders, some forms of muscular dystrophy and other muscle disorders, and diabetes. Urinalysis can reveal abnormal substances in the urine or the presence or absence of certain proteins that cause diseases including the mucopolysaccharidoses.

Genetic testing or counseling can help parents who have a family history of a neurological disease determine if they are carrying one of the known genes that cause the disorder or find out if their child is affected. Genetic testing can identify many neurological disorders, including spina bifida, in utero (while the child is inside the mother's womb). Genetic tests include the following:

- *Amniocentesis*, usually done at 14–16 weeks of pregnancy, tests a sample of the amniotic fluid in the womb for genetic defects (the fluid and the fetus have the same DNA). Under local anesthesia, a thin needle is inserted through the woman's abdomen and into the womb. About 20 milliliters of fluid (roughly four teaspoons) is withdrawn and sent to a lab for evaluation. Test results often take 1–2 weeks.

- *Chorionic villus sampling*, or CVS, is performed by removing and testing a very small sample of the placenta during early pregnancy. The sample, which contains the same DNA as the fetus, is removed by catheter or fine needle inserted through the cervix, or by a fine needle inserted through the abdomen. It is tested for genetic abnormalities and results are usually available within two weeks. CVS should not be performed after the tenth week of pregnancy.

• *Uterine ultrasound* is performed using a surface probe with gel. This noninvasive test can suggest the diagnosis of conditions such as chromosomal disorders.

Neurological Examinations

A neurological examination assesses motor and sensory skills, the functioning of one or more cranial nerves, hearing and speech, vision, coordination and balance, mental status, and changes in mood or behavior, among other abilities. Items including a tuning fork, flashlight, reflex hammer, ophthalmoscope, and needles are used to help diagnose brain tumors, infections such as encephalitis and meningitis, and diseases such as Parkinson disease, Huntington disease, amyotrophic lateral sclerosis (ALS), and epilepsy. Some tests require the services of a specialist to perform and analyze results.

X-rays of the patient's chest and skull are often taken as part of a neurological work-up. X-rays can be used to view any part of the body, such as a joint or major organ system. In a conventional x-ray, also called a radiograph, a technician passes a concentrated burst of low-dose ionized radiation through the body and onto a photographic plate. Since calcium in bones absorbs x-rays more easily than soft tissue or muscle, the bony structure appears white on the film. Any vertebral misalignment or fractures can be seen within minutes. Tissue masses such as injured ligaments or a bulging disc are not visible on conventional x-rays. This fast, noninvasive, painless procedure is usually performed in a doctor's office or at a clinic.

Fluoroscopy is a type of x-ray that uses a continuous or pulsed beam of low-dose radiation to produce continuous images of a body part in motion. The fluoroscope (x-ray tube) is focused on the area of interest and pictures are either videotaped or sent to a monitor for viewing. A contrast medium may be used to highlight the images. Fluoroscopy can be used to evaluate the flow of blood through arteries.

Tests Used to Diagnose Neurological Disorders

Based on the result of a neurological exam, physical exam, patient history, x-rays of the patient's chest and skull, and any previous screening or testing, physicians may order one or more of the following diagnostic tests to determine the specific nature of a suspected neurological disorder or injury. These diagnostics generally involve either nuclear medicine imaging, in which very small amounts of radioactive materials are used to study organ function and structure, or diagnostic imaging, which uses magnets and electrical charges to study human anatomy.

The following list of available procedures—in alphabetical rather than sequential order—includes some of the more common tests used to help diagnose a neurological condition.

Angiography is a test used to detect blockages of the arteries or veins. A cerebral angiogram can detect the degree of narrowing or obstruction of an artery or blood vessel in the brain, head, or neck. It is used to diagnose stroke and to determine the location and size of a brain tumor, aneurysm, or vascular malformation. This test is usually performed in a hospital outpatient setting and takes up to three hours, followed by a 6- to 8-hour resting period. The patient, wearing a hospital or imaging gown, lies on a table that is wheeled into the imaging area. While the patient is awake, a physician anesthetizes a small area of the leg near the groin and then inserts a catheter into a major artery located there. The catheter is threaded through the body and into an artery in the neck. Once the catheter is in place, the needle is removed and a guide wire is inserted. A small capsule containing a radiopaque dye (one that is highlighted on x-rays) is passed over the guide wire to the site of release. The dye is released and travels through the bloodstream into the head and neck. A series of x-rays is taken and any obstruction is noted. Patients may feel a warm or hot sensation, or slight discomfort, as the dye is released.

Biopsy involves the removal and examination of a small piece of tissue from the body. Muscle or nerve biopsies are used to diagnose neuromuscular disorders and may also reveal if a person is a carrier of a defective gene that could be passed on to children. A small sample of muscle or nerve is removed under local anesthetic and studied under a microscope. The sample may be removed either surgically through a slit made in the skin, or by needle biopsy in which a thin hollow needle is inserted through the skin and into the muscle. A small piece of muscle or nerve remains in the hollow needle when it is removed from the body. The biopsy is usually performed at an outpatient testing facility. A brain biopsy, used to determine tumor type, requires surgery to remove a small piece of the brain or tumor. Performed in a hospital, this operation is riskier than a muscle biopsy and involves a longer recovery period.

Brain scans are imaging techniques used to diagnose tumors, blood vessel malformations, or hemorrhage in the brain. These scans are used to study organ function or injury or disease to tissue or muscle. Types of brain scans include computed tomography, magnetic resonance imaging, and positron emission tomography.

Cerebrospinal fluid (CSF) analysis involves the removal of a small amount of the fluid that protects the brain and spinal cord. The fluid is tested to detect any bleeding or brain hemorrhage, diagnose infection in the brain or spinal cord, identify some cases of multiple sclerosis and other neurological conditions, and measure intracranial pressure.

The procedure is usually done in a hospital. The sample of fluid is commonly removed by a procedure known as a lumbar puncture, or spinal tap. The patient is asked to either lie on one side, in a ball position with knees close to the chest, or lean forward while sitting on a table or bed. The doctor will locate a puncture site in the lower back, between two vertebrate, then clean the area and inject a local anesthetic. The patient may feel a slight stinging sensation from this injection. Once the anesthetic has taken effect, the doctor will insert a special needle into the spinal sac and remove a small amount of fluid (usually about three teaspoons) for testing. Most patients will feel a sensation of pressure only as the needle is inserted.

A common after-effect of a lumbar puncture is headache, which can be lessened by having the patient lie flat. Risk of nerve root injury or infection from the puncture can occur, but it is rare. The entire procedure takes about 45 minutes.

Computed tomography, also known as a CT scan, is a noninvasive, painless process used to produce rapid, clear, two-dimensional images of organs, bones, and tissues. Neurological CT scans are used to view the brain and spine. They can detect bone and vascular irregularities, certain brain tumors and cysts, herniated discs, epilepsy, encephalitis, spinal stenosis (narrowing of the spinal canal), a blood clot or intracranial bleeding in patients with stroke, brain damage from head injury, and other disorders. Many neurological disorders share certain characteristics and a CT scan can aid in proper diagnosis by differentiating the area of the brain affected by the disorder.

Scanning takes about 20 minutes (a CT of the brain or head may take slightly longer) and is usually done at an imaging center or hospital on an outpatient basis. The patient lies on a special table that slides into a narrow chamber. A sound system built into the chamber allows the patient to communicate with the physician or technician. As the patient lies still, x-rays are passed through the body at various angles and are detected by a computerized scanner. The data is processed and displayed as cross-sectional images, or slices, of the internal structure of the body or organ. A light sedative may be given to patients who are unable to lie still, and pillows may be used to support and stabilize the head and body. Persons who are claustrophobic may have difficulty taking this imaging test.

Occasionally a contrast dye is injected into the bloodstream to highlight the different tissues in the brain. Patients may feel a warm or cool sensation as the dye circulates through the bloodstream or they may experience a slight metallic taste.

Although very little radiation is used in CT, pregnant women should avoid the test because of potential harm to the fetus from ionizing radiation.

Electroencephalography, or EEG, monitors brain activity through the skull. EEG is used to help diagnose certain seizure disorders, brain tumors, brain damage from head injuries, inflammation of the brain or spinal cord, alcoholism, certain psychiatric disorders, and metabolic and degenerative disorders that affect the brain. EEG is also used to evaluate sleep disorders, monitor brain activity when a patient has been fully anesthetized or loses consciousness, and confirm brain death.

This painless, risk-free test can be performed in a doctor's office, at a hospital, or at a testing facility. Prior to taking an EEG, the person must avoid caffeine intake and prescription drugs that affect the nervous system. A series of cup-like electrodes are attached to the patient's scalp, either with a special conducting paste or with extremely fine needles. The electrodes (also called leads) are small devices that are attached to wires and carry the electrical energy of the brain to a machine for reading. A very low electrical current is sent through the electrodes and the baseline brain energy is recorded. Patients are then exposed to a variety of external stimuli, including bright or flashing light, noise, or certain drugs. Patients may be asked to open and close their eyes, or to change breathing patterns. The electrodes transmit the resulting changes in brain wave patterns. Since movement and nervousness can change brain wave patterns, patients usually recline in a chair or on a bed during the test. EEG takes up to an hour. Testing for certain disorders requires performing an EEG during sleep, which takes at least three hours.

In order to learn more about brain wave activity, electrodes may be inserted through a surgical opening in the skull and into the brain to reduce signal interference from the skull.

Electromyography, or EMG, is used to diagnose nerve and muscle dysfunction and spinal cord disease. It records the electrical activity from the brain and spinal cord to a peripheral nerve root (found in the arms and legs) that controls muscles during contraction and at rest.

During an EMG, very fine wire electrodes are inserted into a muscle to assess changes in electrical voltage that occur during movement and when the muscle is at rest. The electrodes are attached through a series of wires to a recording instrument. Testing usually takes place at a testing facility and lasts about an hour, but may take longer depending on the number of muscles and nerves to be tested. Most patients find this test to be somewhat uncomfortable.

An EMG is usually done in conjunction with a nerve conduction velocity (NCV) test, which measures electrical energy by assessing the nerve's ability to send a signal. This two-part test is conducted most often in a hospital. A technician tapes two sets of flat electrodes on the skin over the muscles. The first set of electrodes is used to send small pulses of electricity (similar to the sensation of static electricity) to stimulate the nerve that directs a particular muscle. The second set of electrodes transmits the responding electrical signal to a recording machine. The physician then reviews the response to verify any nerve damage or muscle disease. Patients who are preparing to take an EMG or NCV test may be asked to avoid caffeine and not smoke for 2–3 hours prior to the test, as well as to avoid aspirin and non-steroidal anti-inflammatory drugs for 24 hours before the EMG. There is no discomfort or risk associated with this test.

Evoked potentials (also called evoked response) measure the electrical signals to the brain generated by hearing, touch, or sight. These tests are used to assess sensory nerve problems and confirm neurological conditions including multiple sclerosis, brain tumor, acoustic neuroma (small tumors of the inner ear), and spinal cord injury. Evoked potentials are also used to test sight and hearing (especially in infants and young children), monitor brain activity among coma patients, and confirm brain death.

Testing may take place in a doctor's office or hospital setting. It is painless and risk-free. Two sets of needle electrodes are used to test for nerve damage. One set of electrodes, which will be used to measure the electrophysiological response to stimuli, is attached to the patient's scalp using conducting paste. The second set of electrodes is attached to the part of the body to be tested. The physician then records the amount of time it takes for the impulse generated by stimuli to reach the brain. Under normal circumstances, the process of signal transmission is instantaneous.

- *Auditory evoked potentials* (also called brain stem auditory evoked response) are used to assess high-frequency hearing loss, diagnose any damage to the acoustic nerve and auditory pathways in the brainstem, and detect acoustic neuromas. The patient sits in a soundproof room and wears headphones. Clicking sounds are delivered one at a time to one ear while a masking sound is sent to the other ear. Each ear is usually tested twice, and the entire procedure takes about 45 minutes.

- *Visual evoked potentials* detect loss of vision from optic nerve damage (in particular, damage caused by multiple sclerosis). The patient sits close to a screen and is asked to focus on the center of a shifting checkerboard pattern. Only one eye is tested at a time; the other eye is either kept closed or covered with a patch. Each eye is usually tested twice. Testing takes 30–45 minutes.

- *Somatosensory evoked potentials* measure response from stimuli to the peripheral nerves and can detect nerve or spinal cord damage or nerve degeneration from multiple sclerosis and other degenerating diseases. Tiny electrical shocks are delivered by electrode to a nerve in an arm or leg. Responses to the shocks, which may be delivered for more than a minute at a time, are recorded. This test usually lasts less than an hour.

Magnetic resonance imaging (MRI) uses computer-generated radio waves and a powerful magnetic field to produce detailed images of body structures including tissues, organs, bones, and nerves. Neurological uses include the diagnosis of brain and spinal cord tumors, eye disease, inflammation, infection, and vascular irregularities that may lead to stroke. MRI can also detect and monitor degenerative disorders, such as multiple sclerosis, and can document brain injury from trauma.

The equipment houses a hollow tube that is surrounded by a very large cylindrical magnet. The patient, who must remain still during the test, lies on a special table that is slid into the tube. The patient will be asked to remove jewelry, eyeglasses, removable dental work, or other items that might interfere with the magnetic imaging. The patient should wear a sweat shirt and sweat pants or other clothing free of metal eyelets or buckles. MRI scanning equipment creates a magnetic field around the body strong enough to temporarily realign water molecules in the tissues. Radio waves are then passed through the body to detect the relaxation of the molecules back to a random alignment and trigger a resonance signal at different angles within the body. A computer processes this resonance into either a three-dimensional picture or a two-dimensional slice of the tissue being scanned, and differentiates between bone, soft tissues, and fluid-filled spaces by their water content and structural properties. A contrast dye may be used to enhance visibility of certain areas or tissues. The patient may hear grating or knocking noises when the magnetic field is turned on and off. (Patients may wear special earphones to block out the sounds.) Unlike CT scanning, MRI does not use ionizing radiation to produce images. Depending on the part(s) of the body to be scanned, MRI can take up to an hour to complete. The test is painless and risk-free, although persons who are obese or claustrophobic may find it somewhat uncomfortable. (Some centers also use open MRI machines that do not completely surround the person being tested and are less confining. However, open MRI does not currently provide the same picture quality as standard MRI, and some tests may not be available using this equipment). Due to the incredibly strong magnetic field generated by an MRI, patients with implanted medical devices, such as a pacemaker, should avoid the test.

Functional MRI (fMRI) uses the blood's magnetic properties to produce real-time images of blood flow to particular areas of the brain. An fMRI can pinpoint areas of the brain that become active and note how long they stay active. It can also tell if brain activity within a region occurs simultaneously or sequentially. This imaging process is used to assess brain damage from head injury or degenerative disorders, such as Alzheimer disease, and to identify and monitor other neurological disorders, including multiple sclerosis, stroke, and brain tumors.

Positron emission tomography (PET) scans provide two- and three-dimensional pictures of brain activity by measuring radioactive isotopes that are injected into the bloodstream. PET scans of the brain are used to detect or highlight tumors and diseased tissue, measure cellular and tissue metabolism, show blood flow, evaluate patients who have seizure disorders that do not respond to medical therapy and patients with certain memory disorders, and determine brain changes following injury or drug abuse, among other uses. PET may be ordered as a follow-up to a CT or MRI scan to give the physician a greater understanding of specific areas of the brain that may be involved with certain problems. Scans are conducted in a hospital or at a testing facility, on an outpatient basis. A low-level radioactive isotope, which binds to chemicals that flow to the brain, is injected into the blood-stream and can be traced as the brain performs different functions. The patient lies still while overhead sensors detect gamma rays in the body's tissues. A computer processes the information and displays it on a video monitor or on film. Using different compounds, more than one brain function can be traced simultaneously. PET is painless and relatively risk-free. Length of test time depends on the part of the body to be scanned. PET scans are performed by skilled technicians at highly sophisticated medical facilities.

Single photon emission computed tomography (SPECT), a nuclear imaging test involving blood flow to tissue, is used to evaluate certain brain functions. The test may be ordered as a follow-up to an MRI to diagnose tumors, infections, degenerative spinal disease, and stress fractures. As with a PET scan, a radioactive isotope which binds to chemicals that flow to the brain is injected intravenously into the body. Areas of increased blood flow will collect more of the isotope. As the patient lies on a table, a gamma camera rotates around the head and records where the radioisotope has traveled. That information is converted by computer into cross-sectional slices that are stacked to produce a detailed three-dimensional image of blood flow and activity within the brain. The test is performed at either an imaging center or a hospital.

Thermography uses infrared sensing devices to measure small temperature changes between the two sides of the body or within a specific organ. Also known as digital infrared thermal imaging, thermography may be used to detect vascular disease of the head and neck, soft tissue injury, various neuromusculoskeletal disorders, and the presence or absence of nerve root compression. It is performed at an imaging center, using infrared light recorders to take thousands of pictures of the body from a distance of 5 to 8 feet. The information is converted into electrical signals which results in a computer-generated two-dimensional picture of abnormally cold or hot areas indicated by color or shades of black and white. Thermography does not use radiation and is safe, risk-free, and noninvasive.

Ultrasound imaging, also called ultrasound scanning or sonography, uses high-frequency sound waves to obtain images inside the body. Neurosonography (ultrasound of the brain and spinal column) analyzes blood flow in the brain and can diagnose stroke, brain tumors, hydrocephalus (build-up of cerebrospinal fluid in the brain), and vascular problems. It can also identify, or rule out, inflammatory processes causing pain. It is more effective than an x-ray in displaying soft tissue masses and can show tears in ligaments, muscles, tendons, and other soft tissue masses in the back. Transcranial Doppler ultrasound is used to view arteries and blood vessels in the neck and determine blood flow and risk of stroke.

During ultrasound, the patient lies on an imaging table and removes clothing around the area of the body to be scanned. A jelly-like lubricant is applied and a transducer, which both sends and receives high-frequency sound waves, is passed over the body. The sound wave echoes are recorded and displayed as a computer-generated real-time visual image of the structure or tissue being examined. Ultrasound is painless, noninvasive, and risk-free. The test is performed on an outpatient basis and takes between 15 and 30 minutes to complete.

ERCP
(Endoscopic Retrograde Cholangiopancreatography)

Endoscopic retrograde cholangiopancreatography (en-doh-SKAH-pik REH-troh-grayd koh-LAN-jee-oh-PANG-kree-uh-TAH-gruh-fee) (ERCP) enables the physician to diagnose problems in the liver, gallbladder, bile ducts, and pancreas. The liver is a large organ that, among other things, makes a liquid called bile that helps with digestion. The gallbladder is a small, pear-shaped organ that stores bile until it is needed for digestion. The bile ducts are tubes that carry bile from the liver to the gallbladder and small intestine. These ducts are sometimes called the biliary tree. The pancreas is a large gland that produces chemicals that help with digestion and hormones such as insulin.

ERCP is used primarily to diagnose and treat conditions of the bile ducts, including gallstones, inflammatory strictures (scars), leaks (from trauma and surgery), and cancer. ERCP combines the use of x-rays and an endoscope, which is a long, flexible, lighted tube. Through the endoscope, the physician can see the inside of the stomach and duodenum, and inject dyes into the ducts in the biliary tree and pancreas so they can be seen on x-rays.

For the procedure, you will lie on your left side on an examining table in an x-ray room. You will be given medication to help numb the back of your throat and a sedative to help you relax during the exam. You will swallow the endoscope, and the physician will then guide the scope through your esophagus, stomach, and duodenum until it reaches the spot where the ducts of the biliary tree and pancreas open into the duodenum. At this time, you will be turned to lie flat on your stomach, and the physician will pass a small plastic tube through the scope. Through the tube, the physician will inject a dye into the ducts to make them show up clearly on x-rays. X-rays are taken as soon as the dye is injected.

If the exam shows a gallstone or narrowing of the ducts, the physician can insert instruments into the scope to remove or relieve the obstruction. Also, tissue samples (biopsy) can be taken for further testing.

Possible complications of ERCP include pancreatitis (inflammation of the pancreas), infection, bleeding, and perforation of the duodenum. Except for pancreatitis, such problems are uncommon. You may have

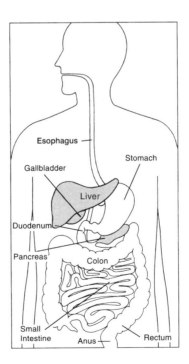

Figure 7.1. *The Digestive System*

74

tenderness or a lump where the sedative was injected, but that should go away in a few days.

ERCP takes thirty minutes to two hours. You may have some discomfort when the physician blows air into the duodenum and injects the dye into the ducts. However, the pain medicine and sedative should keep you from feeling too much discomfort. After the procedure, you will need to stay at the hospital for one to two hours until the sedative wears off. The physician will make sure you do not have signs of complications before you leave. If any kind of treatment is done during ERCP, such as removing a gallstone, you may need to stay in the hospital overnight.

Preparation

Your stomach and duodenum must be empty for the procedure to be accurate and safe. You will not be able to eat or drink anything after midnight the night before the procedure, or for 6–8 hours beforehand, depending on the time of your procedure. Also, the physician will need to know whether you have any allergies, especially to iodine which is in the dye. You must also arrange for someone to take you home—you will not be allowed to drive because of the sedatives. The physician may give you other special instructions.

Skin Biopsy for Diagnosis of Metabolic Diseases

What Is a Skin Biopsy?

A skin biopsy is a procedure in which a physician removes a small sample of tissue to have it tested. This skin sample may help your doctor diagnose a metabolic disease. The skin sample may be removed by a technique known as a punch biopsy.

Before the Procedure

Generally, there is no special preparation needed before a skin biopsy.

During the Procedure

The doctor will first cleanse the biopsy site. He or she will then numb the skin by using an anesthetic (pain-relieving) spray, cream, or injection to minimize pain during the procedure and will then remove two small (3 mm) pieces of skin. A nurse may apply pressure to the area to stop the bleeding. The doctor will then close the incision, using adhesive Steri-Strips™ (which look like small pieces of tape). The entire biopsy procedure lasts about 15 minutes.

After the Procedure

- You will remain in the treatment area for a short time for observation.
- You may have some soreness around the biopsied area for one to two weeks.
- If Steri-Strips™ were used to close the incision, do not remove them. They will gradually fall off on their own.
- You should expect a small scar from the biopsy.
- Ask your doctor when you should come back for a follow-up visit.

How Is the Skin Sample Tested?

The skin sample will usually be sent to labs for microscopic examination (electron microscopy) and fibroblast culture. The electron microscopy report is usually available ten working days after the procedure. Call your doctor's office to get the results.

The fibroblast culture is a way of establishing a "clone" of skin cells that can be used for specific biochemical testing. Skin tissue is different from muscle, brain, heart, and liver tissue, so any results obtained may or may not be helpful in aiding in the diagnosis. Further testing on this clone of cells is not always done. If appropriate, the cells may be frozen for further testing.

Skin cells in culture can stop growing or die at any time. If they die, the entire biopsy procedure will need to be repeated to attempt to establish a clone of skin cells.

Skin cells grow at their own pace, and nothing can be done to make them grow any faster. Sometimes the skin cells grow fast enough to be sent to another lab in approximately two weeks; other times it may take three months or longer. Once the cells have grown enough to be sent to another lab, they must be first tested to make sure they are not contaminated with any bacteria. This can take another five to seven working days.

The specific biochemical testing on the clone of skin cells is not done in many clinics. Depending on which test is ordered, the skin sample will be sent to one of several laboratories that specialize in that specific test. Skin samples are sent by courier service or by overnight mail service to the specialized laboratory. Note: Overnight mail services do not guarantee the safe arrival of human tissues, so if the specimen gets lost, misrouted, or otherwise destroyed, there is nothing that can be done. Unfortunately, there is no practical alternative to using a commercial carrier.

When the cells arrive at the testing laboratory, they must be further grown to a volume that can be used for the test. Depending on the growth rate of the cells, this can take one week to several months. Once the cells have grown to a necessary volume, the test is run. The lab will keep a small amount of cells aside in case your doctor requests more tests. The lab will fax the test results to your doctor as soon as the report is generated. The test results may or may not be diagnostic.

If your doctor determines that the test results are not diagnostic, he or she may order a second test. In this case, the cells used for the first test cannot be used over again, and the cells not used for the first test would be regrown.

When to Call the Doctor

- Call your doctor if you have bleeding that can't be stopped by applying pressure.

- Call your doctor if you have any questions or concerns after the procedure.

Muscle Biopsy for Diagnosis of Metabolic Diseases

What Is a Muscle Biopsy?

A muscle biopsy is an outpatient surgical procedure in which a surgeon removes small samples of muscle tissue for testing. These tissue samples can help your doctor diagnose a metabolic disease, even when other laboratory tests are normal.

Should I Have this Test?

Because a muscle biopsy is an invasive test requiring anesthesia, the risks and costs of the procedure must be considered with the potential of the test yielding positive results, as well as the potential benefits gained by a diagnosis (such as making treatment decisions and family planning). Be sure to discuss all of these variables with your doctor before you decide to have the procedure.

Before the Procedure

Before a muscle biopsy is done, your doctor needs to arrange a plan for how the muscle samples will be distributed to the different labs for testing. The testing laboratories will be contacted before the biopsy is done so that preparation of the muscle is done correctly.

Before the procedure, you will have an opportunity to ask any questions about the procedure. The patient will be given general anesthesia before the procedure. This will make the patient very relaxed and he or she will then be sedated (in a sleep-like state) for the procedure.

During the Procedure

The doctor will first cleanse the biopsy site. The doctor will then make a small incision (1- to 2-inch cut) usually in the top of the thigh. Up to three one-cubic centimeter samples are removed from the rectus muscle. The doctor will then close the incision, usually with stitches. The entire biopsy procedure lasts about 30 minutes.

After the Procedure

- You will remain in the treatment area for a short time for observation.

- There will be some muscle soreness around the biopsied area for 1 to 2 weeks. Patients who have had the procedure describe the pain like a pulled muscle or like pain from a muscle strain.

- Your doctor may prescribe medication to relieve pain for a few days after the procedure.

- Keep the incision area as clean and as dry as possible. Your doctor will tell you when the stitches should be removed (usually within 4 to 7 days).

- You should expect a small scar from the biopsy.

- Ask your doctor when you should come back for a follow-up visit.

When to Call the Doctor

- Call your doctor if you have bleeding that can't be stopped by applying pressure.

- Call your doctor if you have any questions or concerns after the procedure.

Additional Information

American College of Radiology
1891 Preston White Dr.
Reston, VA 20191-4397
Toll-Free: 800-227-5463
Phone: 703-648-8900
Fax: 703-295-6773
Website: http://www.acr.org
E-mail: info@acr.org

American Gastroenterological Association (AGA)
4930 Del Ray Ave.
Bethesda, MD 20814
Phone: 301-654-2055
Fax: 301-654-5920
Website: http://www.gastro.org
E-mail: info@gastro.org

National Digestive Diseases Information Clearinghouse
2 Information Way
Bethesda, MD 20892-3570
Toll-Free: 800-891-5389
Fax: 703-738-4929
Website: http://digestive.niddk.nih.gov
E-mail: nddic@info.niddk.nih.gov

National Institute of Neurological Disorders and Stroke (NINDS)
P.O. Box 20824
Bethesda, MD 20824
Toll-Free: 800-352-9424
Phone: 301-496-5751
Fax: 301-468-5981
Website: http://www.ninds.nih.gov
E-mail: braininfo@ninds.nih.gov

National Library of Medicine (NLM)
8600 Rockville Pike
Bethesda, MD 20894
Toll Free: 888-FIND-NLM (888-346-3656)
Phone: 301-594-5983

Fax: 301-402-1384
Website: http://www.nlm.nih.gov
E-mail: custserv@nlm.nih.gov

Radiological Society of North America
820 Jorie Boulevard
Oak Brook, IL 60523-2251
Toll-Free: 800-381-6660
Phone: 630-571-2670
Fax: 630-571-7837
Website: http://www.rsna.org
E-mail: webmaster@rsna.org

Chapter 8

Prenatal Tests

Every parent-to-be hopes for a healthy baby. But these dreams often are accompanied by moments of worry. What if the baby has a serious or untreatable health problem? What would I do? Would it be my fault?

Concerns like these are completely natural. Fortunately, though, a wide array of prenatal tests for pregnant women can help to reassure them and keep them informed throughout their pregnancies.

Prenatal tests can serve a useful function in terms of identifying—and sometimes treating—health problems that could endanger both you and your unborn child. However, they do have limitations. As an expectant parent, it's important to take the time to educate yourself about these tests and to think about what you would do if a health problem is detected in either you or your baby.

Why Are Prenatal Tests Performed?

Prenatal tests can identify several different things:

- treatable health problems in the mother that can affect the baby's health;

- characteristics of the baby, including size, sex, age, and placement in the uterus;

This information was provided by KidsHealth, one of the largest resources online for medically reviewed health information written for parents, kids, and teens. For more articles like this one, visit www.KidsHealth.org, or www.TeensHealth.org. © 2005 The Nemours Foundation.

- the chance that a baby has certain congenital, genetic, or chromosomal problems;

- certain types of fetal abnormalities, including heart problems.

The last two items on this list may seem the same, but there's a key difference. Some prenatal tests are screening tests and only reveal the possibility of a problem existing. Other prenatal tests are diagnostic, which means they can determine—with a fair degree of certainty—whether a fetus has a specific problem. In the interest of making the more specific determination, the screening test may be followed by a diagnostic test.

Prenatal testing is further complicated by the fact that approximately 250 birth defects can be diagnosed in a fetus—many more than can be treated or cured.

What Do Prenatal Tests Find?

Among other things, routine prenatal tests can determine key things about the mother's health including:

- her blood type;

- whether she has gestational diabetes;

- her immunity to certain diseases;

- whether she has a sexually transmitted disease (STD) or cervical cancer.

All of these conditions can affect the health of the fetus.

Prenatal tests also can determine things about the fetus' health, including whether it's one of the 2% to 3% of babies in the United States that the American College of Obstetricians and Gynecologists (ACOG) says have major congenital birth defects. The different categories of defects screened by prenatal tests include:

Dominant Gene Disorders

In dominant gene disorders, there's a 50–50 chance a child will inherit the gene from the affected parent and have the disorder. Dominant gene disorders include:

- **Achondroplasia:** A rare abnormality of the skeleton that causes a form of dwarfism.

- **Huntington disease:** A disease of the nervous system that causes a combination of mental deterioration and a movement disorder affecting people in their 30s and 40s.

Recessive Gene Disorders

Because there are so many genes in each cell, everyone carries some abnormal genes, but most people don't have a defect because the normal gene overrules the abnormal recessive one. But if a fetus has a pair of abnormal recessive genes (one from each parent), the child will have the disorder. It's more likely for this to happen in children born to certain ethnic groups. Recessive gene disorders include:

- **Cystic fibrosis:** A disease most common among people of northern European descent that is life threatening and causes severe lung damage and nutritional deficiencies.

- **Sickle cell disease:** A disease most common among people of African descent in which red blood cells form a "sickle" shape (rather than the typical donut shape), which can get caught in blood vessels and cause damage to organs and tissues.

- **Tay-Sachs disease:** A disorder most common among people of European (Ashkenazi) Jewish descent that causes mental retardation, blindness, seizures, and death.

- **Beta thalassemia:** A disorder most common among people of Mediterranean descent that causes anemia.

X-Linked Disorders

These disorders are determined by genes on the X chromosome. The X and Y chromosomes are the chromosomes that determine sex. These disorders are much more common in boys because the pair of sex chromosomes in males contains only one X chromosome (the other is a Y chromosome). If the disease gene is present on the one X chromosome, the X-linked disease shows up because there's no other paired gene to "overrule" the disease gene. One such X-linked disorder is hemophilia, which prevents the blood from clotting properly.

Chromosomal Disorders

Some chromosomal disorders are inherited, but most are caused by a random error in the genetics of the egg or sperm. The chance of a child having these disorders increases with the age of the mother. For example, according to ACOG, 1 in 1,667 live babies born to 20-year-olds have Down syndrome, which causes mental retardation and physical defects. That number changes to 1 in 378 for 35-year-olds, and 1 in 106 for 40-year-olds.

Multifactorial Disorders

This final category includes disorders that are caused by a mix of genetic and environmental factors. Their frequency varies from country to country, and some can be detected during pregnancy. Multifactorial disorders include neural tube defects, which occur when the tube enclosing the spinal cord doesn't form properly. Neural tube defects, which often can be prevented by taking folic acid during the early part of pregnancy, include:

• **Spina bifida:** Also called "open spine," this defect happens when the lower part of the neural tube doesn't close during embryo development, leaving the spinal cord and nerve bundles exposed.

• **Anencephaly:** This defect occurs when the brain and head don't develop properly, and the top half of the brain is completely absent.

Other multifactorial disorders include:

• congenital heart defects;
• obesity;
• diabetes;
• cancer.

Who Has Prenatal Tests?

Certain prenatal tests are considered routine—that is, almost all pregnant women receiving prenatal care get them. Other non-routine tests are recommended only for certain women, especially those with high-risk pregnancies. These include women who:

• are age 35 or older;
• have had a premature baby;
• have had a baby with a birth defect—especially heart or genetic problems;

- have high blood pressure, diabetes, lupus, asthma, or a seizure disorder;

- have an ethnic background in which genetic disorders are common (or a partner who does);

- have a family history of mental retardation (or a partner who does).

Although your health care provider (which may be your OB-GYN, family doctor, or a certified nurse-midwife) may recommend these tests, it's ultimately up to you to decide whether to have them. Also, if you or your partner has a family history of genetic problems, you may want to consult with a genetic counselor to help you construct a family tree going back as far as three generations.

To decide which tests are right for you, it's important to carefully discuss with your health care provider:

- what these tests are supposed to measure;

- how reliable they are;

- the potential risks;

- your options and plans if the results indicate a disorder or defect.

Prenatal Tests during the First Visit

During your first visit to your health care provider for prenatal care, you can expect to have a full physical, including a pelvic and rectal examination, and you'll undergo certain tests regardless of your age or genetic background.

Blood tests check for:

- Your blood type and Rh factor. If your blood is Rh negative and your partner's is Rh positive, you may develop antibodies that prove dangerous to your fetus. This can be treated through a course of injections.

- Anemia (a low red blood cell count) to make sure you're not iron deficient.

- Hepatitis B, syphilis, and human immunodeficiency virus (HIV).

- Immunity to German measles (rubella) and chickenpox (varicella).

- Cystic fibrosis. Health care providers now routinely check for this even when there's no family history of the disorder.

Cervical tests (also called Pap smears) check for:

- sexually transmitted disease (STD) such as chlamydia and gonorrhea, and

- cervical cancer.

To do a Pap smear, your health care provider uses what looks like a very long mascara wand or cotton swab to gently scrape the inside of your cervix (the opening to the uterus that's located at the very top of the vagina). This doesn't hurt at all; some women say they feel a little twinge, but it only lasts a second.

Prenatal Tests Performed Throughout or Later in Pregnancy

After the initial visit, your health care provider will order other tests based on, among other things, your personal medical history and needs. Some of these tests may include:

- Urine tests for sugar, protein, and signs of infection. The sugar in urine indicates gestational diabetes—diabetes that occurs during pregnancy; the protein can indicate preeclampsia—a condition that develops in late pregnancy and is characterized by a sudden rise in blood pressure and excessive weight gain, with fluid retention and protein in the urine.

- Group B streptococcus (GBS) infection. GBS bacteria are found naturally in the vaginas of many women and can cause serious infections in newborns. This test involves swabbing the vagina, usually between the 35th and 37th weeks of pregnancy.

- Sickle cell trait tests for women of African or Mediterranean descent, who are at higher risk for having sickle cell anemia—a chronic blood disease—or carrying the trait, which can be passed on to their children.

Other Tests

Following is a list of other tests that are now performed almost routinely in the United States as well as those that are performed only in high-risk pregnancies or if the health care provider suspects an abnormality in the fetus.

Ultrasound

Why is this test performed?

In this test, sound waves are bounced off the baby's bones and tissues to construct an image showing the baby's shape and position in the uterus. Ultrasounds were once used only in high-risk pregnancies but have become so common that they're often part of routine prenatal care.

Also called a sonogram, sonograph, echogram, or ultrasonogram, an ultrasound is used:

- to determine whether the fetus is growing at a normal rate;

- to verify the expected date of delivery;

- to record fetal heartbeat or breathing movements;

- to see whether there might be more than one fetus;

- to identify a variety of abnormalities that might affect the remainder of the pregnancy or delivery;

- to make sure the amount of amniotic fluid in the uterus is adequate;

- to indicate the position of the placenta in late pregnancy (which may be blocking the baby's way out of the uterus);

- to detect pregnancies outside the uterus;

- as a guide during other tests such as amniocentesis.

Ultrasounds also are used to detect:

- structural defects such as spina bifida and anencephaly,

- congenital heart defects,

- gastrointestinal and kidney malformations, or

- cleft lip or palate.

Should I have this test?

Most women have at least one ultrasound. The test is considered to be safe; however, it is wise to find out from your health care provider if it's the most appropriate test for you.

When should I have this test?

An ultrasound is usually performed at 18 to 20 weeks to look at your baby's anatomy. If you want to know your baby's gender, you may be able to find out during this time—that is, if his or her genitals are in a visible position.

Ultrasounds also can be done sooner or later and sometimes more than once, depending on the health care provider. For example, some will order an ultrasound to date the pregnancy, usually during the first two months. And others may want to order one during late pregnancy to make sure the baby's turned the right way before delivery.

Women with high-risk pregnancies may need to have multiple ultrasounds using more sophisticated equipment. Results can be confirmed when needed using special three-dimensional (3-D) equipment that allows the technician to get a more detailed look at the baby.

How is this test performed?

Women need to have a full bladder for a transabdominal ultrasound (an ultrasound of the belly) to be performed in the early months—you may be asked to drink a lot of water and not urinate. You'll lie on an examining table and your abdomen will be coated with a special ultrasound gel. A technician will pass a wand-like instrument called a transducer back and forth over your abdomen. High-frequency sound waves "echo" off your body and create a picture of the fetus inside on a computer screen.

You may want to ask to have the picture interpreted for you, even in late pregnancy—it often doesn't look like a baby to the untrained eye.

Sometimes, if the technician isn't getting a good enough image from the ultrasound, he or she will determine that a transvaginal ultrasound is necessary. This is especially common in early pregnancy. For this procedure, your bladder should be empty. Instead of a transducer being moved over your abdomen, a slender probe called an endovaginal transducer is placed inside your vagina. This technique often provides improved images of the uterus and ovaries.

Some health care providers may have the equipment and trained personnel necessary to provide in-office ultrasounds, whereas others may have you go to a local hospital or radiology center. Depending on where you have the ultrasound done, you may be able to get a printed picture (or multiple pictures) of your baby or a disc of images you can view on your computer and even send to friends and family.

When are the results available?

Immediately, but a full evaluation may take up to one week. A radiologist (a physician experienced in obstetric ultrasound) will analyze the images and send a signed report with his or her interpretation to your doctor.

Depending on where you have the ultrasound done, the technician may be able to tell you that day whether everything looks okay. However, most radiology centers or health care providers prefer that technicians not comment until a specialist has taken a look—especially if an abnormality is detected, but even when everything is okay.

Glucose Screening

Why is this test performed?

Glucose screening checks for gestational diabetes, a short-term form of diabetes that develops in some women during pregnancy. Gestational diabetes occurs in 1% to 3% of pregnancies and can cause health problems for the baby.

Should I have this test?

Most women have this test.

When should I have this test?

Screening for gestational diabetes usually takes place at 12 weeks for women at higher risk of having the condition, including those who:

- have previously had a baby that weighs more than nine pounds (4.1 kilograms);
- have a family history of diabetes;
- are obese;
- are older than age 30.

All other pregnant women are tested for diabetes at around 24 to 28 weeks. But if you've had high sugar in two routine urine tests, your health care provider may order it earlier.

How is the test performed?

This test involves drinking a sugary liquid and then having your blood drawn after an hour. If the sugar level in the blood is high, you'll have a glucose-tolerance test, which means you'll drink a glucose solution on an empty stomach and have your blood drawn once every hour for three hours. The American Diabetes Association suggests that in order to confirm diabetes, these tests be performed at different times.

When are the results available?

The results are usually available within a day, although your health care provider probably won't call you unless the reading is high and you need to come in for another test.

Chorionic Villus Sampling (CVS)

Why is this test performed?

Chorionic villi are tiny finger-like units that make up the placenta (a disk-like structure that sticks to the inner lining of the uterus and provides nutrients from the mother to the fetus through the umbilical cord). They have the same chromosomes and genetic makeup as the fetus.

This newer alternative to an amniocentesis removes some of the chorionic villi and tests them for chromosomal abnormalities, such as Down syndrome. Its advantage over an amniocentesis is that it can be performed earlier, allowing more time for expectant parents to receive counseling and make decisions.

Should I have this test?

Your health care provider may recommend this test if you:

- are older than age 35;
- have a family history of genetic disorders (or a partner who does);
- have a previous child with a birth defect;
- have had an earlier screening test that indicates that there may be a concern.

Possible risks of this test include:

- between a 0.5% and 1% risk of miscarriage
- prematurity
- early labor

- infection
- spotting or bleeding (this is more common with the transcervical method)

When should I have this test?

At 10 to 12 weeks.

How is this test performed?

This test is done in one of two ways:

- *Transcervical:* Using ultrasound as a guide, a thin tube is passed from the vagina into the cervix. Gentle suction removes a sample of tissue from the chorionic villi. No anesthetic is used, although some women do experience a pinch and cramping.

- *Transabdominal:* A needle is inserted through the abdominal wall—this minimizes the chances of intrauterine infection, and in a woman whose uterus is in a bent position, reduces the chance of miscarriage. After the sample is taken, the doctor will check the fetus' heart rate. You should rest for several hours afterward.

When are the results available?

Less than one week for Down syndrome and about two weeks for a thorough analysis.

Maternal Blood Screening/Triple Screen/Quadruple Screen

Why is this test performed?

Doctors use this to test the mother's blood only for alpha-fetoprotein (AFP). AFP is the protein produced by the fetus, and it appears in varying amounts in the mother's blood and the amniotic fluid at different times during pregnancy. A certain level in the mother's blood is considered normal, but higher or lower levels may indicate a problem. The test typically is used to determine risk for Down syndrome.

This test has been expanded, however, to also detect two pregnancy hormones—estriol and human chorionic gonadotropin (HCG)—which is why it's now sometimes called a "triple screen" or "triple marker." The test is called a "quadruple screen" (quad screen) or "quadruple marker" (quad marker) when the level of an additional substance—

inhibin-A—is also measured. The greater number of markers increases the accuracy of the screening and better identifies the possibility of a birth defect.

This test, which also is called a multiple-marker screening, or maternal serum screening, calculates a woman's individual risk of birth defects based on the levels of the three (or more) substances plus:

- her age,
- her weight,
- her race, and
- whether she has diabetes requiring insulin treatment.

It's important to note, though, that this screening test determines risk only—it doesn't diagnose a condition.

Should I have this test?

All women are offered this test. Remember that this is a screening, not a definitive test—it indicates whether a woman is likely to be carrying an affected fetus. It's also not foolproof—spina bifida may go undetected, and some women with high levels have been found to be carrying a healthy baby. Further testing is recommended to confirm a positive result.

When should I have this test?

At 16 to 18 weeks.

How is the test performed?

Blood is drawn from the mother.

When are the results available?

Three to five days, although it may take up two weeks.

Amniocentesis

Why is this test performed?

This test is most often used to detect:

- Down syndrome and other chromosome abnormalities;

- structural defects such as spina bifida and anencephaly; or
- inherited metabolic disorders.

Late in the pregnancy, this test can reveal if a baby's lungs are strong enough to allow the baby to breathe normally after birth. This can help the health care provider make decisions about inducing labor or trying to prevent labor, depending on the situation. For instance, if a mother's water breaks early, the health care provider may want to try to hold off on delivering the baby as long as possible to allow for the baby's lungs to mature.

Other common birth defects, such as heart disorders and cleft lip and palate, can't be determined using this test.

Should I have this test?

Your health care provider may recommend this test if you:

- are older than age 35;
- have a family history of genetic disorders (or a partner who does);
- have a previous child with a birth defect.

This test can be very accurate—close to 100%—but only certain disorders can be detected. According to the Centers for Disease Control and Prevention (CDC), the rate of miscarriage with this procedure is between 1 in 400 and 1 in 200. The procedure also carries a low risk of uterine infection (less than 1 in 1,000), which can cause miscarriage.

When should I have this test?

At 16 to 18 weeks.

How is the test performed?

A needle is inserted through the abdominal wall into the uterus to remove some (about one ounce) of the amniotic fluid. A local anesthetic may be used. Some women report that they experience cramping when the needle enters the uterus or pressure while the doctor retrieves the sample.

The doctor will check the fetus' heartbeat after the procedure to make sure it's normal. Most doctors recommend rest for several hours after the procedure.

The cells in the withdrawn fluid are grown in a special culture and then analyzed (the specific tests conducted on the fluid depend on personal and family medical history).

When are the results available?

Timing varies; it can take up to one month, with the possibility that the lab will ask for a repeat. Tests of lung maturity are available immediately.

Nonstress Test

Why is this test performed?

A nonstress test (NST) can determine if the baby is responding normally to a stimulus. Used mostly in high-risk pregnancies or when a health care provider is uncertain of fetal movement, an NST can be performed at any point in the pregnancy after the 26th to 28th week when fetal heart rate can appropriately respond by accelerating and decelerating.

If you've gone beyond your due date, this test also uses external fetal monitoring to determine fetal movement. The NST can help a doctor make sure that the baby is receiving enough oxygen and that the nervous system is responding. However, a nonresponsive baby doesn't necessarily mean that the baby is in danger.

Should I have this test?

Your health care provider may recommend this if you have a high-risk pregnancy or if you have a low-risk pregnancy but are past your due date.

When should I have this test?

At one week after the due date.

How is the test performed?

The health care provider will measure the response of the fetus' heart rate to each movement the fetus makes as reported by the mother or observed by the doctor on an ultrasound screen. If the fetus doesn't move during the test, he or she may be asleep and the health care provider may use a buzzer to wake the baby.

When are the results available?

Immediately.

Contraction Stress Test

Why is this test performed?

This test stimulates the uterus with Pitocin, a synthetic form of oxytocin (a hormone secreted during childbirth), to determine the effect of contractions on fetal heart rate. It's usually recommended when a nonstress test indicates a problem and can determine whether the baby's heart rate remains stable during contractions.

Should I have this test?

This test is usually ordered if the nonstress test indicates a problem. It does have a high false-positive rate, though, and can induce labor.

When should I have this test?

Your doctor will schedule it if he or she is concerned about how the baby will respond to contractions or feels that it is the appropriate test to determine the fetal heart rate response to a stimulus.

How is the test performed?

Mild contractions are brought on either by injections of Pitocin or by squeezing the mother's nipples (which causes oxytocin to be secreted). The fetus' heart rate is then monitored.

When are the results available?

Immediately.

Percutaneous Umbilical Blood Sampling (PUBS)

Why is this test performed?

This test obtains fetal blood by guiding a needle into the umbilical vein. It's primarily used in addition to an ultrasound and amniocentesis if your health care provider needs to quickly check your baby's chromosomes for defects or disorders, or if he or she is concerned that your baby may be anemic.

The advantage to this test is its speed. There are situations (such as when a fetus shows signs of distress) in which it's helpful to know whether the fetus has a fatal chromosomal defect. If the fetus is suspected to be anemic or to have a platelet disorder, this test is the only way to confirm this because it provides a blood sample rather than amniotic fluid. It also allows transfusion of blood or needed fluids into the baby while the needle is in place.

Should I have this test?

This test is used:

- after an abnormality has been noted on an ultrasound;
- when amniocentesis results aren't conclusive;
- if the fetus may have Rh disease;
- if you've been exposed to an infectious disease that could potentially affect fetal development.

When should I have this test?

Between 18 and 36 weeks.

How is the test performed?

A fine needle is passed through your abdomen and uterus into the fetal vein in the umbilical cord and blood is withdrawn for testing.

When are the results available?

In three days.

Talking to Your Health Care Provider

Some prenatal tests can be stressful, and because many aren't definitive, even a negative result may not ease any anxiety you may be experiencing. Because many women who have abnormal tests end up having healthy babies, and because many of the problems that are detected can't be treated, some women decide not to have some of the tests.

One important thing to consider is what you'll do in the event that a birth defect is discovered. Your health care provider or a genetic counselor can help you establish priorities, give you the facts, and discuss your options.

It's also important to remember that tests are offered to women—they are not mandatory. You should feel free to ask your health care provider why he or she is ordering a certain test, what the risks and benefits are, and, most important, what the results will—and won't—tell you.

If you think that your health care provider isn't answering your questions adequately, you should say so. You don't have to accept the answer, "I do this test on all of my patients." Things you might want to ask include:

- How accurate is this test?
- What are you looking to get from these test results? What do you hope to learn?
- How long before I get the results?
- Is the procedure painful?
- Is the procedure dangerous to me or the fetus?
- Do the potential benefits outweigh the risks?
- What could happen if I don't undergo this test?
- How much will the test cost?
- Will the test be covered by insurance?
- What do I need to do to prepare?

You also can ask your health care provider for literature about each type of test.

Preventing Birth Defects

The best thing that mothers-to-be can do to avoid birth defects is to take care of their bodies during pregnancy by:

- not smoking (and avoiding second-hand smoke),
- avoiding alcohol,
- eating a healthy diet,
- taking prenatal vitamins,
- getting exercise,
- getting plenty of rest, and
- getting prenatal care.

Chapter 9

Newborn Screening for Metabolic Disorders

Newborn Screening Tests

Newborn screening is the practice of testing every newborn for certain harmful or potentially fatal disorders that aren't otherwise apparent at birth. Many of these are metabolic disorders, often called "inborn errors of metabolism," which interfere with the body's use of nutrients to maintain healthy tissues and produce energy. Other disorders that may be detected through screening include problems with hormones) or the blood.

In general, metabolic and other inherited disorders can hinder an infant's normal physical and mental development in a variety of ways. And parents can pass along the gene for a certain disorder without even knowing that they're carriers.

With a simple blood test, doctors can often tell whether newborns have certain conditions that could eventually cause problems. Even though these conditions are considered rare and most babies are given

"Newborn Screening Tests," information provided by KidsHealth, one of the largest resources online for medically reviewed health information written for parents, kids, and teens. For more articles like this one, visit www.KidsHealth.org, or www.TeensHealth.org. © 2006 The Nemours Foundation. Tables 9.1, 9.2, and 9.3 are from the "National Newborn Screening Status Report," reprinted with permission from the National Newborn Screening and Genetics Resource Center (NNSGRC). For additional information, contact the NNSGRC at 1912 W. Anderson Lane, Suite 210, Austin, TX 78757, 512-454-6419, or visit their website at http://genes-r-us.uthscsa.edu.

a clean bill of health, early diagnosis and proper treatment can make the difference between lifelong impairment and healthy development.

Newborn Screening: Past, Present, and Future

In the early 1960s, scientist Robert Guthrie, PhD, developed a blood test that could determine whether newborn babies had a metabolic disorder known as phenylketonuria (PKU). People with PKU lack an enzyme needed to process the amino acid phenylalanine. This amino acid is necessary for normal growth in infants and children and for normal protein use throughout life. However, if too much of it builds up, it damages the brain tissue and can eventually cause mental retardation.

When babies with PKU are put on a special diet right away, they can often avoid the mental retardation that children with PKU experienced in the past. By following certain dietary restrictions, these children can lead normal lives.

Since the development of the PKU test, researchers have developed additional blood tests that can screen newborns for other disorders that, unless detected and treated early, can cause physical problems, mental retardation, and in some cases, death.

Most states, the District of Columbia, Puerto Rico, and the U.S. Virgin Islands now have their own mandatory newborn screening programs (in some states, such as Wyoming and Maryland, the screening is not mandatory). Because the federal government has set no national standard, screening requirements vary from state to state, as determined by individual state public health departments.

Consequently, the comprehensiveness of these programs varies, with states routinely screening for anywhere from four to 30 disorders. The average state program tests from four to 10 disorders.

State requirements tend to change periodically as well. In fact, the pace of change is speeding up, thanks to the development of a new screening technique known as tandem mass spectrometry (often abbreviated as MS/MS). This technology can detect the blood components that are elevated in certain disorders, and is capable of screening for more than 20 inherited metabolic disorders with a single test.

About half of the states are offering expanded screening with tandem mass spectrometry on every baby. However, there's some controversy over whether the new technology has been tested adequately. Also, some experts want more evidence that early detection of every disease tested for will actually offer babies some long-term benefit. Equally important, parents may not want to know ahead of time that their child will develop a serious condition when there are no medical treatments or dietary changes that can improve the outcome. And some questions about who will pay (states, insurance companies, or parents) for the newer technology have yet to be resolved.

The American Academy of Pediatrics (AAP) and the federal government's Health Resources and Services Administration convened a task force of experts to grapple with these issues and recommend next steps. Their report identified some flaws and inconsistencies in the current state-driven screening system and proposed the following:

- All state screening programs should reflect current technology.

- All states should test for the same disorders.

- Parents should be informed about screening procedures and have the right to refuse screening, as well as the right to keep the results private and confidential.

- Parents should be informed about the benefits and risks associated with newborn screening.

All of this can be a little confusing (and anxiety-provoking) for a new parent. The inconsistencies among state requirements mean that there's no clear consensus on what's really necessary. On the one hand, it's important to keep in mind that the disorders being screened for are rare. On the other hand, no parent wants to take any unnecessary chances with the quality of his or her child's life—no matter how small the risk.

How Do States and Hospitals Determine Which Tests They Offer?

Traditionally, state decisions about what to screen for have been based on weighing the costs against the benefits. "Cost" considerations include:

- the risk of false positive results (and the unnecessary anxiety they cause);

- the availability of treatments proven to help the condition;

- financial costs.

And states often face conflicting priorities when determining their budgets. For instance, a state may face a choice between expanding newborn screening and ensuring that all expectant mothers get sufficient prenatal care. Of course, this offers little comfort to parents whose children have a disorder that could have been found through a screening test but wasn't.

So what can you do? Your best strategy is to stay informed. Discuss this issue with both your obstetrician or health care provider and your future baby's doctor before you give birth. Know what tests are routinely done in your state and in the hospital where you'll deliver (some hospitals go beyond what's required by state law).

If your state isn't offering screening for the expanded panel of disorders, you may want to ask your doctors about supplemental screening. Keep in mind, though, that you'll probably have to pay for the additional tests out of your own pocket.

If you're the parent of an infant and are concerned about whether your child was screened for certain conditions, ask your child's doctor for information about which tests were performed and whether further tests are recommended.

What Disorders Will Be Screened for in My Newborn?

Newborn screening varies by state and is subject to change, especially given advancements in technology. However, the disorders listed here are the ones typically included in newborn screening programs and are listed in order from the most common (all states screen for the first two) to least common (ranging from three-fourths or one-half of states to just a few). Incidence figures included in this list are according to a 1996 AAP policy statement.

PKU: When this disorder is detected early, feeding an infant a special formula low in phenylalanine can prevent mental retardation. A low-phenylalanine diet will need to be followed throughout childhood and adolescence and perhaps into adult life. This diet cuts out all high-protein foods, so people with PKU often need to take a special artificial formula as a nutritional substitute. Incidence: 1 in 10,000 to 25,000.

Congenital hypothyroidism: This is the disorder most commonly identified by routine screening. Affected babies don't have enough thyroid hormone and so develop retarded growth and brain development. (The thyroid, a gland at the front of the neck, releases chemical substances that control metabolism and growth.) If the disorder is detected early, a baby can be treated with oral doses of thyroid hormone to permit normal development. Incidence: 1 in 4,000.

Galactosemia: Babies with galactosemia lack the enzyme that converts galactose (one of two sugars found in lactose) into glucose, a sugar the body is able to use. As a result, milk (including breast milk) and other dairy products must be eliminated from the diet. Otherwise, galactose can build up in the system and damage the body's cells and organs, leading to blindness, severe mental retardation, growth deficiency, and even death. Incidence: 1 in 60,000 to 80,000. There are several less severe forms of galactosemia that may be detected by newborn screening. These may not require any intervention.

Sickle cell disease: Sickle cell disease is an inherited blood disease in which red blood cells stretch into abnormal "sickle" shapes and can cause episodes of pain, damage to vital organs such as the lungs and kidneys, and even death. Young children with sickle cell disease are especially prone to certain dangerous bacterial infections, such as pneumonia (inflammation of the lungs) and meningitis (inflammation of the brain and spinal cord). Studies suggest that newborn screening can alert doctors to begin antibiotic treatment before infections occur and to monitor symptoms of possible worsening more closely. The screening test can also detect other disorders affecting hemoglobin (the oxygen-carrying substance in the blood). Incidence: about 1 in every 500 African-American births and 1 in every 1,000 to 1,400 Hispanic-American births; also occurs with some frequency among people of Hispanic, Mediterranean, Middle Eastern, and South Asian descent.

Biotinidase deficiency: Babies with this condition don't have enough biotinidase, an enzyme that recycles biotin (one of the B vitamins) in the body. The deficiency may cause seizures, poor muscle control, immune system impairment, hearing loss, mental retardation, coma, and even death. If the deficiency is detected in time, however, problems can be prevented by giving the baby extra biotin. Incidence: 1 in 72,000 to 126,000.

Congenital adrenal hyperplasia: This is actually a group of disorders involving a deficiency of certain hormones produced by the adrenal gland. It can affect the development of the genitals and may cause death due to loss of salt from the kidneys. Lifelong treatment through supplementation of the missing hormones manages the condition. Incidence: 1 in 12,000.

Maple syrup urine disease (MSUD): Babies with MSUD are missing an enzyme needed to process three amino acids that are essential for the body's normal growth. When these are not processed properly, they can build up in the body, causing urine to smell like maple syrup or sweet, burnt sugar. These babies usually have little appetite and are extremely irritable. If not detected and treated early, MSUD can cause mental retardation, physical disability, and even death. A carefully controlled diet that cuts out certain high-protein foods containing those amino acids can prevent these outcomes. Like people with PKU, those with MSUD are often given a formula that supplies the necessary nutrients missed in the special diet they must follow. Incidence: 1 in 250,000.

Homocystinuria: This metabolic disorder results from a deficiency of one of several enzymes for normal development. If untreated, it can lead to dislocated lenses of the eyes, mental retardation, skeletal abnormalities, and abnormal blood clotting. However, a special diet combined with dietary supplements may help prevent most of these problems. Incidence: 1 in 50,000 to 150,000.

Tyrosinemia: Babies with this disorder have trouble processing the amino acid tyrosine. If it accumulates in the body, it can cause mild retardation, language skill difficulties, liver problems, and even death from liver failure. A special diet and sometimes a liver transplant are needed to treat the condition. Early diagnosis and treatment seem to offset long-term problems, although more information is needed. Incidence: not yet determined. Some babies have a mild self-limited form of tyrosinemia

Cystic fibrosis: Cystic fibrosis is an inherited disorder expressed in the various organs that causes cells to release a thick mucus, which can lead to chronic respiratory disease, problems with digestion, and poor growth. There is no known cure—treatment involves trying to prevent the serious lung infections associated with it and providing adequate nutrition. Some infections may be prevented with antibiotics. Detecting the disease early may help doctors reduce the lung and nutritional problems associated with cystic fibrosis, but the real impact of newborn screening is yet to be determined. Incidence: 1 in 2,000 Caucasian babies; less common in African-Americans, Hispanics, and Asians.

Toxoplasmosis: Toxoplasmosis is a parasitic infection that can be transmitted through the mother's placenta to an unborn child. The disease-causing organism, which is found in uncooked or undercooked meat, can invade the brain, eye, and muscle, possibly resulting in blindness and mental retardation. The benefit of early detection and treatment is uncertain. Incidence: 1 in 1,000. But only one or two states screen for toxoplasmosis.

These aren't the only disorders that can be detected through newborn screening. Certain other rare disorders of body chemistry can also be detected. Other conditions that are candidates for newborn screening include:

- Duchenne muscular dystrophy, a childhood form of muscular dystrophy that can be detected through a blood test;

- Human immunodeficiency virus (HIV);

- neuroblastoma, a type of cancer that can be detected with a urine test.

Hearing Screening

Most, but not all states require newborns' hearing to be screened before they are discharged from the hospital. If your infant isn't examined at that time, it's important to make sure that he or she does get screened within the first three weeks of life. A child develops critical speaking and language skills in the first few years of life, and if a hearing loss is caught early, doctors can treat it so that it doesn't interfere with that development.

Should I Request Additional Tests?

If you answer "yes" to any of the questions below, talk to your child's future doctor and perhaps a genetic counselor about requesting additional tests.

- Do you have a positive family history of an inherited disorder?

- Have you previously given birth to a child who's affected by a disorder?

- Did an infant in your family die because of a suspected metabolic disorder?

- Do you have another reason to believe that your child may be at risk for a certain condition?

If your hospital can't or won't make expanded screening available to you, and your doctors believe additional testing would be worthwhile,

Table 9.1. National Newborn Screening Status Report (Updated March 6, 2007); reprinted with permission from the National Newborn Screening and Genetics Resource Center (NNSGRC).

The U.S. National Screening Status Report lists the status of newborn screening in the United States.

Dot "●" indicates that screening for the condition is universally required by Law or Rule and fully implemented

A = universally offered but not yet required, B = offered to select populations, or by request, C = testing required but not yet implemented
D = likely to be detected (and reported) as a by-product of MRM screening (MS/MS) targeted by Law or Rule

STATE	Hearing HEAR	Endocrine CH	Endocrine CAH	Core[1] Conditions Hemoglobin Hb S/S	Hb S/A	Hb S/C	Other BIO	GALT	CF	Additional Conditions Included in Screening Panel (universally required unless otherwise indicated)
Alabama	A	●	●	●	●	●	●	●		
Alaska	●	●	●	●	●	●	●	●	C	
Arizona	A	●	●	●	●	●	●	●	C	
Arkansas	●	●	●	●	●	●	●	●		
California	B	●	●	●	●	●	C	●	C	HHH; PRO; EMA
Colorado	●	●	●	●	●	●	●	●	●	
Connecticut	●	●	●	●	●	●	●	●	B	HHH; HIV[2]; NKH
D.C.	●	●	●	●	●	●	●	●	●	
Delaware	●	●	●	●	●	●	●	●	●	G6PD
Florida	●	●	●	●	●	●	●	●	C	
Georgia	A	●	●	●	●	●	●	●	●	
Hawaii	A	●	●	●	●	●	●	●		
Idaho	A	●	●	●	●	●	●	●		
Illinois	●	●	●	●	●	●	●	●	●	5-OXO, HIV[2]
Indiana	●	●	●	●	●	●	●	●	●	
Iowa	●	●		●	●	●	●	●	●	HHH; NKH
Kansas	●	●	●	●	●	●	●	●		
Kentucky	●	●	●	●	●	●	●	●	●	
Louisiana	●	●	●	●	●	●	●	●		
Maine	A	●	●	●	●	●	●	●	●	
Maryland	●	●	●	●	●	●	●	●		HHH; CPS (D)
Massachusetts	●	●	●	●	●	●	●	●	A	TOXO; HHH (A); CPS (D)
Michigan	●	●	●	●	●	●	●	●	C	
Minnesota	A	●	●	●	●	●	●	●	●	
Mississippi	●	●	●	●	●	●	●	●	●	5-OXO; CPS; HHH
Missouri	●	●	●	●	●	●	C	●	C	
Montana	A	●	B	●	●	●	B	●	B	
Nebraska	A	●	●	●	●	●	●	●	●	5-OXO; HHH; NKH (A)

Main screening table (rotated in original). States listed with markers and additional condition notes:

State	BIO	Additional conditions / notes
Nevada	A	
New Hampshire	A	
New Jersey		
New Mexico		
New York		HIV; HHH; Krabbe Disease
North Carolina		
North Dakota	A	HHH; NKH
Ohio		
Oklahoma		
Oregon	A	
Pennsylvania		5-OXO; CPS; G6PD; HHH; NKH (B)
Rhode Island		
South Carolina	A	
South Dakota	A	5-OXO; EMA; HHH; NKH
Tennessee	B	5-OXO; HHH; NKH
Texas		
Utah		
Vermont		CPS
Virginia		
Washington	A	
West Virginia		
Wisconsin	A	
Wyoming	A	

[1] Terminology consistent with ACMG report - Newborn Screening; Towards a Uniform Screening Panel and System. Genet Med. 2006; 8(5) Suppl: S12-S252

[2] Newborn screened for HIV only if mother was not screened during pregnancy

Additional Conditions/Abbreviations and Names

BIO	Biotinidase	CF	Cystic fibrosis	G6PD	Glucose 6 phosphate dehydrogenase	HB S/C	Sickle – C disease	HEAR	Hearing screening
CAH	Congenital adrenal hyperplasia	CH	Congenital hypothyroidism	HHH	Hyperammonemia/ornithinemia/ citrullinemia (Ornithine transporter defect)	HB S/A	S-β thalassemia		
		GALT	Transferase deficient galactosemia (Classical)	HIV	Human immunodeficiency virus				
		HB S/S	Sickle cell disease						

Other Disorders

Abbr	Name	Abbr	Name
5-OXO	5-oxoprolinuria (pyroglutamic aciduria)	NKH	Nonketotic hyperglycinemia
CPS	Carbamoylphosphate synthetase	PRO	Prolinemia
EMA	Ethylmalonic encephalopathy	TOXO	Toxoplasmosis

Table 9.2. National Newborn Screening Status Report: Core Conditions–Metabolic; reprinted with permission from the National Newborn Screening and Genetics Resource Center (NNSGRC).

Dot "●" indicates that screening for the condition is universally required by Law or Rule and fully implemented

A = universally offered but not yet required, B = offered to select populations, or by request, C = testing required but not yet implemented

D = likely to be detected (and reported) as a by-product of MRM screening (MS/MS) targeted by Law or Rule

STATE	Fatty Acid Disorders					Organic Acid Disorders									Amino Acid Disorders					
	CUD	LCHAD	MCAD	TFP	VLCAD	GA-I	HMG	IVA	3-MCC	CbI-A,B	BKT	MUT	PROP	MCD	ASA	CIT	HCY	MSUD	PKU	TYR-I
Alabama	●	●	●			●	●	●	●	●	●	●	●		D	●	●	●	●	●
Alaska	●	●	●	●	●	●	●	●	●	●	●	●	●	●	●	●	●	●	●	●
Arizona	●	●	●	●	●	●	●	●	●	●	●	●	●	●	●	●	●	●	●	●
Arkansas	●		●																●	
California	●	●	●	●	●	●	●	●	●	●	●	●	●	●	●	●	●	●	●	●
Colorado	●	●	●	●	●	●	●	●	●	●	●	●	●	●	●	●	●	●	●	●
Connecticut	●	●	●	●	●	●	●	●	●	●	●	●	●	●	●	●	●	●	●	●
D. of Columbia	●	●	●	●	●	●	●	●	●	●	●	●	●	●	●	●	●	●	●	●
Delaware		●	●	●	●	●	●	●	●	●	●	●	●	●	●	●	●	●	●	●
Florida	●	●	●	●	●	●	●	●	●	●	●	●	●	●	●	●	●	●	●	●
Georgia	●	●	●	●	●	●	●	●	●	●	●	●	●	●	●	●	●	●	●	●
Hawaii	●	●	●	●	●	●	●	●	C	●	●	●	●	●	●	●	●	●	●	●
Idaho	●	●	●	●	●	●	●	●	●	●	●	●	●	●	●	●	●	●	●	●
Illinois	●	●	●	●	●	●	●	●	●	●	●	●	●	D	●	●	●	●	●	●
Indiana	●	●	●	●	●	●	●	●	●	●	●	●	●	D	●	●	●	●	●	●
Iowa	●	●	●	●	●	●	●	●	●	●	●	●	●	●	●	●	●	●	●	●
Kansas																				
Kentucky	●	●	●	●	●	●	●	●	●	●	●	●	●	●	●	●	●	●	●	●
Louisiana	D	●	●	●	●	●	●	●	●	●	●	●	●	●	●	●	●	●	●	●
Maine	D	●	●	D	●	●	●	●	●	●	●	●	●	D	●	●	●	●	●	●
Maryland	D	●	●	●	●	●	●	●	●	●	●	●	●	●	●	●	●	●	●	●
Massachusetts	D	A	●	D	A	A	A	A	A	A	●	A	A	D	A	A	●	●	●	A
Michigan	●	●	●	●	●	●	●	●	●	●	●	●	●	D	●	●	●	●	●	●
Minnesota	●	●	●	●	●	●	●	●	●	●	●	●	●	●	●	●	●	●	●	●
Mississippi	●	●	●	●	●	●	●	●	●	●	●	●	●	●	●	●	●	●	●	●

Core¹ Conditions - Metabolic

Deficiency/Disorder Abbreviations and Names (optional nomenclature)

Abbrev.	Disorder
3-MCC	3-Methylcrotonyl-CoA carboxylase
ASA	Argininosuccinate acidemia
BKT	Beta ketothiolase (mitochondrial acetoacetyl-CoA thiolase ; short-chain ketoacyl thiolase; T2)
CBL A,B	Methylmalonic acidemia (Vitamin B12 Disorders)
CIT I	Citrullinemia type I (Argininosuccinate synthetase)
CUD	Carnitine uptake defect (Carnitine transport defect)
GA-1	Glutaric acidemia type 1
HCY	Homocystinuria (cystathionine beta synthase)
HMG	3-Hydroxy 3 - methylglutaric aciduria (3-Hydroxy 3- methylglutaryl-CoA lyase)
IVA	Isovaleric acidemia (Isovaleryl-CoA dehydrogenase)
LCHAD	Long-chain L-3- hydroxyacyl-CoA dehydrogenase
MCAD	Medium-chain acyl-CoA dehydrogenase
MCD	Multiple carboxylase (Holocarboxylase synthetase)
MSUD	Maple syrup urine disease (branched-chain ketoacid dehydrogenase)
MUT	Methylmalonic Acidemia (methylmalonyl-CoA mutase)
PKU	Phenylketonuria/ hyperphenylalaninemia
PROP	Propionic acidemia (Propionyl-CoA carboxylase)
TFP	Trifunctional protein deficiency
TYR-1	Tyrosinemia Type 1
VLCAD	Very long-chain acyl-CoA dehydrogenase

[1] Terminology consistent with ACMG report - Newborn Screening; Towards a Uniform Screening Panel and System. Genet Med. 2006; 8(5) Suppl: S12-S252

States listed (row labels) in the accompanying screening matrix: Missouri, Montana, Nebraska, Nevada, New Hampshire, New Jersey, New Mexico, New York, North Carolina, North Dakota, Ohio, Oklahoma, Oregon, Pennsylvania, Rhode Island, South Carolina, South Dakota, Tennessee, Texas, Utah, Vermont, Virginia, Washington, West Virginia, Wisconsin, Wyoming.

Table 9.3. National Newborn Screening Status Report–Secondary Target Conditions; reprinted with permission from the National Newborn Screening and Genetics Resource Center (NNSGRC).

Dot "●" indicates that screening for the condition is universally required by Law or Rule and fully implemented
A = universally offered but not yet required, B = offered to select populations, or by request, C = testing required but not yet implemented
D = likely to be detected (and reported) as a by-product of MRM screening (MS/MS) targeted by Law or Rule

STATE	CACT	CPT-Ia	CPT-II	DE-RED.	GA-II	MCKAT	M/SCHAD	SC AD	2M3HBA	2MBG	3MGA	CbP-C,D	IBG	MAL	ARG	BIOPT-BS	BIOPT-RG	CIT-II	H-PHE	MET	TYR-II	TYR-III	GALE	GALK	Variant Hbg's
Alabama	●	●	●						●	●	●	●	●	●	●	D	D	●	●	●	●	●			D
Alaska	●	●	●		●			●	●		●	●	●	●		B	B	●	●	●	D		B	B	●
Arizona																		D	●		D	D			●
Arkansas																									A
California	●	●	●		●			●	●	●	●	●	●	●	●		●	●	●	●	●	●	●	●	●
Colorado	●	●	●	●	●			●	●	●	●	●	●	●	●		●	●	●	●	●	●	●	●	●
Connecticut	●	●	●	●	●		●	●	●	●	●	●	●	●	●		●	●	●	●	●	●	●	●	●
D. of Columbia	●	●	●	●		A	●	●	●		A					A	A	●	●	●	●	●	●	●	●
Delaware	●				●		●	●							●		A	●	●	●	●	●	●	●	●
Florida	●	●					●	●	●	D					●				●	●	●	●			●
Georgia	●	●	●		●			●	●	●	●	●	●	●	●	B	B		●	●	●	●	●	●	●
Hawaii	●	●	●		●			●	●	●	●	●	●	●	●	D	D	●	●	●	●	D	B	B	●
Idaho	●	D	●	D	●	D	●	●	●		●	●	●	●	●	B	B	D	●	●	●	●	B	B	●
Illinois	●	●	●	●	●		●	●	●		●	●	●	●	●			●	●	●	●	●		●	●
Indiana	●	●	●		●	●	●	●	●		●	●	●	●	●	●	●	D	●	●	●	●			●
Iowa	●																		●						●
Kansas		A	A	A					A						A	B	B	A	●	A	A		●		●
Kentucky							●		D										●			D	●	●	●
Louisiana															A				●						●
Maine	D	D						●	D	D	D	●	D	D	●			●	●	D	●	D	●	●	●
Maryland	●	D	●	D	●	D	●	●	D		D	●	●	●	A	B	B	A	●	●	●	●	●	●	●
Massachusetts	D	D	A	●	A	D	●	A	D		D	A	D	●	A	D	D	●	●	D	A	D	●	●	●
Michigan	●	●	●	●	●	●	●	●	●	●	●	●	●	●	●	●	●	●	●	●	●	A	●	●	●
Minnesota	●	●	●	A	●		●	●	●		●	●	●	●	●		●	A	●	●	●	●	●	●	●
Mississippi	●	●	●	A	●	A	A	●	A		D	●	D	D	A	A	A	●	●	●	●	A	●	●	●
Missouri	B	D	B	B	B	D	D	B	D	B	B	●	B	D	●	D	D	D	●	B	B	D	●	●	●
Montana	A		A	A		B		A	B	A	B	A	A	B	●	B	B	B	●	A	B	B			●
Nebraska	A		●	●				●				A	A	A	●			A	●	●	A				●
Nevada	●	●	●		●		●	●	●		●	●	●	●	●	B	B	●	●	●	●		B	B	A

States listed (rows of the screening matrix): New Hampshire, New Jersey, New Mexico, New York, North Carolina, North Dakota, Ohio, Oklahoma, Oregon, Pennsylvania, Rhode Island, South Carolina, South Dakota, Tennessee, Texas, Utah, Vermont, Virginia, Washington, West Virginia, Wisconsin, Wyoming.

[1]Terminology consistent with ACMG report - Newborn Screening: Towards a Uniform Screening Panel and System. Genet Med. 2006; 8(5) Suppl: S12-S252

Deficiency/Disorder Abbreviations and Names (optional nomenclature)

Abbr.	Name	Abbr.	Name
2M3HBA	2-Methyl-3-hydroxy butyric aciduria	CACT	Carnitine acylcarnitine translocase
2MBG	2-Methylbutyryl-CoA dehydrogenase	CBL-C,D	Methylmalonic acidemia (Cbl C,D)
3MGA	3-Methylglutaconic aciduria	CIT-II	Citrullinemia type II
ARG	Arginemia (Arginase deficiency)	CPT-Ia	Carnitine palmitoyltransferase I
BIOPT-BS	Defects of biopterin cofactor biosynthesis	CPT-II	Carnitine palmitoyltransferase II
BIOPT-REG	Defects of biopterin cofactor regeneration	De-Red	Dienoyl-CoA reductase

Abbr.	Name	Abbr.	Name
GA-II	Glutaric acidemia Type II	MAL	Malonic acidemia (Malonyl-CoA decarboxylase)
GALE	Galactose epimerase	MCKAT	Medium-chain ketoacyl-CoA thiolase
GALK	Galactokinase	MET	Hypermethioninemia
H-PHE	Benign hyperphenylalaninemia	SCAD	Short-chain acyl-CoA dehydrogenase
IBG	Isobutyryl-CoA dehydrogenase	TYR-II	Tyrosinemia type II
M/SCHAD	Medium/Short chain L-3-hydroxy acyl-CoA dehydrogenase	TYR-III	Tyrosinemia type III

you may want to contact outside laboratory services that provide supplemental testing for more than 30 metabolic disorders through a mail-order service available anywhere in the United States. The labs send out kits that are used to collect additional blood at the time of your baby's regular screening, and this sample is then mailed back for analysis. The cost ranges from $25 to $50.

How Is Newborn Screening Performed?

Within the first 2 or 3 days of life, your baby's heel will be pricked and a small sample of her blood will then be applied to a filter paper. Most states have identified a state or regional laboratory to which hospitals should send the samples for analysis. (If your hospital offers expanded screening that uses the new technology, your baby's sample may be sent to a private laboratory. Some states use a private lab for all of their studies.)

It's generally recommended that the sample be taken after the first 24 hours of life. Some tests, such as the one for PKU, may not be as sensitive if they're done too soon after birth. However, because mothers and newborns are often discharged within a day, some babies may be tested within the first 24 hours. If this happens, the AAP recommends that a repeat sample be taken no more than 1 to 2 weeks later. It's especially important that the PKU screening test be run again for accurate results. Some states routinely do two tests on all infants.

Getting the Results

Different labs have different procedures for notifying families and pediatricians of the results. Some may send them to the hospital where your child was born and not directly to your child's doctor, which may mean a delay in getting the results to you. And although some states have a system that allows doctors to access the results via phone or computer, others may not. Ask your child's doctor how you will get the results and when you should expect them.

If a test result should come back abnormal, try not to panic. This does not necessarily mean that your child has the disorder in question. A screening test is not the same as diagnostic test. The initial screening provides only preliminary information that must be followed up with more specific diagnostic testing.

If testing confirms that your child does have a disorder, your child's doctor may refer you to a specialist for further evaluation and treatment. Keep in mind that dietary restrictions and supplements, along with proper medical supervision, can often avert most of the serious physical and mental problems that were associated with metabolic disorders in the past.

You may also wonder whether the disorder can be passed on to any future children. This is a matter you'll want to discuss with your child's doctor and perhaps a genetic counselor. Also, if you have other children who weren't screened for the disorder, you may want to have this done. Again, talk this over with your children's doctor.

Know Your Options

Because state programs are subject to change, you'll want to find up-to-date information about your state's (and individual hospital's) program. Talk to your child's doctor or contact your state's department of health for more information.

Chapter 10

Chromosome Abnormalities

Chromosomes are the structures that hold our genes. Genes are the individual instructions that tell our bodies how to develop and function; they govern our physical and medical characteristics, such as hair color, blood type and susceptibility to disease. Each chromosome has a p and q arm; p is the shorter arm and q is the longer arm. The arms are separated by a pinched region known as the centromere.

Where are chromosomes found in the body?

The body is made up of individual units called cells. Your body has many different kinds of cells, such as skin cells, liver cells, and blood cells. In the center of most cells is a structure called the nucleus. This is where chromosomes can be found.

How many chromosomes do humans have?

The typical number of chromosomes in a human cell is 46—two pairs of 23—holding an estimated 30,000 to 35,000 genes. One set of 23 chromosomes is inherited from the biological mother (from the egg), and the other set is inherited from the biological father (from the sperm).

How do scientists study chromosomes?

In order for chromosomes to be seen with a microscope, they need to be stained. Once stained, the chromosomes look like strings with

Excerpted from "Chromosome Abnormalities Fact Sheet," National Human Genome Research Institute, October 2006.

light and dark bands and their picture can be taken. A picture, or chromosome map, of all 46 chromosomes is called a karyotype. The karyotype can help identify chromosome abnormalities that are evident in either the structure or the number of chromosomes.

To help identify chromosomes, the pairs have been numbered from one to twenty-two, with the 23rd pair labeled X and Y. In addition, each chromosome arm is defined further by numbering the bands that appear after staining; the higher the number, the further that area is from the centromere. The first 22 pairs of chromosomes are called autosomes and the final pair is called the sex chromosomes. The sex chromosomes an individual has determines that person's gender; females have two X chromosomes (XX), and males have an X and a Y chromosome (XY).

What are chromosome abnormalities?

A chromosome abnormality reflects an abnormality of chromosome number or structure. There are many types of chromosome abnormalities. However, they can be organized into two basic groups:

Numerical abnormalities: When an individual is missing either a chromosome from a pair (monosomy) or has more than two chromosomes of a pair (trisomy). An example of a condition caused by numerical abnormalities is Down syndrome, also known as Trisomy 21 (an individual with Down syndrome has three copies of chromosome 21, rather than two). Turner syndrome is an example of monosomy, where the individual—in this case a female—is born with only one sex chromosome, an X.

Structural abnormalities: When the chromosome's structure is altered. This can take several forms:

- **Deletions:** A portion of the chromosome is missing or deleted.

- **Duplications:** A portion of the chromosome is duplicated, resulting in extra genetic material.

- **Translocations:** When a portion of one chromosome is transferred to another chromosome. There are two main types of translocations. In a reciprocal translocation, segments from two different chromosomes have been exchanged. In a Robertsonian translocation, an entire chromosome has attached to another at the centromere.

- **Inversions:** A portion of the chromosome has broken off, turned upside down, and reattached; therefore, the genetic material is inverted.

- **Rings:** A portion of a chromosome has broken off and formed a circle or ring. This can happen with, or without, loss of genetic material.

Most chromosome abnormalities occur as an accident in the egg or sperm. Therefore, the abnormality is present in every cell of the body. Some abnormalities, however, can happen after conception, resulting in mosaicism (where some cells have the abnormality and some do not).

Chromosome abnormalities can be inherited from a parent (such as a translocation) or be de novo (new to the individual). This is why chromosome studies are often performed on parents when a child is found to have an abnormality.

How do chromosome abnormalities happen?

Chromosome abnormalities usually occur when there is an error in cell division. There are two kinds of cell division.

- **Mitosis** results in two cells that are duplicates of the original cell. In other words, one cell with 46 chromosomes becomes two cells with 46 chromosomes each. This kind of cell division occurs throughout the body, except in the reproductive organs. This is how most of the cells that make up our body are made and replaced.

- **Meiosis** results in cells with half the number of chromosomes, 23 instead of the normal 46. These are the eggs and sperm.

In both processes, the correct number of chromosomes is supposed to end up in the resulting cells. However, errors in cell division can result in cells with too few or too may copies of a chromosome. Errors can also occur when the chromosomes are being duplicated.

Other factors that can increase the risk of chromosome abnormalities are:

- **Maternal Age:** Women are born with all the eggs they will ever have. Therefore, when a woman is 30 years old, so are her eggs. Some researchers believe that errors can crop up in the eggs' genetic material as they age over time. Therefore, older women are more at risk of giving birth to babies with chromosome abnormalities than younger women. Since men produce new sperm throughout their life, paternal age does not increase risk of chromosome abnormalities.

- **Environment:** Although there is no conclusive evidence that specific environmental factors cause chromosome abnormalities, it is still a possibility that the environment may play a role in the occurrence of genetic errors.

Chapter 11

Genetic Counseling

If you and your partner are newly pregnant, you may be amazed at the number and variety of prenatal tests available to you. Blood tests, urine tests, monthly medical exams, diet questionnaires, and family history forms crowd your schedule and your desk, but each of these tests helps to assess the health of you and your baby—and to predict any potential health risks.

Unlike your parents, you may also have the option of genetic testing. These tests identify the likelihood of passing certain genetic diseases or disorders (those caused by a defect in the genes—the tiny, DNA-containing units of heredity that determine the characteristics and functioning of the entire body) to your children.

Some of the more familiar genetic disorders are:

- Down syndrome;

- cystic fibrosis;

- sickle cell anemia;

- Tay-Sachs disease (a fatal disease affecting the central nervous system).

This information was provided by KidsHealth, one of the largest resources online for medically reviewed health information written for parents, kids, and teens. For more articles like this one, visit www.KidsHealth.org, or www .TeensHealth.org. © 2004 The Nemours Foundation.

If your history suggests that genetic testing would be helpful, you may be referred to a genetic counselor. Or, you might decide to seek out genetic counseling yourself. But what do genetic counselors do, and how can they help your family-to-be?

What Is Genetic Counseling?

Genetic counseling is the process of:

• evaluating family history and medical records;

• ordering genetic tests;

• evaluating the results of this investigation;

• helping parents understand and reach decisions about what to do next.

Genetic tests are done by analyzing small samples of blood or body tissues. They determine whether you, your partner, or your baby carry genes for certain inherited disorders.

Genes are made up of DNA molecules, which are the simplest building blocks of heredity. They're grouped together in specific patterns within a person's chromosomes, forming the unique "blueprint" for every physical and biological characteristic of that person.

Humans have 46 chromosomes, arranged in pairs in every living cell of our bodies. When the egg and sperm join at conception, half of each chromosomal pair is inherited from each parent. This newly formed combination of chromosomes then copies itself again and again during fetal growth and development, passing identical genetic information to each new cell in the growing fetus. Current science suggests that human chromosomes carry from 25,000 to 35,000 genes. An error in just one gene (and in some instances, even the alteration of a single piece of DNA) can sometimes be the cause for a serious medical condition.

Some diseases, such as Huntington disease (a degenerative nerve disease) and Marfan syndrome (a connective tissue disorder), can be inherited from just one parent. Most disorders cannot occur unless both the mother and father pass along the gene. Some of these are cystic fibrosis, sickle cell anemia, and Tay-Sachs disease. Other genetic conditions, such as Down syndrome, are not inherited. In general, they result from an error (mutation) in the cell division process during conception or fetal development. Still others, such as achondroplasia (the most common form of dwarfism), may either be inherited or the result of a genetic mutation.

Genetic tests don't yield easy-to-understand results. They can reveal the presence, absence, or malformation of genes or chromosomes. Deciphering what these complex tests mean is where a genetic counselor comes in.

Who Are Genetic Counselors?

Genetic counselors are professionals who have completed a master's program in medical genetics and counseling skills. They then pass a certification exam administered by the American Board of Genetic Counseling. Genetic counselors can help identify and interpret the risks of an inherited disorder, explain inheritance patterns, suggest testing, and lay out possible scenarios. (They refer you to a doctor or a laboratory for the actual tests.) They will explain the meaning of the medical science involved, provide support, and address any emotional issues often raised by the results of the genetic testing.

Who Should See One?

Most couples planning a pregnancy or who are expecting don't need genetic counseling. About 3% of babies are born with birth defects each year, according to the U.S. Centers for Disease Control and Prevention—and of the malformations that do occur, the most common are also among the most treatable. Cleft palate and clubfoot, two of the more common birth defects, can be surgically repaired, as can many heart malformations.

The best time to seek genetic counseling is before becoming pregnant, when a counselor can help assess your risk factors. But even after you become pregnant, a meeting with a genetic counselor can still be helpful. For example, several babies have been diagnosed with spina bifida before birth. Recent research suggests that delivering a baby with spina bifida via cesarean section (avoiding the trauma of travel through the birth canal) can minimize damage to the baby's spine—and perhaps reduce the likelihood that the child will need a wheelchair.

You should consider genetic counseling if any of the following risk factors apply to you:

- if a standard prenatal screening test (such as the alpha fetoprotein test) yields an abnormal result;

- if an amniocentesis yields an unexpected result (such as a chromosomal defect in the unborn baby);

- if either parent or a close relative has an inherited disease or birth defect;

- if either parent already has children with birth defects or genetic disorders;

- if the mother-to-be has had two or more miscarriages or babies that died in infancy;

- if the mother-to-be will be 35 or older when the baby is born (Chances of having a child with Down syndrome increase with the mother's age: a 35-year-old woman has a one in 350 chance of conceiving a child with Down syndrome. This chance increases to one in 110 by age 40 and one in 30 by age 45.);

- if parents are concerned about genetic defects that occur frequently in their ethnic or racial group (For example, couples of African descent are most at risk for having a child with sickle cell anemia; couples of central or eastern European Jewish (Ashkenazi), Cajun, or Irish descent may be carriers of Tay-Sachs disease; and couples of Italian, Greek, or Middle Eastern descent may carry the gene for thalassemia, a red blood cell disorder.).

What to Expect during a Visit with a Genetic Counselor

Before you meet with a genetic counselor in person, you'll be asked to gather information about your family history. The counselor will want to know of any relatives with genetic disorders, multiple miscarriages, and early or unexplained deaths. The counselor will also want to look over your medical records, including any ultrasounds, prenatal test results, past pregnancies, and medications you may have taken before or during pregnancy.

If more tests are necessary, the counselor will help you set up those appointments and track the paperwork. When the results come in, the counselor will call you with the news. Often, the counselor will encourage you to come in for a discussion.

The counselor will study your records before meeting with you, so you can make the best use of your time together. During your session, he or she will go over any gaps or potential problem areas in your family or medical history. The counselor can then help you understand the inheritance patterns of any potential disorders and help assess your chances of having a child with those disorders.

He or she will distinguish between risks that every pregnancy faces and risks that you personally face. Even if you discover you have a particular problem gene, science can't always predict the severity of the related disease. For instance, a child with cystic fibrosis can have debilitating lung problems or, less commonly, milder respiratory symptoms.

After Counseling

You and your family will have to decide what to do next. Genetic counselors help you to understand your options and adjust to the difficulties and uncertainties you face.

If you've learned prior to conception that you and/or your partner are at high risk for having a child with a severe or fatal defect, your options might include:

- pre-implantation diagnosis, which occurs when eggs that have been fertilized in vitro (in a laboratory, outside of the womb) are tested for defects at the 8-cell (blastocyst) stage—and only unaffected blastocysts are implanted in the uterus to establish a pregnancy;

- using donor sperm or donor eggs;

- adoption.

If you've received a prenatal diagnosis of a severe or fatal defect, your options might include:

- preparing yourself for the challenges you'll face when you have your baby;

- fetal surgery to repair the defect before birth (surgery can only be used to treat some defects, such as spina bifida or congenital diaphragmatic hernia, a hole in the diaphragm that can cause severely underdeveloped lungs. Most defects cannot be surgically repaired.);

- ending the pregnancy.

For some families, knowing that they'll have an infant with a severe or fatal genetic condition seems too much to bear. Other families are able to adapt to the news—and to the birth—remarkably well.

Genetic counselors can share the experiences they've had with other families in your situation. But they will not suggest a particular course of action. A good genetic counselor understands that what is right for one family may not be right for another.

Genetic counselors can, however, refer you to specialists for further help. For instance, many babies with Down syndrome are born with heart defects. Your counselor might encourage you to meet with a cardiologist to discuss heart surgery, and a neonatologist to discuss the care of a post-operative newborn. Genetic counselors can also refer you to social workers, support groups, or mental health professionals to help you adjust to and prepare for your complex new reality.

Finding a Genetic Counselor

Working with a genetic counselor can be reassuring and informative, especially if you or your partner have known risk factors. Talk to your doctor if you feel you would benefit from genetic counseling. Many doctors have a list of local genetic counselors with whom they work. You can also contact the National Society of Genetic Counselors for more information.

Part Two

The Pituitary Gland and Growth Disorders

Chapter 12

Growth Disorders in Children

What Is a Growth Disorder?

Lately, it seems as though your child is looking up to classmates—literally. The other kids in the class have been getting taller and developing into young adults, but your child's growth seems to be lagging behind. Classmates now tower over your child.

Is something wrong? Maybe or maybe not. Some kids may just grow more slowly than others simply because their parents did, too. But other children may have an actual growth disorder. This can be any type of problem in infants, kids, or teens that prevents them from meeting realistic expectations of growth, from failure to gain height and weight in young children to short stature or delayed sexual development in teens.

Variations of Normal Growth Patterns in Children

A couple of differences seen in the growth patterns of normal children include these common conditions, which are not growth disorders:

Constitutional growth delay: This condition describes children who are small for their ages but who are growing at a normal rate. They usually have a delayed "bone age," which means that their skeletal

"What Is a Growth Disorder?" was provided by KidsHealth, one of the largest resources online for medically reviewed health information written for parents, kids, and teens. For more articles like this one, visit www.KidsHealth.org, or www.TeensHealth.org. © 2005 The Nemours Foundation.

maturation is younger than their age in years. (A child's bone age is measured by taking an x-ray of a child's hand and wrist and comparing it to standard x-ray findings seen in children of the same age.) These children don't have any signs or symptoms of diseases that affect growth. They tend to reach puberty later than their peers do, with delay in the onset of sexual development and the pubertal growth spurt. But because they continue to grow until an older age, they tend to catch up to their peers when they reach adult height. One or both parents or other close relatives of these children often experienced a similar "late-bloomer" growth pattern.

Familial (or genetic) short stature: This is a condition in which shorter parents tend to have shorter children. This term applies to short children who don't have any symptoms of diseases that affect their growth. Children with familial short stature still have growth spurts and enter puberty at normal ages, but they usually will only reach a height similar to that of their parents.

With both constitutional growth delay and familial short stature, children and families need to be reassured that the child does not have a disease or medical condition that poses a threat to health or that requires treatment. However, because they may be short or may not enter puberty when their classmates do, some kids with these growth patterns may need extra help coping with teasing by their peers, or they may need reassurance that they will go through full sexual development eventually. In a few normal children who are very short or very late entering puberty, hormone treatment may be helpful.

Growth Disorders

Diseases of the kidneys, heart, gastrointestinal tract, lungs, bones, or other body systems may affect growth. Other symptoms or physical signs in children with these illnesses usually give clues as to the disease causing the growth delay. However, poor growth may be the first sign of a problem in some of these conditions. Here are a few examples of growth disorders:

Failure to thrive isn't a specific growth disorder itself, but it can be a sign of an underlying condition causing growth problems. Although it's common for newborns to lose a little weight in the first few days, failure to thrive is a condition in which some infants continue to show slower than expected weight gain and growth. Usually caused by inadequate nutrition or a feeding problem, failure to thrive is most common in children younger than age three. It may also be a symptom of another problem, such as an infection, a digestive problem, child neglect, or abuse.

Endocrine diseases (diseases involving hormones, the chemical messengers of the body) involve a deficiency or excess of hormones and can be responsible for growth failure during childhood and adolescence. Growth hormone deficiency is a disorder that involves the pituitary gland (the small gland at the base of the brain that secretes several hormones, including growth hormone). A damaged or malfunctioning pituitary gland may not produce enough hormones for normal growth. Hypothyroidism is a condition in which the thyroid gland fails to make enough thyroid hormone, which is essential for normal bone growth.

Turner syndrome, one of the most common genetic growth disorders, occurs in girls and is a syndrome in which there's a missing or abnormal X chromosome. In addition to short stature, girls with Turner syndrome usually don't undergo normal sexual development because their ovaries (the sex organs that produce eggs and female hormones) fail to mature and function normally.

How Is a Growth Disorder Diagnosed?

The tests a doctor may recommend to detect a growth disorder depend on the findings at each step of evaluation. A short child who's healthy and growing at a normal rate may just be observed throughout childhood, but a child who has stopped growing, or is growing more slowly than expected, will often need additional testing.

Your child's doctor or endocrinologist will look for signs of the many possible causes of short stature and growth failure. Blood tests may be performed to look for hormone and chromosome abnormalities as well as to rule out other diseases associated with growth failure. A bone age x-ray is frequently done, and special scans (such as an MRI) can check the pituitary gland for abnormalities.

To measure the ability of the child's pituitary gland to produce growth hormone, the doctor (usually a pediatric endocrinologist) may perform a growth hormone stimulation test. This involves giving the child certain medications that cause the pituitary gland to secrete growth hormone, and then drawing several small blood samples to check growth hormone levels over a period of time after the medications are given.

How Is a Growth Disorder Treated?

Although the treatment of a growth problem usually isn't an urgent situation, earlier diagnosis and treatment of some conditions may help kids catch up with peers and increase the final height they attain.

If an underlying medical condition is identified, specific treatment may result in improved growth. Growth failure due to hypothyroidism, for example, is usually simply treated by giving the child thyroid hormone replacement therapy in pill form.

Growth hormone injections for children with growth hormone deficiency, Turner syndrome, and chronic kidney failure may help children with these conditions reach a more normal height. Human growth hormone is generally considered safe and effective, although full treatment may take many years and not all children will have a good response. And the treatment can be quite costly (approximately $20,000 to $30,000 per year), although most health insurance plans will cover the costs.

What about growth hormone treatment for short children who aren't growth hormone deficient when tested? The Food and Drug Administration (FDA) has approved the use of growth hormone therapy for non-growth hormone deficient children who are predicted to reach a very short final height (under 4 feet 11 inches [150 centimeters] for a girl, or 5 feet 4 inches [163 centimeters] for a boy). Talk with your child's doctor for more information about this and other treatment options if you're concerned.

How Can I Help My Child?

You can boost your child's self-esteem by providing positive reinforcement and emphasizing other characteristics, like intelligence, personality, and talents. Try to de-emphasize the focus on height as a measure of social acceptance.

Kids who are very self-conscious about their size may need some additional help in coping. In some cases, evaluation and treatment by a mental health professional may be needed.

What Do I Do if I Suspect a Problem?

If you're concerned about your child's growth, visit his or her doctor. Depending on the findings of the examination, the doctor may refer your child to a pediatric endocrinologist, who can help diagnose and treat specific growth disorders.

It's also important to be on the lookout for the social and emotional problems that kids with growth disorders face. It's not easy being the shortest kid in the class, and it's never any fun being teased. Helping your child build self-esteem and emphasizing his or her abilities—regardless of how tall he or she may grow—might be just what the doctor ordered.

Chapter 13

Growth Hormone Deficiency in Adults

This information is based on clinical guidelines that were written to help physicians who are evaluating and treating patients with growth hormone deficiency (GHD). It summarizes information about the best way to diagnose GHD in adults, how physicians will begin care and follow-up with patients who have a diagnosis of GHD, and the potential benefits of growth hormone (GH) treatment. This chapter also provides information for patients with GHD to help them improve the outcome of their treatment. The guidelines do not apply to people who want to take GH to prevent aging or to improve their strength or athletic performance. Claims about using GH to slow down the aging process or help build muscle in athletes have not been shown to be true and such use may cause harm.

How were the guidelines developed?

The clinical guidelines were developed after an extensive review of the best clinical studies about GHD and treatment with GH. An expert panel of The Endocrine Society examined evidence from studies that had been published in peer-reviewed medical journals (that is, the studies were carefully evaluated by the journal's scientists and editors). The panel rated the quality of the studies and gave the most weight to studies that were randomized and placebo controlled. This means that the people in the study were assigned into groups at random. One group took the study drug and the other took the placebo (an injection that did not contain the GH). This allows physicians to learn whether the GH injection is more effective than no treatment at all.

The panel developed recommendations based on these types of studies or suggestions based on studies that were less rigorously designed or carried out. Once the panel reached an agreement about their recommendations and suggestions, the guideline was reviewed and approved by several committees and, finally, by the general membership of The Endocrine Society. No funding for the guidelines came from any pharmaceutical company.

What are the causes of GHD?

Adults with GHD fall into two categories:

1. Those who developed GHD during childhood; or,

2. Those who developed GHD after reaching adulthood.

The actual causes of GHD include inherited causes that are present at birth. These might involve problems of GH production in the pituitary gland and other disorders of pituitary development (for example, defects in the gene responsible for producing GH). Other causes that can take place at any age involve damage to the pituitary, which may be from tumors, surgery, irradiation, and other types of trauma. Rarely, GHD is of unknown origin (idiopathic GHD).

What are the goals of GH therapy?

The panel recommended that if you had childhood GHD with structural lesions (for example, tumor or surgery in the area of the pituitary) and other pituitary hormone deficiencies, or if you have proven genetic causes, a low insulinlike growth factor-1 (IGF-1) level at least one month off of GH therapy shows that you have GHD, and therefore, you won't need further testing. (IGF-1 is regulated by GH from the pituitary gland to cause growth.) On the other hand, if you had childhood GHD without structural lesions or other pituitary hormone deficiencies, the panel recommended that you should be retested as an adult. The panel also recommended that as little time as possible go by between the end of your childhood treatment and the testing.

Therapeutic goals of GH therapy include:

- building muscle mass;

- lowering fat levels;

- building stronger, healthier bones;

- improving heart function; and

- increasing energy.

Diagnosing GH deficiency in adults can be difficult. It requires one or more tests to determine if the deficiency is present and if it is severe enough to require treatment. The panel found that the insulin tolerance test and the growth hormone-releasing hormone (GHRH) arginine test are the most specific and sensitive tests for diagnosing GHD in adults. Doctors need to work with each individual to determine the most appropriate tests and to determine the best treatment.

The primary goal when prescribing growth hormone injections is always to replace the normal amount of growth hormone the individual would have if he or she did not have a deficiency of the hormone. Taking too much growth hormone over a prolonged period of time can be harmful. Your doctor can best explain all the risks and benefits of GH replacement and other treatments that you may need.

The panel found evidence that treatment of adult GHD achieved the following therapeutic goals:

- Building muscle mass and decreasing fat levels in your body.

- Building stronger, healthier bones. GH stimulates both bone formation and bone resorption (the breakdown process of old bone, essential to health). Patients should have a dual energy x-ray absorptiometry (DXA) bone scan to measure bone mineral density (BMD) before treatment. If it is abnormal, a BMD test should be done about every two years after starting GH treatment.

- Improving heart function. Replacing GH sometimes helps by improving heart functioning and reducing the markers of inflammation, which indicate risk for heart and blood vessel damage. GH also improves metabolism of lipoproteins (fat molecules), and decreases the amount of bad cholesterol (low-density lipoprotein) and total cholesterol as seen in blood tests.

- Increased energy. Energy, vitality, and exercise capacity increase in some people who are treated with GH. The degree of improvement depends on the individual's status before treatment. Not everyone will see an improvement.

How will your doctor help you get to your treatment goals?

Your endocrinologist, a specialist in growth hormone treatment, will carefully evaluate you and determine whether or not you need GH and, if you do, what is the right dose of GH for you. The panel recommended that GH should not be given if you have a diagnosis of cancer. In addition, they suggested that for those patients who also have diabetes mellitus that their diabetes medications may need to be adjusted because GH treatment can raise blood sugar.

The panel recommended that the dose of GH should be individualized. Your weight, gender, age, and other medications you might be taking should be taken into account. The dose of GH may be adjusted over time. Doctors usually start by giving a low amount of GH. This may be increased if your blood tests show you could benefit from more GH to reach your health goals. Doctors adjust GH doses based on how you are responding and on any side effects you may have.

While GH is always prescribed on a case by case basis that looks at the entire individual, most doctors who provide GH treatment want to see their patient for a check-up every one to two months to check for progress and any side effects. Once the right dose is established and tests show that the GH is benefiting you as much as possible, you may only need to follow up every six months.

Your doctor will also take into account any other medications you need and make sure that all of your medications are working together as well as possible. If you are taking more than one medication, make sure your endocrinologist and primary care physician know about all of the medications you take.

If you feel different or worse after you begin a drug, call your doctor. Your new symptoms may be a side effect of the drug or an interaction from taking more than one drug.

What can you do to help your treatment process?

Treatment for GHD usually needs to be continued for many years and possibly for a lifetime. One of the most important things you can do as a patient is to keep taking your recommended dose of GH and medications you might be taking to treat other conditions. Another is to report any side effects you may have to your doctor. You also will improve your health by having a healthy lifestyle that includes regular exercise, good nutrition, limited alcohol consumption, not smoking, and losing weight if you are overweight. You and your doctor should be partners in your care. Keep regular appointments with your endocrinologist, ask questions and participate in your care to ensure the success of your GH treatment. And remember, if you have not been diagnosed with GHD, using GH can be dangerous to your health.

Additional Information

The Hormone Foundation
8401 Connecticut Ave., Suite 900
Chevy Chase, MD 20815-5817
Toll-Free: 800-Hormone (467-6663)
Website: http://www.hormone.org
E-mail: hormone@endo-society.org

The Hormone Foundation provides a physician referral directory on their website.

Chapter 14

Growth Hormone
Evaluation Process

Evaluation Process of Adults with Growth Hormone Deficiency

You have been referred to an endocrinologist, a doctor who specializes in the diagnosis and treatment of disorders of the endocrine glands. Endocrine glands release chemicals into the blood, which tell parts of the body to do certain jobs. These chemicals are referred to as hormones. Endocrine disorders are those that involve deficiencies or excesses of hormones. A deficiency exists when there is not enough of a hormone in the body. In order for your doctor to make an accurate diagnosis, some testing may be necessary. This section was written to help you and your family understand the evaluation process of hormone deficiencies.

Control of Hormones and Hormone Deficiency

The hypothalamus controls the pituitary gland; both are located in the brain. The pituitary gland releases or controls many hormones in

This chapter begins with: "Evaluation Process of Adults with Growth Hormone Deficiency," © 2006 The MAGIC Foundation (www.magicfoundation.org). Reprinted with permission. All rights reserved. Additional information under the heading, "Growth Hormone: The Test," is © 2006 American Association for Clinical Chemistry. Reprinted with permission. For additional information about clinical lab testing, visit the Lab Tests Online website at www.labtestsonline.org.

the body. The hormones are released in very small amounts into the bloodstream and then travel to parts of the body (referred to as target organs) to perform a specific job. These hormones control many of the body's functions, which are the following: Thyroid-stimulating hormone (TSH) turns the thyroid gland "on" in order to control your metabolism. Adrenocorticotropic hormone (ACTH) stimulates cortisol production to assist your body in daily function and stress. Vasopressin assists in the salt and water regulation of the body. Gonadotropins (follicle-stimulating hormone, luteinizing hormone [FSH, LH]) stimulate the ovaries (in women) or testes (in men) to release sex hormones (estradiol or testosterone). Growth hormone is released from the pituitary gland to cause growth in children and affects bone density, lipid metabolism, and muscle in children and adults.

Deficiencies of these hormones may occur alone or in combination with one or more other hormone deficiencies. The hormone deficiency may be congenital, resulting from a defect in the brain. The deficiency may also be acquired, stemming from the damage to the brain after a sever head injury, serious illness (such as meningitis or encephalitis), brain tumor, and/or radiation. Sometimes no cause for the hormone deficiency can be identified.

Evaluation and Testing

In order to confirm or determine the possibility of hormone deficiencies, your doctor will perform an examination and ask you some questions. Past records may have to be reviewed. Screening blood tests will usually be done. The blood tests will check the secretion of the pituitary hormones and their target organs.

Possible tests that may be done include:

- Thyroxine/thyroid-stimulating hormone (T_4/TSH) to test thyroid function.

- Cortisol FSH/LH to test stimulation ability of the ovaries or testes.

- Insulinlike growth factor-1 (IGF-1), an indirect measure of growth hormone.

- Electrolytes to measure water and salt balance.

- Imaging tests. You may need to have a picture of the brain; this is done by a computed tomography (CT) scan or magnetic resonance image (MRI). A CT scan gives a detailed picture of the brain using x-rays and a computer. A MRI gives a detailed picture of the brain using a magnet, radio waves, and a computer. These tests are not painful, but you will have to hold still for approximately one hour during the test.

Growth Hormone

If there is a possibility that you have growth hormone deficiency, more testing will have to be performed. Growth hormone is secreted by the pituitary gland in quick bursts and does not last long in the blood, so checking a single blood sample for growth hormone will not be helpful. Deep sleep, vigorous exercise, and certain drugs are known to stimulate the secretion of growth hormone. The amount of growth hormone in the blood is measured by taking blood samples over a period of time. This is done by performing a stimulation test. This refers to drawing baseline hormone levels, stimulating growth hormone release by giving a drug, and drawing intermittent growth hormone levels for one to three hours. The specifics of the tests, such as type of drug, length of test, and amount of the samples, will be determined by your doctor.

The doctor will need to make sure you are on adequate hormone replacement for other hormone deficiencies prior to stimulation testing. You will be given instructions. You should not have anything to eat or drink, except for water, after midnight the night before the test. You should have minimal activity before the test (no exercise that morning). An indwelling venous line (IV) will be started and baseline hormone levels drawn. You will be given a medication. The medication and its effects will be reviewed by your doctor or nurse. Growth hormone levels will be drawn intermittently from the IV at specified times for a period of two hours. If the IV stops working during the test, it is important that it be restarted so the samples may be obtained at the specified times.

The purpose of the testing is to determine if you are growth hormone deficient and/or eligible for growth hormone therapy. In order to start growth hormone treatment you will have one to two simulation tests performed. The number of tests will be decided by your doctor. Adults with peak growth hormone levels less than 3–5 mcg/L are identified as growth hormone deficient. Please keep in mind that these numbers are not definitive; your doctor will make the final diagnosis. It may take several weeks for your doctor to receive and review the test results. You should discuss the results and the possibility of growth hormone therapy with your doctor.

Summary

Hormone replacement will be prescribed by your doctor if you are deficient in pituitary hormones. Remember that each hormone has a specific function in your body, replacement medication is very important.

Growth Hormone: The Test

GH testing is usually provocative, using either a GH stimulation test or a GH suppression test to track GH levels over time. GH testing may be used to screen for abnormal pituitary function, and to help diagnose the condition causing the abnormality, its severity, and the complications that have arisen because of it.

Often other blood tests that reflect pituitary function, such as thyroxine (T_4), thyroid-stimulating hormone (TSH), cortisol, follicle-stimulating hormone (FSH), luteinizing hormone (LH), and testosterone (in men), are also ordered. These tests are usually done prior to GH testing to make sure that they are normal and/or controlled with medication before GH testing is done. Glucose levels are run on the samples collected during the GH suppression test (which is an oral glucose tolerance test), both to track glucose levels, and to make sure that the patient's system is sufficiently challenged by the glucose solution given.

IGF-1 (insulinlike growth factor-1) is often measured once during GH provocation testing and often used by itself or with GH as a monitoring tool. Produced in the liver, IGF-1 mirrors GH excesses and deficiencies, but its level is stable throughout the day—making it a useful indicator of average GH levels.

GH testing is usually ordered on those with symptoms of growth hormone abnormalities or as a follow-up to other abnormal test results. It is not recommended for general screening. GH tests may be ordered to help evaluate pituitary function:

• GH stimulation tests are used to screen for hypopituitarism.

• GH suppression tests are used to screen for hyperpituitarism.

GH testing may be ordered to evaluate the long-term effects of chemotherapy on pituitary function in children who undergo such treatment. Growth hormone tests also help identify excess and diminished GH production, give your doctor information about the severity of your condition, and are part of the diagnostic workup to find the reason for the abnormal hormone production.

- GH stimulation tests help diagnose growth hormone deficiency (GHD) in children and adults.

- GH suppression tests help diagnose gigantism in children and acromegaly in adults. Along with other blood tests and imaging scans, they help identify and locate pituitary tumors.

GH and IGF-1 levels are often monitored for extended periods of time following treatment for GHD, gigantism, and acromegaly, and are monitored following surgery, drug treatment, and/or radiation for a pituitary tumor. GH testing may also be done to test for the use of performance enhancing steroids.

When is it ordered?

GH stimulation testing is ordered when your child has symptoms of GHD, such as when:

- his growth rate slows down in early childhood and he is significantly shorter than others his age;

- TSH tests show that your child is not hypothyroid (low thyroid levels can also cause slowed growth);

- x-rays show that his bones are showing delayed development; or,

- your doctor suspects that your child's pituitary gland is underactive.

Once GHD is diagnosed your doctor may use stimulation testing to confirm the diagnosis, along with IGF-1 to monitor the effectiveness of GH replacement (if indicated), and as a child reaches adulthood, to see if continued supplementation is necessary.

Stimulation testing is ordered in adults when patients have symptoms of GHD and/or hypopituitarism such as: decreased bone density, fatigue, adverse lipid changes, and reduced exercise tolerance. Other hormone testing is done first to rule out other conditions that may cause similar symptoms.

GH suppression testing is done when children show signs of gigantism, adults show signs of acromegaly, and/or when their doctor suspects hyperpituitarism. Suppression testing may be done when a pituitary tumor is suspected, and may be used along with IGF-1 levels and other hormone levels to monitor the effectiveness of treatment for these conditions. Monitoring may continue at regular intervals for many years to watch for recurrence.

What does the test result mean?

Note: A standard reference range is not available for this test. Because reference values are dependent on many factors, including patient age, gender, sample population, and test method, numeric test results have different meanings in different labs. Your lab report should include the specific reference range for your test. It is strongly recommended that you discuss your test results with your doctor.

Since GH is released by the pituitary in bursts, random GH levels are not very useful. There is too much overlap between abnormal results and normal daily variation. GH levels will be higher first thing in the morning, and will increase with exercise and stress.

If your GH levels are not significantly suppressed during a GH suppression test (they stay higher than they should), and:

• you have symptoms of gigantism or acromegaly;

• other pituitary hormone levels are normal and/or controlled; or

• your IGF-1 levels are high;

then it is likely that you are producing too much GH, and it is causing complications. If you have other pituitary hormones that are abnormal, then you may have a condition causing hyperpituitarism. If a mass shows up on an x-ray, CT scan, or MRI, then you may have a pituitary tumor (or very rarely a malignancy). If you are being monitored for a previous tumor, then you may be having a recurrence.

If your GH levels are not significantly stimulated during a GH stimulation test (they stay lower than they should), and:

• you have symptoms of GHD;

• other pituitary hormone levels are normal and/or controlled;

• your IGF-1 level is low;

then it is likely that you have a deficiency of GH that your doctor may treat. If your TSH level is low then that should be addressed first as thyroid deficiencies can cause symptoms similar to GHD. You may also have a more general decrease in pituitary function.

Is there anything else I should know?

Pituitary tumors are the most common cause of excess GH production but may also cause deficiencies. If the tumor produces another of the pituitary hormones (such as ACTH or prolactin), then it may inhibit GH secretion. If the tumor is relatively large, it may inhibit all pituitary hormone production and cause damage to the surrounding tissues.

Some other conditions can also cause general hyper- or hypopituitarism. They may be genetic, due to disease, or to trauma. Interfering factors include:

- stress, exercise, and low blood glucose levels;

- drugs that can increase GH include: amphetamines, arginine, dopamine, estrogens, glucagon, histamine, insulin, levodopa, methyldopa, and nicotinic acid;

- drugs that can decrease levels: corticosteroids and phenothiazines; and

- radioactive scan within week of test (with some laboratory methods).

Abnormal GH levels can usually be modified once they are identified. Synthetic GH is available to alleviate deficiencies in children (treatment of adults with GHD is more controversial). Combinations of surgery, medication, and radiation can be used to treat pituitary tumors that are causing excess GH production. The important thing is to identify GH abnormalities as soon as possible for good outcomes. The bone growth changes associated with gigantism and acromegaly are permanent, and if left untreated, the GH deficient child's short stature will remain.

There can be long-term complications from GH abnormalities. Acromegaly, for instance, can cause colon polyps (increasing a patient's risk of developing colon cancer), diabetes, high blood pressure, and visual abnormalities. If a pituitary tumor permanently damages pituitary cells, then multiple hormone replacement may be necessary. Increased bone growth may also lead to trapped nerves (carpal tunnel), arthritis, and weak bones.

Chapter 15

Growth Hormone Therapy

Growth Hormone Therapy Questions

What is growth hormone?

Growth hormone is a protein hormone secreted by the pituitary which promotes linear growth.

Is growth hormone a steroid?

No. It is a protein hormone made up of amino acids.

Are there any side effects when using growth hormone?

Growth hormone does not have any significant side effects when used as a replacement therapy for growth hormone inadequacy or deficiency. Children with hypopituitarism (multiple pituitary hormone deficiencies) sometimes experience fasting hypoglycemia that improves with treatment. Growth hormone results in reduction in body fat with increased muscle growth development.

The recommended doses of growth hormone do not lead to problems, but long-term over-dosage, could result in signs and symptoms of acromegaly consistent with the known effects of excessive human growth hormone. This is not to be expected with properly prescribed growth hormone replacement therapy. Consult your physician or pharmaceutical company for further detail.

Why is growth hormone necessary?

Growth hormone is a natural hormone which is necessary for normal linear growth. Growth hormone is indicated for the long-term therapy of children who have growth failure due to inadequate growth hormone secretion.

How do you determine the dosage and will the dosage remain the same throughout therapy?

Growth hormone is generally prescribed in a dosage of 0.3 milligrams per kilogram of weight per week (mg/kg/week). Higher doses may benefit some teenage growth hormone deficient patients, especially those who are most growth retarded during puberty.

What changes, if any, should I expect to see in my child during therapy (for example, moodiness or hyperactivity)?

There should be no specific changes in your child's mood or activity on growth hormone therapy. However, children generally will have an improvement in self-esteem which may lead to other improved psychological aspects.

What are the different types of growth hormone, and how often are the injections given?

Growth hormone is available as a powder, or as a premixed liquid. It is also available in devices which use a vial that you will mix or that will mix itself when readied for use. Growth hormone is usually administered 6–7 days per week.

Should I worry when bubbles appear in the syringe that has been prepared for my child's injection?

A few bubbles may be of no consequence. One needs to practice to improve technique. Mixing and drawing require training and practice.

How long will my child be on growth hormone?

Growth hormone is utilized for until full growth has been attained with a bone maturation of 16 years, or more for males and 14 years or more in females, or the growth rate is less than two centimeters per year.

Consult your physician for continuing growth hormone therapy under the guidelines for adult growth hormone deficiency. Growth hormone therapy may be indicated in adults with growth hormone deficiency and teenagers after full growth has been attained. Growth hormone stimulation tests are necessary. Peak growth hormone values of less than five milligrams per milliliter (mg/ml) qualify for continued replacement therapy. Adult growth hormone deficiency patients have impaired quality of life, reduced exercise capacity, high cholesterol, increased body fat, reduced muscle mass, and reduced bone density.

Should my child give his own injections?

Children can share in the administration of their injections with supervision. Children eight years of age and older may decide to give their own injections. Sharing part of the injection technique may be important to self-esteem.

What kind of growth should I expect to see in my child?

Generally, growth prior to therapy is less than five centimeters (cm), or 2.5 inches per year. Growth may be 8–12 cm during the initial year of growth hormone therapy. The second and third year may be closer to seven cm per year. Growth is approximately 1½ inches or less prior to therapy and 3–4 inches per year after initiation of therapy.

I left the growth hormone at room temperature for several hours. What shall I do?

Growth hormone is a protein which can be destroyed by extreme temperatures. Prior to mixing growth hormone, a vial can be left out for 72 hours and then reconstituted with full effectiveness. Once a vial is reconstituted, it could be left out at normal temperatures up to 24 hours. Manufactures have devices which protect medicine for a short time. Always refer to the information provided by them regarding the safety of your medications. Growth hormone is a protein hormone, which can be destroyed by heat or extreme temperatures, but there are some general recommendations to follow. Prior to reconstitution (mixing) of your growth hormone, a vial can be left out for 72 hours and then reconstituted with full effectiveness. Once a vial is reconstituted it could be left out inadvertently at normal temperatures up to 24 hours.

If my child prefers injections in the legs instead of the arms, is it okay to inject in the legs only?

Rotation of injection site is encouraged in the arms and legs; other areas may also be utilized. Avoidance of the same location is important to avoid local bumps in the skin called lipohypertrophy.

Is it advisable to give the injection when my child is sleeping?

This is a question only parents can decide. Injections are generally preferred at bedtime. Each child has an individual response or fear of injections.

I don't feel I can give the injections to my child. Is this a normal reaction?

This is a normal reaction of conscientious parents who have concern of hurting their children. Children may express discomfort following an injection. Utilizing smaller needles and quicker subcutaneous injections are recommended. The child needs reassurance that the discomfort will diminish when they become used to the injections. The parent can reinforce the benefit of the injection by maintaining a positive attitude. Ask your child's physician about your options.

What if I forget an injection?

One can make up for missed injections by adding extra doses on other days. Remember the total weekly dose remains the same.

What if my child wants to discontinue the injections, but there is a potential for more growth?

Children need to be encouraged to continue their therapy for full effectiveness. Only an individual family can make a final decision regarding what is best for their child. One needs to examine the child's motive for wanting to discontinue injections when they are obtaining a definite benefit.

What should I do if I run out of growth hormone?

It is recommended that you be aware of your growth hormone supply and contact the source of supply prior to running out. Make sure the prescription is refillable and the insurance company has continued the approval. It is advisable to restart the injections as promptly as possible.

How often will my child need to visit the endocrinologist, and what additional tests need to be taken during the course of therapy?

The number of visits to the endocrinologist depend upon the age of the child and if there are other conditions or hormone deficiencies. The general recommendation is for visits every three months. Periodically, blood testing is necessary such as thyroid function studies and a bone age assessment is recommended yearly. There is an increased incidence for the need of thyroid replacement as well, and indeed, other deficiencies may be coexisting.

Information for People Treated with Human Growth Hormone (hGH)

How did the problem of Creutzfeldt-Jakob Disease (CJD) occur in people who were treated with hGH?

Before scientists learned how to make synthetic hormones, many animal hormones, such as insulin, were used to treat human disorders. Growth hormone (GH) from animals did not work in humans. Human growth hormone (hGH) was made from human pituitary glands by the National Hormone and Pituitary Program (NHPP), funded by the U.S. Public Health Service (PHS). From 1963 to 1985, the NHPP sent hGH to hundreds of doctors across the country. Doctors used the hormone to treat nearly 7,700 children for failure to grow.

In 1985, the PHS learned that three young men treated with hGH died of CJD, a rare and incurable brain disease. The PHS believed these illnesses were related to hGH. PHS doctors immediately stopped distributing the hormone. They began a national study to learn more about how hGH treatment caused this problem. The PHS continues to contact people who have been treated with hGH to provide information to them and to their doctors about health risks linked to hGH.

How many people treated with hGH in the U.S. got CJD?

The Public Health Service has identified 26 cases of CJD among the 7,700 people in the United States who received NHPP hGH. As of October 2005, none of these people began treatment with hGH after 1977, when Dr. Albert Parlow's laboratory began producing NHPP GH and a new purification step was added.

Six people in New Zealand and two people in Brazil who received U.S.-made hGH also got CJD. All together, 34 people who were treated with hGH made in the U.S. have gotten CJD.

What about other diseases?

Many people treated with hGH also have problems making other pituitary hormones. One pituitary hormone tells the adrenal gland to make cortisol, a hormone necessary for life. People lacking this hormone are at risk of death from adrenal crisis, but this can be prevented. More people treated with hGH have died from adrenal crisis than from CJD.

Besides CJD, other serious or fatal health risks from hGH treatment have not been found. People who received hGH are not at higher risk for variant CJD (vCJD) called mad cow disease, neither do they have a higher risk for acquired immunodeficiency syndrome (AIDS).

Deficient GH in Adults: Some people who received hGH as children may have low levels of GH as adults. Symptoms vary, but may include the following:

• more body fat

• less muscle

• less bone mass

• less strength

• less energy

If you have these problems, ask your doctor whether they might be due to low GH. Since these conditions are common in lots of people, they are not always due to low amounts of GH. Studies have shown that GH administration in adults with low GH results in reductions in fat and increments in muscle mass. Effects on strength, energy, and bone fractures in GH-deficient adults receiving GH replacement are not as clear. Today GH is completely synthetic. It poses no threat of contamination.

Cancer: Many people who received NHPP hGH had brain tumors that caused their lack of GH. People who have had one tumor have an increased risk for getting other tumors. Studies of people who received NHPP hGH show no higher overall risk of death from cancer than is seen in the general population in those who did not have tumors before hGH treatment.

What about other problems?

The NHPP has no evidence that hGH causes changes in personality, emotional problems, or suicide.

What are the early symptoms of CJD?

CJD does not cause the same symptoms in everyone. In most people treated with hGH, the first signs of CJD were difficulty with walking, dizziness, clumsiness, and problems with balance. Later, a person with CJD may begin to slur words, lose muscle control, or have problems with vision, memory, or thinking. Once symptoms begin, CJD usually gets worse quickly. Within two to three months, patients could not walk or do other simple tasks.

Headaches are not a symptom of CJD. Mild symptoms that come and go over a long time, such as feeling clumsy, irritable, or forgetful, probably do not mean that you have CJD. Discuss concerns with your doctor if you are not sure.

CJD is a rare disease, and most cases of CJD are not linked to hGH. When CJD is not linked to hGH, the first symptoms are usually mental changes such as confusion, problems thinking, memory loss, behavior changes, and dementia. Though symptoms may differ, there are similar changes in the brain tissue of all patients with CJD.

What is my risk for getting CJD?

No one can say what an individual person's risk is. Of the approximately 7,700 people who received NHPP hGH, 26 people got CJD. The two greatest risk factors are how long a person was treated, and when the person was treated.

How Long a Person Was Treated

- In the United States, the average length of time for hGH treatment was about three years. For the people who later got CJD, the average length of treatment was about nine years.

- Even though the longer treatment time increased the risk for CJD in the U.S., in other countries CJD has developed after shorter treatment periods.

When a Person Was Treated

- There is still no CJD in Americans who began treatment after new methods of purifying hormone began in the United States in 1977.

- A purification step used to make NHPP hGH after 1977 greatly reduced and may have gotten rid of possible CJD infection.

- No CJD has been reported in people who were treated with commercial hGH from human pituitaries. The new preparation step used after 1977 by the NHPP was also used for commercial hGH.

- It can take 30 years or more for a person to develop CJD. This means that more time must pass before it is known if someone who began treatment after 1977 could still develop CJD. With each year that goes by with no CJD in people who only received the newer hormone, we are more encouraged about the safety of hGH.

- Overall, one person out of about 300 people, or 26 out of 7,700 people, who were treated with hGH in the U.S. got CJD.

- Not all who received hGH are at equal risk. The risk in those who began treatment before 1977 is about one in 104 people or a little less than one percent.

- People who started treatment before 1970 are at higher risk. In that early group, one in 52 people got CJD (about two percent of the early group). Because there was no new CJD in the past five years in those who began treatment before 1970, these patients may be moving out of the incubation period for CJD. However, it is still too soon to be sure whether there will be additional reports of CJD in this group.

- The longest time from the start of hGH treatment to first signs of CJD is 33 years in U.S. patients, according to reports. One person in Holland got CJD attributed to hGH 38 years after a very brief use of hGH. Research studies indicate that the time it takes to get CJD depends, in part, on how much infectious material is given and how it is given. The disease generally takes longer to develop when a small amount of infectious material is given. The patient in Holland with the long incubation time received a very brief exposure to hGH.

When was I treated and for how long?

The best person to give you details on your treatment is the doctor who gave you hGH or a doctor who has access to your treatment records. To protect patients' privacy, the PHS did not ask for the names of those treated with hGH until 1985. In 1985, doctors and treatment centers were asked for names and addresses so people could be informed of the risk of CJD.

We know which hGH preparations were sent to each treatment center and when they were sent. But because individual doctors administered the hGH, we don't know which preparation each person might have gotten. The doctor who treated you is the best person to tell you about your treatment.

Which hormone preparations caused CJD?

No particular preparation of hGH has been found that is especially likely to carry CJD. It is believed that CJD did not come from a single infected pituitary gland or preparation. Prior to 1977, in an effort to extract as much hormone as possible from pituitaries, the pituitaries were often processed repeatedly. Hormone extracted from the same pituitaries was often included in many hormone preparations. Also, patients who got CJD were treated on average for nearly nine years and received many different hormone preparations. This makes it very difficult to identify any preparation associated with transmitting CJD.

If I have CJD can I pass it to my spouse or children?

- Scientists do not believe that CJD is transmitted through casual contact or sexual contact.

- Spouses and children of patients with CJD are not at increased risk.

- Except for rare genetic forms of CJD, a pregnant woman does not pass CJD on to her child.

- CJD from hGH does not affect the genes and is not passed on to future generations.

Is there a test to predict if I will get CJD?

Although researchers are trying to develop a test that will predict who might get CJD, there is currently no test that can identify who will, or will not, get CJD. There are variations in the structure of the gene for the brain protein that becomes abnormal in CJD. These differences may make some people more likely to get CJD than others. While a person's genetics may affect the risk of CJD, researchers cannot accurately predict the risk of developing CJD in individuals from genetic or other tests.

Why can't I donate blood or organs?

There have been two reports of the agent that causes variant CJD (vCJD) being transmitted through blood. Variant CJD is the disease that occurs in people who ate tainted beef or were exposed to products from cattle with mad cow disease. Variant CJD is different from the classic type of CJD that occurred in hGH recipients. It is not known if the type of CJD that occurred in GH recipients can be transmitted by blood. Nevertheless, doctors want to be especially careful because there is no test they can use to screen blood supplies.

Until more is known, the following people should not donate blood:

- Anyone who was treated with pituitary hGH. People who have been treated only with biosynthetic GH, in use since 1985, can donate blood.

- Relatives of patients with CJD. It is important to prevent donation by people from families with rare genetic forms of CJD. They could harbor CJD even if they do not have symptoms. Family members of people treated with hGH are not affected by this policy and can donate blood.

- Those who lived in Europe when cattle products may have spread the agent responsible for vCJD.

How is CJD diagnosed?

CJD is usually diagnosed based on signs and symptoms of the illness, how severe they are, and how quickly they become worse. Laboratory test results can suggest CJD as well. However, doctors must study brain tissue from a biopsy or autopsy in order to diagnose CJD for sure. In 1996, researchers developed a test that helps doctors diagnose CJD in patients with symptoms. This test detects an abnormal protein in a sample of spinal fluid. When this protein is found it helps make a diagnosis of CJD. It is much easier and safer to take a sample of spinal fluid than to do a brain biopsy. Unfortunately, this test cannot identify CJD in patients who do not have symptoms. The test cannot predict who may develop CJD in the future.

British researchers reported success using magnetic resonance imaging (MRI) to diagnose variant CJD in people with symptoms of the disease. MRI is a safe and painless tool that does not take brain or spinal fluid samples. (Zeidler M, et al. The pulvinar sign on magnetic resonance imaging in variant Creutzfeldt-Jakob disease. *Lancet.* 2000; 355:1412–1418, available online or at a medical library.)

What does research tell us about CJD?

- Although CJD is a rare disorder, some of the world's leading researchers are working hard to learn more about this disease. The most common type of CJD occurs all over the world and is very rare. Only one in a million people develop CJD per year. Most people who develop CJD get it after age 55.

About ten percent of the people who get CJD have inherited it. Some people have gotten CJD from medical procedures such as hGH injections, tissue grafts, or corneal transplants. Scientists don't fully understand what causes CJD. Evidence suggests that a unique infectious agent called a prion [pree'-on] may be the cause. A prion is an unusual infectious agent because it contains no genetic material. It is a protein that takes on different forms. In its normal, harmless form the protein is curled into a spiral. In its infectious form, the protein folds into an abnormal shape. Somehow, these abnormal proteins change the shape of normal proteins. This change begins a serious chain reaction that results in brain problems.

People with inherited CJD have an abnormal gene that leads to changes in their prion protein. This gene makes the protein likely to assume the abnormal shape. Exposure to the abnormal form of the protein can also occur through injection of contaminated hGH, tissue grafts, corneal transplants, or other exposures to infected brain tissue.

If CJD results from a defect in protein folding, it may be possible to identify drugs that can help the prion protein assume its proper shape. Such drugs would slow or stop the progress of the disease. Treatments like these are being studied in animal models and early clinical trials. Researchers both in Europe and the U.S. are trying to develop a test that will identify CJD before symptoms appear.

Support and Additional Information

Creutzfeldt-Jakob Disease Foundation Inc.
P.O. Box 5312
Akron, OH 44334
Toll-Free: 800-659-1991
Phone: 330-665-5590
Website: http://www.cjdfoundation.org
E-mail: help@cjdfoundation.org

Endocrine and Metabolic Diseases Information Service
6 Information Way
Bethesda, MD 20892-3569
Toll-Free: 888-828-0904
Fax: 703-738-4929
Website: http://www.endocrine.niddk.nih.gov
E-mail: endoandmeta@info.niddk.nih.gov

Human Growth Foundation (HGF)
997 Glen Cove Ave., Suite 5
Glen Head, NY 11545
Toll-Free: 800-451-6434
Fax: 516-671-4055
Website: http://www.hgfound.org.
E-mail: hgf1@hgfound.org

Chapter 16

Acromegaly

Acromegaly is a hormonal disorder that results when the pituitary gland produces excess growth hormone (GH). It most commonly affects middle-aged adults and can result in serious illness and premature death. Once recognized, acromegaly is treatable in most patients, but because of its slow and often insidious onset, it frequently is not diagnosed correctly.

The name acromegaly comes from the Greek words for "extremities" and "enlargement" and reflects one of its most common symptoms, the abnormal growth of the hands and feet. Soft tissue swelling of the hands and feet is often an early feature, with patients noticing a change in ring or shoe size. Gradually, bony changes alter the patient's facial features: the brow and lower jaw protrude, the nasal bone enlarges, and spacing of the teeth increases.

Overgrowth of bone and cartilage often leads to arthritis. When tissue thickens, it may trap nerves, causing carpal tunnel syndrome, characterized by numbness and weakness of the hands. Other symptoms of acromegaly include thick, coarse, oily skin; skin tags; enlarged lips, nose, and tongue; deepening of the voice due to enlarged sinuses and vocal cords; snoring due to upper airway obstruction; excessive sweating and skin odor; fatigue and weakness; headaches; impaired vision; abnormalities of the menstrual cycle and sometimes breast

National Institute of Diabetes and Digestive and Kidney Diseases (NIDDK), NIH Publication No. 02–3924, June 2002. Updated in January 2007 by Dr. David A. Cooke, M.D., Diplomate, American Board of Internal Medicine.

discharge in women; and impotence in men. There may be enlargement of body organs, including the liver, spleen, kidneys, and heart. The most serious health consequences of acromegaly are diabetes mellitus, hypertension, and increased risk of cardiovascular disease. Heart failure may also occur. Patients with acromegaly are also at increased risk for benign uterine tumors, and possibly for polyps of the colon that can develop into cancer.

When GH-producing tumors occur in childhood, the disease that results is called gigantism rather than acromegaly. Fusion of the growth plates of the long bones occurs after puberty so that development of excessive GH production in adults does not result in increased height. Prolonged exposure to excess GH before fusion of the growth plates causes increased growth of the long bones and increased height.

Causes of Acromegaly

Acromegaly is caused by prolonged overproduction of GH by the pituitary gland. The pituitary is a small gland at the base of the brain that produces several important hormones to control body functions such as growth and development, reproduction, and metabolism. GH is part of a cascade of hormones that, as the name implies, regulates the physical growth of the body. This cascade begins in a part of the brain called the hypothalamus, which makes hormones that regulate the pituitary. One of these, growth hormone-releasing hormone (GHRH), stimulates the pituitary gland to produce GH. Another hypothalamic hormone, somatostatin, inhibits GH production and release. Secretion of GH by the pituitary into the bloodstream causes the production of another hormone, called insulin-like growth factor-1 (IGF-1), in the liver. IGF-1 is the factor that actually causes the growth of bones and other tissues of the body. IGF-1, in turn, signals the pituitary to reduce GH production. GHRH, somatostatin, GH, and IGF-1 levels in the body are tightly regulated by each other and by sleep, exercise, stress, food intake, and blood sugar levels. If the pituitary continues to make GH independent of the normal regulatory mechanisms, the level of IGF-1 continues to rise, leading to bone growth and organ enlargement. The excess GH also causes changes in sugar and lipid metabolism and can cause diabetes.

Pituitary Tumors

In over 90 percent of acromegaly patients, the overproduction of GH is caused by a benign tumor of the pituitary gland, called an adenoma. These tumors produce excess GH and, as they expand, compress surrounding brain tissues, such as the optic nerves. This expansion causes the headaches and visual disturbances that are often symptoms of acromegaly. In addition, compression of the surrounding normal pituitary tissue can alter production of other hormones, leading to changes in menstruation and breast discharge in women and impotence in men.

There is a marked variation in rates of GH production and the growth of the tumor. Some adenomas grow slowly and symptoms of GH excess are often not noticed for many years. Other adenomas grow rapidly and compress surrounding brain areas or the sinuses, which are located near the pituitary. In general, younger patients tend to have more rapidly growing tumors.

Most pituitary tumors arise spontaneously and are not genetically inherited. Many pituitary tumors arise from a genetic alteration in a single pituitary cell which leads to increased cell division and tumor formation. This genetic change, or mutation, is not present at birth, but is acquired during life. The mutation occurs in a gene that regulates the transmission of chemical signals within pituitary cells; it permanently switches on the signal that tells the cell to divide and secrete GH. The events within the cell that cause disordered pituitary cell growth and GH oversecretion currently are the subject of intensive research.

Non-Pituitary Tumors

In a few patients, acromegaly is caused not by pituitary tumors but by tumors of the pancreas, lungs, and adrenal glands. These tumors also lead to an excess of GH, either because they produce GH themselves or, more frequently, because they produce GHRH, the hormone that stimulates the pituitary to make GH. In these patients, the excess GHRH can be measured in the blood and establishes that the cause of the acromegaly is not due to a pituitary defect. When these non-pituitary tumors are surgically removed, GH levels fall and the symptoms of acromegaly improve.

In patients with GHRH-producing, non-pituitary tumors, the pituitary still may be enlarged and may be mistaken for a tumor. Therefore, it is important that physicians carefully analyze all "pituitary tumors" removed from patients with acromegaly in order not to overlook the possibility that a tumor elsewhere in the body is causing the disorder.

How Common Is Acromegaly?

Small pituitary adenomas are common. During autopsies, they are found in up to 25 percent of the U.S. population. However, these tumors

161

rarely cause symptoms or produce excessive GH or other pituitary hormones. Scientists estimate that about three out of every million people develop acromegaly each year and that 40 to 60 out of every million people suffer from the disease at any time. However, because the clinical diagnosis of acromegaly often is missed, these numbers probably underestimate the frequency of the disease.

Diagnosis of Acromegaly

If a doctor suspects acromegaly, he or she can measure the GH level in the blood after a patient has fasted overnight, to determine if it is elevated. However, a single measurement of an elevated blood GH level is not enough to diagnose acromegaly because GH is secreted by the pituitary in spurts and its concentration in the blood can vary widely from minute to minute. At a given moment, a patient with acromegaly may have a normal GH level, whereas a GH level in a healthy person may be five times higher.

Because of these problems, more accurate information can be obtained when GH is measured under conditions in which GH secretion is normally suppressed. Physicians often use the oral glucose tolerance test to diagnose acromegaly because ingestion of 75 grams (g) of the sugar glucose lowers blood GH levels less than two nanograms per milliliter (ng/ml) in healthy people. In patients with GH overproduction, this reduction does not occur. The glucose tolerance test is the most reliable method of confirming a diagnosis of acromegaly.

Physicians also can measure IGF-1 levels in patients with suspected acromegaly. As mentioned earlier, elevated GH levels increase IGF-1 blood levels. Because IGF-1 levels are much more stable over the course of the day, they are often a more practical and reliable measure than GH levels. Elevated IGF-1 levels almost always indicate acromegaly. However, a pregnant woman's IGF-1 levels are two to three times higher than normal. In addition, physicians must be aware that IGF-1 levels decline in aging people and may be abnormally low in patients with poorly controlled diabetes mellitus.

After acromegaly has been diagnosed by measuring GH or IGF-1, imaging techniques, such as computed tomography (CT) scans or magnetic resonance imaging (MRI) scans of the pituitary are used to locate the tumor that causes the GH overproduction. Both techniques are excellent tools to visualize a tumor without surgery. If scans fail to detect a pituitary tumor, the physician should look for non-pituitary tumors in the chest, abdomen, or pelvis as the cause for excess GH.

162

The presence of such tumors usually can be diagnosed by measuring GHRH in the blood and by a CT scan of possible tumor sites.

Treatment of Acromegaly

The goals of treatment are to reduce GH production to normal levels, to relieve the pressure that the growing pituitary tumor exerts on the surrounding brain areas, to preserve normal pituitary function, and to reverse or ameliorate the symptoms of acromegaly. Currently, treatment options include surgical removal of the tumor, drug therapy, and radiation therapy of the pituitary.

Surgery

Surgery is a rapid and effective treatment. The surgeon reaches the pituitary through an incision in the nose and, with special tools, removes the tumor tissue in a procedure called transsphenoidal surgery. This procedure promptly relieves the pressure on the surrounding brain regions and leads to a lowering of GH levels. If the surgery is successful, facial appearance and soft tissue swelling improve within a few days. Surgery is most successful in patients with blood GH levels below 40 nanograms per milliliter (ng/ml) before the operation and with pituitary tumors no larger than ten millimeters (mm) in diameter. Success depends on the skill and experience of the surgeon. The success rate also depends on what level of GH is defined as a cure. The best measure of surgical success is normalization of GH and IGF-1 levels. Ideally, GH should be less than two ng/ml after an oral glucose load. A review of GH levels in 1,360 patients worldwide immediately after surgery revealed that 60 percent had random GH levels below five ng/ml. Complications of surgery may include cerebrospinal fluid leaks, meningitis, or damage to the surrounding normal pituitary tissue, requiring lifelong pituitary hormone replacement.

Even when surgery is successful and hormone levels return to normal, patients must be carefully monitored for years for possible recurrence. More commonly, hormone levels may improve, but not completely return to normal. These patients may then require additional treatment, usually with medications.

Drug Therapy

Two medications currently are used to treat acromegaly. These drugs reduce both GH secretion and tumor size. Medical therapy is sometimes used to shrink large tumors before surgery. Bromocriptine (Parlodel®) in divided doses of about 20 milligrams (mg) daily reduces GH secretion from some pituitary tumors. Side effects include gastrointestinal upset, nausea, vomiting, light-headedness when standing, and nasal congestion. These side effects can be reduced or eliminated if medication is started at a very low dose at bedtime, taken with food, and gradually increased to the full therapeutic dose.

Because bromocriptine can be taken orally, it is an attractive choice as primary drug or in combination with other treatments. However, bromocriptine lowers GH and IGF-1 levels and reduces tumor size in less than half of patients with acromegaly. Some patients report improvement in their symptoms although their GH and IGF-1 levels still are elevated.

The second medication used to treat acromegaly is octreotide (Sandostatin®). Octreotide is a synthetic form of a brain hormone, somatostatin, which stops GH production. This drug must be injected under the skin every eight hours for effective treatment. Most patients with acromegaly respond to this medication. In many patients, GH levels fall within one hour and headaches improve within minutes after the injection. Several studies have shown that octreotide is effective for long-term treatment. Octreotide also has been used successfully to treat patients with acromegaly caused by non-pituitary tumors.

Because octreotide inhibits gastrointestinal and pancreatic function, long-term use causes digestive problems such as loose stools, nausea, and gas in one-third of patients. In addition, approximately 25 percent of patients develop gallstones, which are usually asymptomatic. In rare cases, octreotide treatment can cause diabetes. On the other hand, scientists have found that in some acromegaly patients who already have diabetes, octreotide can reduce the need for insulin and improve blood sugar control.

Radiation Therapy

Radiation therapy has been used both as a primary treatment and combined with surgery or drugs. It is usually reserved for patients who have tumor remaining after surgery. Often, these patients also receive medication to lower GH levels. Radiation therapy is given in divided doses over four to six weeks. This treatment lowers GH levels by about 50 percent over 2–5 years. Patients monitored for more than five years show significant further improvement. Radiation therapy causes a gradual loss of production of other pituitary hormones with time. Loss of vision and brain injury, which have been reported, are very rare complications of radiation treatments.

No single treatment is effective for all patients. Treatment should be individualized depending on patient characteristics, such as age and tumor size. If the tumor has not yet invaded surrounding brain tissues, removal of the pituitary adenoma by an experienced neurosurgeon is usually the first choice. After surgery, a patient must be monitored for a long time for increasing GH levels. If surgery does not normalize hormone levels or a relapse occurs, a doctor will usually begin additional drug therapy. The first choice should be bromocriptine because it is easy to administer; octreotide is the second alternative. With both medications, long-term therapy is necessary because their withdrawal can lead to rising GH levels and renewed tumor expansion. Radiation therapy is generally used for patients whose tumors are not completely removed by surgery; for patients who are not good candidates for surgery because of other health problems; and for patients who do not respond adequately to surgery and medication.

Additional Information

Pituitary Network Association
P.O. Box 1958
Thousand Oaks, CA 91358
Phone: 805-499-9973
Fax: 805-480-0633
Website: http://www.pituitary.org
E-mail: pna@pituitary.org

Endocrine and Metabolic Diseases Information Service
6 Information Way
Bethesda, MD 20892-3569
Toll-Free: 888-828-0904
Fax: 703-738-4929
Website: http://www.endocrine.niddk.nih.gov
E-mail: endoandmeta@info.niddk.nih.gov

Chapter 17

Pituitary Cushing Disease

Cushing disease is a condition in which the pituitary gland releases too much adrenocorticotropic hormone (ATCH). The pituitary gland is an organ of the endocrine system. Cushing disease is a form of Cushing syndrome.

Causes, Incidence, and Risk Factors

Cushing disease is caused by a tumor or hyperplasia (excess growth) of the pituitary gland. This gland is located at the base of the brain.

People with Cushing disease have too much ACTH. ACTH stimulates the production and release of cortisol, a stress hormone. Too much ACTH means too much cortisol. Cortisol is normally released during stressful situations. It controls the body's use of carbohydrates, fats, and proteins and also helps reduce the immune system's response to inflammation (swelling).

Symptoms

- moon face (round, red, and full)
- buffalo hump (a collection of fat on the back of the neck)
- central obesity (person has an abdomen that sticks out and thin arms and legs)

"Pituitary Cushing's (Cushing's Disease)," © 2007 A.D.A.M., Inc. Reprinted with permission.

- weight gain
- weakness
- backache
- headache
- acne or other skin infections
- thirst
- increased urination
- purple streaks on the skin of the abdomen, thighs, and breasts
- mental changes
- impotence
- stopping of menstruation
- excessive hair growth in females

Signs and Tests

Tests are done to confirm there is too much cortisol in the body, then to determine the cause. In general, the fasting glucose may be high, and serum potassium may be low.

These tests confirm too much cortisol:

- 24-hour urine cortisol
- 24-hour urine creatinine
- dexamethasone suppression test (low dose)
- serial serum cortisol levels that do not show diurnal (night / day) variation
- nighttime saliva cortisol levels

These tests determine cause:

- serum ACTH levels
- cranial MRI scan that shows a pituitary tumor
- CRH (corticotropin-releasing hormone) test—CRH acts on the pituitary gland to bring about the release of ACTH
- petrosal sinus sampling—this test measures ACTH levels in the veins that drain the pituitary gland
- dexamethasone suppression test (high dose)

Treatment

Treatment is surgery to remove the pituitary tumor, if possible. After surgery, the pituitary may slowly start to work again and return to normal.

During the recovery process, cortisol replacement treatments may be necessary. Radiation treatment of the pituitary gland may also be used.

If the tumor does not respond to surgery or radiation, medications to stop the body from making cortisol are given.

Expectations (Prognosis)

Untreated, Cushing disease can cause severe illness, even death. Removal of the tumor may lead to full recovery, but the tumor can grow back.

Complications

- high blood pressure
- diabetes
- infections
- compression fractures
- kidney stones
- psychosis

Calling Your Health Care Provider

Call your health care provider if you develop symptoms of pituitary Cushing.

If you have had a pituitary tumor removed, call if signs of complications occur, including signs of recurrence (return) of the tumor.

Chapter 18

Diabetes Insipidus

Diabetes insipidus (DI) causes frequent urination. The large volume of urine is diluted, mostly water. To make up for lost water, you may feel the need to drink large amounts. You are likely to urinate frequently, even at night, which can disrupt sleep or, on occasion, cause bedwetting. Because of the excretion of abnormally large volumes of dilute urine, you may quickly become dehydrated if you do not drink enough water. Children with DI may be irritable or listless and may have fever, vomiting, or diarrhea. In its clinically significant forms, DI is a rare disease.

Diabetes Insipidus versus Diabetes Mellitus

DI should not be confused with diabetes mellitus, which results from insulin deficiency or resistance leading to high blood glucose. Diabetes insipidus and diabetes mellitus are unrelated, although they can have similar signs and symptoms, like excessive thirst and excessive urination.

Diabetes mellitus (DM) is far more common than DI and receives more news coverage. DM has two forms, referred to as type 1 diabetes (formerly called juvenile diabetes, or insulin-dependent diabetes mellitus, or IDDM) and type 2 diabetes (formerly called adult-onset diabetes, or noninsulin-dependent diabetes mellitus, or NIDDM). DI is a different form of illness altogether.

National Institute of Diabetes and Digestive and Kidney Diseases (NIDDK), NIH Publication No. 05–4620, August 2005.

Normal Fluid Regulation in the Body

Your body has a complex system for balancing the volume and composition of body fluids. Your kidneys remove extra body fluids from your bloodstream. This fluid waste is stored in the bladder as urine. If your fluid regulation system is working properly, your kidneys make less urine to conserve fluid when the body is losing water. Your kidneys also make less urine at night when the body's metabolic processes are slower.

In order to keep the volume and composition of body fluids balanced, the rate of fluid intake is governed by thirst, and the rate of excretion is governed by the production of antidiuretic hormone (ADH), also called vasopressin. This hormone is made in the hypothalamus, a small gland located in the base of the brain. ADH is stored in the nearby pituitary gland and released from it into the bloodstream when necessary. When ADH reaches the kidneys, it directs the kidneys to concentrate the urine by returning excess water to the bloodstream and therefore make less urine.

DI occurs when this precise system for regulating the kidneys' handling of fluids is disrupted. The most common form of clinically serious DI, central DI, results from damage to the pituitary gland, which disrupts the normal storage and release of ADH. Another form, nephrogenic DI, results when the kidneys are unable to respond to ADH. Rarer forms occur because of a defect in the thirst mechanism (dipsogenic DI) or during pregnancy (gestational DI). A specialist should determine which form of DI is present before starting any treatment.

Central DI

Damage to the pituitary gland can be caused by different diseases as well as by head injuries, neurosurgery, or genetic disorders. To treat the ADH deficiency that results from any kind of damage to the hypothalamus or pituitary, a synthetic hormone called desmopressin can be taken by an injection, a nasal spray, or a pill. While taking desmopressin, you should drink fluids or water only when you are thirsty and not at other times. This is because the drug prevents water excretion and water can build up now that your kidneys are making less urine and are less responsive to changes in body fluids.

Nephrogenic DI

The kidneys' ability to respond to ADH can be impaired by drugs (like lithium, for example) and by chronic disorders including polycystic

172

kidney disease, sickle cell disease, kidney failure, partial blockage of the ureters, and inherited genetic disorders. Sometimes the cause of nephrogenic DI is never discovered. Desmopressin will not work for this form of DI. Instead, you may be given a drug called hydrochlorothiazide (also called HCTZ) or indomethacin. HCTZ is sometimes combined with another drug called amiloride. The combination of HCTZ and amiloride is sold under the brand name Moduretic. Again, with this combination of drugs, you should drink fluids only when you are thirsty and not at other times.

Dipsogenic DI

A third type of DI is caused by a defect in or damage to the thirst mechanism, which is located in the hypothalamus. This defect results in an abnormal increase in thirst and fluid intake that suppresses ADH secretion and increases urine output. Desmopressin or other drugs should not be used to treat dipsogenic DI because they may decrease urine output but not thirst and fluid intake. This fluid "overload" can lead to water intoxication, a condition that lowers the concentration of sodium in the blood and can seriously damage the brain.

Gestational DI

A fourth type of DI occurs only during pregnancy. Gestational DI occurs when an enzyme made by the placenta destroys ADH in the mother. The placenta is the system of blood vessels and other tissue that develops with the fetus. The placenta allows exchange of nutrients and waste products between mother and fetus.

Most cases of gestational DI can be treated with desmopressin. In rare cases, however, an abnormality in the thirst mechanism causes gestational DI, and desmopressin should not be used.

Diagnosis

Because DM is more common and because DM and DI have similar symptoms, a health care provider may suspect that a patient with DI has DM. But testing should make the diagnosis clear.

Your physician must determine which type of DI is involved before proper treatment can begin. Diagnosis is based on a series of tests, including urinalysis and a fluid deprivation test.

Urinalysis is the physical and chemical examination of urine. The urine of a person with DI will be less concentrated. Therefore, the salt and waste concentrations are low, and the amount of water excreted is high. A physician evaluates the concentration of urine by measuring how many particles are in a kilogram of water (osmolality) or by comparing the weight of the urine to an equal volume of distilled water (specific gravity).

A fluid deprivation test helps determine whether DI is caused by (1) excessive intake of fluid, (2) a defect in ADH production, or (3) a defect in the kidneys' response to ADH. This test measures changes in body weight, urine output, and urine composition when fluids are withheld. Sometimes measuring blood levels of ADH during this test is also necessary.

In some patients, a magnetic resonance image (MRI) of the brain may be necessary as well.

Additional Information

National Kidney and Urologic Diseases Information Clearinghouse
3 Information Way
Bethesda, MD 20892-3580
Toll-Free: 800-891-5390
Fax: 703-738-4929
Website: http://kidney.niddk.nih.gov
E-mail: nkudic@info.niddk.nih.gov

National Organization for Rare Disorders (NORD)
P.O. Box 1968
Danbury, CT 06813-1968
Toll-Free: 800-999-NORD (6673)
Phone: 203-744-0100
Fax: 203-798-2291
Website: http://www.rarediseases.org
E-mail: orphan@rarediseases.org

Chapter 19

Prolactinomas

A prolactinoma is a benign tumor of the pituitary gland that produces a hormone called prolactin. It is the most common type of pituitary tumor. Symptoms of prolactinoma are caused by too much prolactin in the blood (hyperprolactinemia) or by pressure of the tumor on surrounding tissues.

Prolactin stimulates the breast to produce milk during pregnancy. After delivery of the baby, a mother's prolactin levels fall unless she breast feeds her infant. Each time the baby nurses, prolactin levels rise to maintain milk production.

The pituitary gland, sometimes called the master gland, plays a critical role in regulating growth and development, metabolism, and reproduction. It produces prolactin and a variety of other key hormones. These include growth hormone, which regulates growth; adrenocorticotropic hormone, or ACTH (corticotropin), which stimulates the adrenal glands to produce cortisol; thyrotropin, which signals the thyroid gland to produce thyroid hormone; and luteinizing hormone (LH) and follicle-stimulating hormone (FSH), which regulate ovulation and estrogen and progesterone production in women, and sperm formation and testosterone production in men.

The pituitary gland sits in the middle of the head in a bony box called the sella turcica. The eye nerves sit directly above the pituitary gland. Enlargement of the gland can cause local symptoms such as

National Institute of Diabetes and Digestive and Kidney Diseases (NIDDK), NIH Publication No. 02–3924, June 2002. Updated in January 2007 by Dr. David A. Cooke, M.D., Diplomate, American Board of Internal Medicine.

175

headaches or visual disturbances. Pituitary tumors may also impair production of one or more pituitary hormones, causing reduced pituitary function (hypopituitarism).

Autopsy studies indicate that 25 percent of the U.S. population have small pituitary tumors. Forty percent of these pituitary tumors produce prolactin, but most are not considered clinically significant. Clinically significant pituitary tumors affect the health of approximately 14 out of 100,000 people.

Causes of Prolactinoma

Although research continues to unravel the mysteries of disordered cell growth, the cause of pituitary tumors remains unknown. Most pituitary tumors are sporadic—they are not genetically passed from parents to offspring.

Symptoms of Prolactinoma

In women, high blood levels of prolactin often cause infertility and changes in menstruation. In some women, periods may disappear altogether. In others, periods may become irregular or menstrual flow may change. Women who are not pregnant or nursing may begin producing breast milk. Some women may experience a loss of libido (interest in sex). Intercourse may become painful because of vaginal dryness.

In men, the most common symptom of prolactinoma is impotence. Because men have no reliable indicator such as menstruation to signal a problem, many men delay going to the doctor until they have headaches or eye problems caused by the enlarged pituitary pressing against nearby eye nerves. They may not recognize a gradual loss of sexual function or libido. Only after treatment do some men realize they had a problem with sexual function.

What else causes prolactin to rise?

In some people, high blood levels of prolactin can be traced to causes other than a pituitary tumor.

Prescription drugs. Prolactin secretion in the pituitary is normally suppressed by the brain chemical, dopamine. Drugs that block the effects of dopamine at the pituitary or deplete dopamine stores in the brain may cause the pituitary to secrete prolactin. These drugs include the major tranquilizers trifluoperazine (Stelazine) and haloperidol

176

(Haldol); metoclopramide (Reglan), used to treat gastroesophageal reflux and the nausea caused by certain cancer drugs; and less often, alpha methyldopa and reserpine, used to control hypertension.

Other pituitary tumors. Other tumors arising in or near the pituitary—such as those that cause acromegaly or Cushing syndrome—may block the flow of dopamine from the brain to the prolactin-secreting cells.

Hypothyroidism. Increased prolactin levels are often seen in people with hypothyroidism, and doctors routinely test people with hyperprolactinemia for hypothyroidism.

Breast stimulation also can cause a modest increase in the amount of prolactin in the blood.

Diagnosis of Prolactinoma

A doctor will test for prolactin blood levels in women with unexplained milk secretion (galactorrhea) or irregular menses or infertility, and in men with impaired sexual function and, in rare cases, milk secretion. If prolactin is high, a doctor will test thyroid function and ask first about other conditions and medications known to raise prolactin secretion. The doctor will also request a magnetic resonance imaging (MRI), which is the most sensitive test for detecting pituitary tumors and determining their size. MRI scans may be repeated periodically to assess tumor progression and the effects of therapy. Computed tomography (CT scan) also gives an image of the pituitary, but it is less sensitive than the MRI.

In addition to assessing the size of the pituitary tumor, doctors also look for damage to surrounding tissues, and perform tests to assess whether production of other pituitary hormones is normal. Depending on the size of the tumor, the doctor may request an eye exam with measurement of visual fields.

Treatment of Prolactinoma

Medical Treatment

The goal of treatment is to return prolactin secretion to normal, reduce tumor size, correct any visual abnormalities, and restore normal pituitary function. In the case of very large tumors, only partial achievement of this goal may be possible. Because dopamine is the chemical that normally inhibits prolactin secretion, doctors may treat prolactinoma with bromocriptine or cabergoline, drugs that act like dopamine. This type of drug is called a dopamine agonist. These drugs shrink the tumor and return prolactin levels to normal in approximately 80 percent of patients. Both have been approved by the Food and Drug Administration for the treatment of hyperprolactinemia. Bromocriptine is the only dopamine agonist approved for the treatment of infertility. Another dopamine agonist, pergolide, is available in the U.S., but is not approved for treating conditions that cause high blood levels of prolactin.

Bromocriptine is associated with side effects such as nausea and dizziness. To avoid these side effects, it is important for bromocriptine treatment to start slowly. An example of a typical approach used by an experienced endocrinologist follows:

- Begin by taking a quarter of a 2.5 milligram tablet of bromocriptine with a snack at bedtime. After three days, increase the dose to a quarter of a tablet with breakfast and a quarter at bedtime. After three more days, take half a tablet twice a day, and three days later, one tablet at night and half with breakfast. Finally, the dose is increased to one tablet twice a day. If prolactin is still high, add half a tablet with lunch. If the medication is well tolerated, increase the dose to a full tablet. If side effects develop with a higher dose, return to the previous dosage. With time, side effects disappear while the drug continues to lower prolactin.

Bromocriptine treatment should not be interrupted without consulting a qualified endocrinologist. Prolactin levels often rise again in most people when the drug is discontinued. In some, however, prolactin levels remain normal, so the doctor may suggest reducing or discontinuing treatment every two years on a trial basis.

Cabergoline is also associated with side effects such as nausea and dizziness, but these may be less common and less severe than with bromocriptine. As with bromocriptine therapy, side effects may be avoided if treatment is started slowly. An example of a typical approach used by an experienced endocrinologist follows:

- Begin by taking 0.25 milligrams (or ½ tablet) twice a week. After four weeks, increase the dose by 0.25 milligrams to 0.50 milligrams (or 1 tablet) twice a week. After four more weeks, increase the dose by 0.25 milligrams to 0.75 milligrams (or 1½ tablets) twice a week. Finally, after four additional weeks, the dose can be increased to 1 milligram (or 2 tablets) twice a week. If side effects develop with a higher dose, the doctor may return to the previous dosage. If a patient's prolactin level remains normal for six months, a doctor may consider stopping treatment.

Cabergoline should not be interrupted without consulting a qualified endocrinologist.

Surgery

Surgery should be considered if medical therapy cannot be tolerated or if it fails to reduce prolactin levels, restore normal reproduction and pituitary function, and reduce tumor size. If medical therapy is only partially successful, this therapy should continue, possibly combined with surgery or radiation.

The results of surgery depend a great deal on tumor size and prolactin level as well as the skill and experience of the neurosurgeon. The higher the prolactin level, the lower the chance of normalizing serum prolactin. In the best medical centers, surgery corrects prolactin levels in 80 percent of patients with a serum prolactin less than 250 nanograms per milliliter (ng/ml). Even in patients with large tumors that cannot be completely removed, drug therapy may be able to return serum prolactin to the normal range after surgery. Depending on the size of the tumor and how much of it is removed, studies show that 20 to 50 percent will recur, usually within five years.

Frequently Asked Questions

How do I choose a skilled neurosurgeon?

Because the results of surgery are so dependent on the skill and knowledge of the neurosurgeon, a patient should ask the surgeon about the number of operations he or she has performed to remove pituitary tumors, and for success and complication rates in comparison to major medical centers. The best results come from surgeons who have performed many hundreds or even thousands of such operations.

How does prolactinoma affect pregnancy and oral contraceptives?

If a woman has a small prolactinoma, there is no reason that she cannot conceive and have a normal pregnancy after successful medical therapy. The pituitary enlarges and prolactin production increases during normal pregnancy in women without pituitary disorders. Women with prolactin-secreting tumors may experience further pituitary enlargement and must be closely monitored during pregnancy. However, damage to the pituitary or eye nerves occurs in less than one percent of pregnant women with prolactinoma. In women with large tumors, the risk of damage to the pituitary or eye nerves is greater, and some doctors consider it as high as 25 percent. If a woman has completed a successful pregnancy, the chance of her completing further successful pregnancies is extremely high.

A woman with a prolactinoma should discuss her plans to conceive with her physician, so she can be carefully evaluated prior to becoming pregnant. This evaluation will include a magnetic resonance imaging (MRI) scan to assess the size of the tumor and an eye examination with measurement of visual fields. As soon as a patient is pregnant, her doctor will usually advise that she stop taking bromocriptine or cabergoline, the common treatments for prolactinoma. Most endocrinologists see patients every two months throughout the pregnancy. The patient should consult her endocrinologist promptly if she develops symptoms—particularly headaches, visual changes, nausea, vomiting, excessive thirst or urination, or extreme lethargy. Bromocriptine or cabergoline treatment may be renewed and additional treatment may be required if the patient develops symptoms from growth of the tumor during pregnancy. Pituitary apoplexy, which is bleeding inside the pituitary tumor, is known to occur occasionally during delivery, and is also a consideration.

At one time, oral contraceptives were thought to contribute to the development of prolactinomas. However, this is no longer thought to be true. Patients with prolactinoma treated with bromocriptine or cabergoline may also take oral contraceptives. Similarly, post-menopausal estrogen replacement is safe in patients with prolactinoma treated with medical therapy or surgery.

Is osteoporosis a risk in women with high prolactin levels?

Women whose ovaries produce inadequate estrogen are at increased risk for osteoporosis. Hyperprolactinemia can cause reduced estrogen production. Although estrogen production may be restored after treatment for hyperprolactinemia, even a year or two without estrogen can compromise bone strength, and these women should protect themselves from osteoporosis by increasing exercise and calcium intake through diet or supplementation, and by avoiding smoking. Women may want to have bone density measurements to assess the effect of estrogen deficiency on bone density. They may also want to discuss with their physician whether estrogen replacement therapy is advisable in their case, as this has both risks and benefits.

Additional Information

Pituitary Network Association
P.O. Box 1958
Thousand Oaks, CA 91358
Phone: 805-499-9973
Fax: 805-480-0633
Website: http://www.pituitary.org
E-mail: pna@pituitary.org

Endocrine and Metabolic Diseases Information Service
6 Information Way
Bethesda, MD 20892-3569
Toll-Free: 888-828-0904
Fax: 703-738-4929
Website: http://www.endocrine.niddk.nih.gov
E-mail: endoandmeta@info.niddk.nih.gov

Chapter 20

Pituitary Tumors and Treatment Options

What are pituitary tumors?

Pituitary tumors are tumors found in the pituitary gland, a small organ about the size of a pea in the center of the brain just above the back of the nose. The pituitary gland makes hormones that affect growth and the functions of other glands in the body. Pituitary tumors may be grouped as follows:

- *Benign adenomas*, which are noncancer. These grow very slowly and do not spread from the pituitary gland to other parts of the body.

- *Invasive adenomas*, which spread to the outer covering of the brain, bones of the skull, or the sinus cavity below the pituitary gland.

- *Carcinomas*, which are malignant (cancer). These are pituitary tumors that have spread far from the pituitary gland in the central nervous system (brain and spinal cord) or outside of the central nervous system.

These pituitary tumors may be either functioning or nonfunctioning. Tumors that make one or more of the pituitary hormones are

Excerpted from PDQ® Cancer Information Summary. National Cancer Institute, Bethesda, MD. Pituitary Tumors (PDQ®): Treatment–Patient. Updated 02/2006. Available at http://cancer.gov. Accessed 02/06/2007.

called functioning tumors, while those that do not make hormones are called nonfunctioning tumors. Each type of functioning tumor causes different symptoms, depending on the type of hormone that is being made by the tumor. Symptoms may also be caused if the tumor grows large and presses on nearby parts of the brain. A doctor should be seen if there are symptoms such as these:

- Headaches
- Trouble seeing or moving the eyes
- Vomiting
- Any of the symptoms caused by too many hormones, as described under the tumor types in the "Stage Explanation" section

Some cancers in other parts of the body may metastasize (spread) to the pituitary gland, but these pituitary tumors usually do not cause symptoms. Breast and lung cancer are the most common types of cancer that spread to the pituitary.

If there are symptoms, a doctor may order laboratory tests to see what the hormone levels are in the blood. The doctor may also order a magnetic resonance imaging (MRI) scan, which uses magnetic waves to make a picture of the inside of the brain. Other special x-rays may also be done.

Stage Explanation

Pituitary tumors are classified according to size:

- Microadenomas are smaller than 10 millimeters.
- Macroadenomas are 10 millimeters or larger.

Most pituitary adenomas are microadenomas.

Once a pituitary tumor is found, more tests will be done to find out how far the tumor has spread, the type of tumor, and whether or not it makes hormones. A doctor needs to know the type of tumor to plan treatment.

Types of Pituitary Tumors

Prolactin-producing tumors. These tumors make prolactin, a hormone that stimulates a woman's breasts to make milk during and after pregnancy. Prolactin-secreting tumors can cause the breasts to make milk and menstrual periods to stop when a woman is not pregnant. In men, prolactin-producing tumors can cause impotence.

Adrenocorticotropic hormone (ACTH)-producing tumors. These tumors make a hormone called adrenocorticotropic hormone (ACTH), which stimulates the adrenal glands to make glucocorticoids. When the body makes too much ACTH, it causes Cushing disease. In Cushing disease, fat builds up in the face, back, and chest, and the arms and legs become very thin. Another symptom of ACTH-producing tumors is weakened bones.

Growth hormone-producing tumors. These tumors make growth hormone. Too much growth hormone can cause acromegaly (the hands, feet, and face are larger than normal) or gigantism (the whole body grows much larger than normal).

Nonfunctioning pituitary tumors. Nonfunctioning tumors do not produce hormones. Symptoms may include headache or trouble seeing that may be caused by the tumor pressing on nearby brain tissue. If the tumor presses on or destroys parts of the pituitary gland, the pituitary gland may stop making one or more of its hormones. Lack of a certain hormone will affect the work of the gland or organ that the hormone controls. For example, if the pituitary gland stops making the hormone that affects the ovaries, the ovaries will not work normally or will not develop normally in a child.

Thyroid hormone-producing tumors. These tumors make thyrotrophin, which stimulates the thyroid gland to make thyroid hormone. The thyroid hormone helps regulate heart rate, body temperature, the level of calcium in the blood, and the rate at which food is changed into energy. Too much thyroid hormone can cause rapid heartbeat, weight loss, and other symptoms. Thyroid hormone-producing tumors may be large and may spread. They sometimes also make growth hormone and/or prolactin.

Pituitary carcinomas. These tumors usually grow quickly and make hormones, commonly ACTH and prolactin. Symptoms may be caused by the hormone that is made by the tumor and by the tumor pressing on nearby brain tissue.

Recurrent pituitary tumors. Recurrent disease means that the tumor has come back (recurred) after it has been treated. It may come back in the pituitary gland or in another part of the body.

Treatment Option Overview

There are treatments for all patients with pituitary tumors. Three kinds of treatment are used:

- surgery (taking out the tumor in an operation)
- radiation therapy (using high-dose x-rays to kill tumor cells)
- drug therapy

Surgery is a common treatment of pituitary tumors. A doctor may remove the tumor using one of the following operations:

- Transsphenoidal surgery removes the tumor through a cut in the nasal passage.
- A craniotomy removes the tumor through a cut in the front of the skull.

Radiation therapy uses high-energy x-rays to kill cancer cells and shrink tumors. Radiation for pituitary tumors usually comes from a machine outside the body (external radiation therapy). Clinical trials are testing stereotactic radiation surgery, in which radiation is aimed to the tumor only, with less damage to healthy tissue. A computed tomography (CT) scan or MRI is used to find the exact location of the tumor. A rigid head frame is attached to the skull and high-dose radiation is directed to the tumor through openings in the head frame, so only a small amount of normal brain tissue is affected. This procedure does not involve surgery. Radiation therapy may be used alone or in addition to surgery or drug therapy.

Drug therapy is the use of drugs to stop the pituitary gland from making too many hormones.

Treatment by Type

Treatments for pituitary tumors depend on the type of tumor, the symptoms of its hormone activity, how far the tumor has spread into the brain, and the patient's age and overall health.

Standard treatment may be considered because of its effectiveness in patients in past studies, or participation in a clinical trial may be considered. Not all patients are cured with standard therapy, and some standard treatments may have more side effects than are desired. For these reasons, clinical trials are designed to find better ways to treat cancer patients and are based on the most up-to-date information.

Clinical trials are ongoing in some parts of the country for patients with pituitary tumors.

Prolactin-Producing Pituitary Tumors

Treatment may be one of the following:

1. Drug therapy to stop the tumor from making prolactin.

2. Surgery to remove the tumor (transsphenoidal surgery or craniotomy) when the tumor does not respond to drug therapy or when the patient cannot take the drug.

3. Radiation therapy.

ACTH-Producing Pituitary Tumors

Treatment may be one of the following:

1. Surgery to remove the tumor (usually transsphenoidal surgery) with or without radiation therapy.

2. Radiation therapy alone.

3. Drug therapy to stop the tumor from making ACTH.

4. A clinical trial of stereotactic radiation surgery.

Growth Hormone-Producing Pituitary Tumors

Treatment may be one of the following:

1. Surgery to remove the tumor (usually transsphenoidal surgery).

2. Drug therapy to stop the tumor from making growth hormone.

3. Surgery followed by radiation therapy.

Nonfunctioning Pituitary Tumors

Treatment may be one of the following:

1. Surgery to remove the tumor (transsphenoidal surgery or craniotomy) followed by watchful waiting (closely monitoring a patient's condition without giving any treatment until symptoms appear or change). Radiation therapy is given if the tumor comes back.

2. Radiation therapy.

3. Surgery followed by radiation therapy.

Thyroid Hormone-Producing Tumors

Treatment may be one of the following:

1. Surgery to remove the tumor (usually transsphenoidal surgery) with or without radiation therapy.

2. Drug therapy to stop the tumor from making hormones.

Pituitary Carcinomas

Treatment is usually palliative, to relieve symptoms and improve the patient's quality of life. Treatment may be one of the following:

1. Surgery to remove the cancer (transsphenoidal surgery or craniotomy) with or without radiation therapy.

2. Drug therapy to stop the tumor from making hormones.

3. Chemotherapy.

Recurrent Pituitary Tumors

Treatment of recurrent pituitary tumor depends on the type of tumor, the type of treatment the patient has already had, and other factors such as the patient's general condition. Patients may want to take part in a clinical trial of new treatments. Treatment may be one of the following:

1. Radiation therapy.

2. A clinical trial of stereotactic radiation surgery.

Additional Information

National Cancer Institute
Cancer Information Service
6116 Executive Blvd., Room 3036A
Bethesda, MD 20892-8322
Toll-Free: 800-4-CANCER (422-6237)
Toll-Free TTY: 800-332-8615
Website: http://www.cancer.gov
E-mail: cancergovstaff@mail.nih.gov

Information about ongoing clinical trials is available from the NCI website at http://www.cancer.gov/clinicaltrials.

Chapter 21

Pituitary Disorders Treatment Options

Several types of medical therapy can help to relieve pituitary problems. Prolactinomas, for example, respond well to a dopamine agonist drug. If surgery does not remove the entire tumor, sometimes octreotide is used in patients with acromegaly or thyroid-stimulating hormone (TSH)-secreting tumors. Medication is used to lower high hormone levels or to shrink the tumor. Sometimes pegvisomant may be used to block the action of growth hormone. In many cases, medical therapy is combined with surgery and/or radiation treatment.

Hormone Therapy

Hormone replacement therapy is an important part of any treatment for a pituitary disorder. Hormones must be prescribed to meet your exact needs. Sometimes tumors cause a lack of hormone, which can lead to the symptoms you are having. Sometimes lack of hormone is caused by the treatment you have for pituitary tumors. Radiation therapy, for example, can lead to permanent loss of hormone secretion.

Some hormones are absolutely necessary for survival. These hormones must be replaced immediately. The replacement of cortisol is important, because this hormone regulates blood pressure and blood glucose levels. Cortisol replacement is common during tumor surgeries because it helps the body to handle stress.

TSH, or thyroid stimulating hormone, is also vital to survival, because it regulates the body's metabolism. If TSH secretion is low, you may also need to start thyroid hormone replacement.

Antidiuretic hormone (ADH), or vasopressin, needs immediate replacement, because it controls the body's water balance. If it is missing, this can cause excess thirst and urination, which is usually a temporary condition. (Note: This is not the same as diabetes mellitus, a common confusion.)

Other hormones, such as estrogen and progesterone in women and testosterone in men also may need to be replaced. While they are not vital for survival, they help you to live a full and healthy life. In addition to reproductive effects, these hormones are important for many functions such as maintaining normal bone mass. It is important to remember that hormone replacement of estrogen and progesterone in young women for example, replacing hormones back to where they would be if the pituitary works, is not the same as post-menopausal hormone replacement. In the latter case, hormones are being given at a time in life when they are not normally made.

Some hormones may return to normal levels after treatment for a pituitary condition. In other cases, there may be some permanent loss of hormone function. You may need to take certain hormones for the rest of your life. Your doctor will work with you to monitor and adjust your hormone replacement therapy as needed. You should always take your hormone treatment as directed.

Surgery

The most common form of surgery to remove pituitary tumors is transsphenoidal microsurgery. A neurosurgeon approaches the pituitary tumor through the nose, in the sphenoid sinus cavity. Using this natural pathway the surgeon does not need to drill a hole in your skull. With a surgical microscope and special instruments, the surgeon can typically safely remove the tumor without damaging the surrounding pituitary gland.

This surgery is not very painful, and you won't have any outer scars. You may have a sore nose or what feels like a sinus headache. The biggest discomfort usually is from the padding inserted in the nose for 24 to 48 hours after surgery. However with newer techniques, packs are often not required at all. You will probably be in the hospital for two or three days. You should take it easy for a few weeks after the surgery, until your doctor says it is time to resume your usual activities, including exercise.

Radiation Treatments

To treat a pituitary tumor with radiation, doctors may use a variety of techniques depending on the size and location of the tumor. Conventional radiation covers a wide area in and around the tumor and is usually given daily for several weeks. A number of more focused "radiosurgery" therapies are also available and may be appropriate for your case including gamma knife and proton beam. These methods begin with a magnetic resonance imaging (MRI) scan to image your brain. The scan locates the precise location and size of the tumor. After the MRI, you go into a special treatment room. Using the points mapped from the MRI, several narrow beams of high-dose radiation are delivered to the exact tumor location. These beams are so precise that they can avoid the normal tissue surrounding the tumor. All radiation therapy works slowly, and it may take from six months to several years for your condition to improve. This is why radiation therapy is typically used together with other therapies. It is important to have an evaluation for radiation therapy at a center with expertise in treating pituitary tumors.

Part Three

Thyroid and Parathyroid Gland Disorders

Chapter 22

Thyroid Function

What is the thyroid?

The thyroid gland is a butterfly-shaped endocrine gland that is normally located in the lower front of the neck. The thyroid's job is to make thyroid hormone, which is secreted into the blood and then carried to every tissue in the body. Thyroid hormone is essential to help each cell in each tissue and organ to work right. For example, thyroid hormone helps the body use energy, stay warm, and keep the brain, heart, muscles and other organs working as they should.

How does the thyroid gland function?

The major thyroid hormone secreted by the thyroid gland is thyroxine, also called T_4 because it contains four iodine atoms. To exert its effects, T_4 is converted to triiodothyronine (T_3) by the removal of an iodine atom. This occurs mainly in the liver and in certain tissues where T_3 acts, such as in the brain. The amount of T_4 produced by the thyroid gland is controlled by another hormone, which is made in the pituitary gland located at the base of the brain, called thyroid stimulating hormone (abbreviated TSH). The amount of TSH that the pituitary sends

---

This chapter begins with questions and answers from "Thyroid Function Tests," reprinted with permission from The American Thyroid Association, Inc., © 2005. Online Patient Resources at www.thyroid.org. Text under the heading, "When Is a Thyroid Gland Abnormal?" is excerpted from "Thyroid Gland," and is reprinted with permission of the American Academy of Otolaryngology–Head and Neck Surgery Foundation, copyright © 2006. All rights reserved.

into the blood stream depends on the amount of T_4 that the pituitary sees. If the pituitary sees very little T_4, then it produces more TSH to tell the thyroid gland to produce more T_4. Once the T_4 in the blood stream goes above a certain level, the pituitary's production of TSH is shut off. In fact, the thyroid and pituitary act in many ways like a heater and a thermostat. When the heater is off and it becomes cold, the thermostat reads the temperature and turns on the heater. When the heat rises to an appropriate level, the thermostat senses this and turns off the heater. Thus, the thyroid and the pituitary, like a heater and thermostat, turn on and off.

What tests are used to evaluate thyroid function?

Blood tests to measure TSH, T_4 and T_3 are readily available and widely used. These include:

TSH Tests: The best way to initially test thyroid function is to measure the TSH level in a blood sample. A high TSH level indicates that the thyroid gland is failing because of a problem that is directly affecting the thyroid (primary hypothyroidism). The opposite situation, in which the TSH level is low, usually indicates that the person has an overactive thyroid that is producing too much thyroid hormone (hyperthyroidism). Occasionally, a low TSH may result from an abnormality in the pituitary gland, which prevents it from making enough TSH to stimulate the thyroid (secondary hypothyroidism). In most healthy individuals, a normal TSH value means that the thyroid is functioning normally.

T_4 Tests: T_4 circulates in the blood in two forms: 1) T_4 bound to proteins that prevent the T_4 from entering the various tissues that need thyroid hormone, and 2) free T_4, which does enter the various target tissues to exert its effects. The free T_4 fraction is the most important to determine how the thyroid is functioning, and tests to measure this are called the free T_4 (FT_4) and the free T_4 index (FT_4I or FTI). Individuals who have hyperthyroidism will have an elevated FT_4 or FTI, whereas patients with hypothyroidism will have a low level of FT_4 or FTI. Combining the TSH test with the FT_4 or FTI accurately determines how the thyroid gland is functioning. The finding of an elevated TSH and low FT_4 or FTI indicates primary hypothyroidism due to disease in the thyroid gland. A low TSH and low FT_4 or FTI indicates hypothyroidism due to a problem involving the pituitary gland. A low TSH with an elevated FT_4 or FTI is found in individuals who have hyperthyroidism.

T_3 Tests: T_3 tests are often useful to diagnosis hyperthyroidism or to determine the severity of the hyperthyroidism. Patients who are hyperthyroid will have an elevated T_3 level. In some individuals with a low TSH, only the T_3 is elevated and the FT_4 or FTI is normal. T_3 testing rarely is helpful in the hypothyroid patient, since it is the last test to become abnormal. Patients can be severely hypothyroid with a high TSH and low FT_4 or FTI, but have a normal T_3.

Thyroid Antibody Tests: The immune system of the body normally protects us from foreign invaders such as bacteria and viruses by destroying these invaders with substances called antibodies produced by blood cells known as lymphocytes. In many patients with hypothyroidism or hyperthyroidism, lymphocytes make antibodies against their thyroid that either stimulate or damage the gland. Two common antibodies that cause thyroid problems are directed against thyroid cell proteins: thyroid peroxidase and thyroglobulin. Measuring levels of thyroid antibodies may help diagnose the cause of the thyroid problems. For example, positive anti-thyroid peroxidase and/ or anti-thyroglobulin antibodies in a patient with hypothyroidism make a diagnosis of Hashimoto thyroiditis. If the antibodies are positive in a hyperthyroid patient, the most likely diagnosis is autoimmune thyroid disease.

Radioactive Iodine Uptake: Because T_4 contains much iodine, the thyroid gland must pull a large amount of iodine out from the blood stream in order for the gland to make an appropriate amount of T_4. The thyroid has developed a very active mechanism for doing this. Therefore, this activity can be measured by having an individual swallow a small amount of iodine, which is radioactive. The radioactivity allows the doctor to track where the iodine molecules go. By measuring the amount of radioactivity that is taken up by the thyroid gland (radioactive iodine uptake, RAIU), doctors may determine whether the gland is functioning normally. A very high RAIU is seen in individuals whose thyroid gland is overactive (hyperthyroidism), while a low RAIU is seen when the thyroid gland is underactive (hypothyroidism). In addition to the radioactive iodine uptake, a thyroid scan may be obtained, which shows a picture of the thyroid.

When Is a Thyroid Gland Abnormal?

Diseases of the thyroid gland are very common, affecting millions of Americans. The most common diseases are an over- or under-active gland. These conditions are called hyperthyroidism (for example, Graves disease) and hypothyroidism. Sometimes the thyroid gland can become enlarged from over-activity (as in Graves disease) or from under-activity (as in hypothyroidism). An enlarged thyroid gland is often called a goiter. Sometimes an inflammation of the thyroid gland (Hashimoto disease) will cause enlargement of the gland. Patients may develop lumps or masses in their thyroid glands. They may appear gradually or very rapidly.

Patients who had radiation therapy to the head or neck as children for acne, adenoids, or other reasons are more prone to develop thyroid malignancy. A doctor should evaluate all thyroid lumps (nodules).

How Your Doctor Makes the Diagnosis

The diagnosis of a thyroid abnormality in function or a thyroid mass is made by taking a medical history and a physical examination. Specifically, your doctor will examine your neck and ask you to lift up your chin to make your thyroid gland more prominent. You may be asked to swallow during the examination, which helps to feel the thyroid and any mass in it. Other tests your doctor may order include:

- ultrasound examination of the neck and thyroid
- blood tests of thyroid function
- radioactive thyroid scan
- fine needle aspiration biopsy
- chest x-ray
- computed tomography (CT) or magnetic resonance image (MRI) scan

Fine Needle Aspiration

If a lump in your thyroid is diagnosed, your doctor may recommend a fine needle aspiration biopsy. This is a safe, relatively painless procedure. A hypodermic needle is passed into the lump, and samples of tissues are taken. Often several passes with the needle are required. There is little pain afterward, and very few complications from the procedure occur. This test gives the doctor more information on the nature of the lump in your thyroid gland and specifically will help to differentiate a benign from a malignant thyroid mass.

Treatment of Thyroid Disease

Abnormalities of thyroid function (hyper or hypothyroidism) are usually treated medically. If there is insufficient production of thyroid hormone, this may be given in a form of a thyroid hormone pill taken daily. Hyperthyroidism is treated mostly by medical means, but occasionally it may require the surgical removal of the thyroid gland.

If there is a lump of the thyroid or a diffused enlargement (goiter), your doctor will propose a treatment plan based on the examination and your test results. Most thyroid lumps are benign. Often they may be treated with thyroid hormone, and this is called suppression therapy.

The object of this treatment is to attempt shrinkage of the mass over time, usually three to six months. If the lump continues to grow during treatment when you are taking the medication, most doctors will recommend removal of the affected lump.

If the fine needle aspiration is reported as suspicious for, or suggestive of, cancer, then thyroid surgery is required.

Thyroid Surgery

Thyroid surgery is an operation to remove part or all of the thyroid gland. It is performed in the hospital, and general anesthesia is usually required. Usually the operation removes the lobe of the thyroid gland containing the lump and possibly the isthmus. A frozen section (an immediate microscopic reading) may or may not be used to determine if the rest of the thyroid gland should be removed. Sometimes, based on the result of the frozen section, the surgeon may decide to stop and remove no more thyroid tissue, or proceed to remove the entire thyroid gland, and/or other tissue in the neck. This is a decision usually made in the operating room by the surgeon, based on findings at the time of surgery. Your surgeon will discuss these options with you preoperatively.

After surgery, you may have a drain (a tiny piece of plastic tubing), which prevents fluid from building up in the wound. This is removed after the fluid accumulation is minimal. Most patients are discharged one to three days after surgery. Complications after thyroid surgery are rare. They include bleeding, a hoarse voice, difficulty swallowing, numbness of the skin on the neck, and low blood calcium. Most complications go away after a few weeks. Patients who have all of their thyroid gland removed have a higher risk of low blood calcium postoperatively.

Patients who have thyroid surgery may be required to take thyroid medication to replace thyroid hormones after surgery. Some patients may need to take calcium replacement if their blood calcium is low. This will depend on how much thyroid gland remains, and what was found during surgery. If you have any questions about thyroid surgery, ask your doctor and he or she will answer them in detail.

Additional Information

American Academy of Otolaryngology–Head and Neck Surgery
One Prince St.
Alexandria, VA 22314-3357
Phone: 703-836-4444
Website: http://www.entnet.org

American Thyroid Association
6066 Leesburg Pike, Suite 550
Falls Church, VA 22041
Toll-Free: 800-THYROID (849-7643)
Phone: 703-998-8890
Fax: 703-998-8893
Website: http://www.thyroid.org
E-mail: thyroid@thyroid.org

Chapter 23

Thyroiditis

Symptoms

What is thyroiditis?

Thyroiditis is a general term that refers to inflammation of the thyroid gland. Thyroiditis includes a group of individual disorders that all cause thyroidal inflammation and, as a result, cause many different clinical presentations. For example, Hashimoto thyroiditis is the most common cause of hypothyroidism in the United States. Postpartum thyroiditis, which causes transient thyrotoxicosis (high thyroid hormone levels in the blood) followed by transient hypothyroidism, is a common cause of thyroid problems after the delivery of a baby. Subacute thyroiditis is the major cause of pain in the thyroid. Thyroiditis can also be seen in patients taking the drugs interferon and amiodarone.

What are the clinical symptoms of thyroiditis?

There are no symptoms unique to thyroiditis. If the thyroiditis causes slow and chronic thyroid cell damage and destruction, leading to a fall in thyroid hormone levels in the blood, the symptoms would be those of hypothyroidism. Typical hypothyroid symptoms include fatigue, weight gain, constipation, dry skin, depression, and poor exercise tolerance. This would be the case in patients with Hashimoto thyroiditis. If the thyroiditis causes rapid thyroid cell damage and destruction, the

Reprinted with permission from The American Thyroid Association, Inc., © 2005. Online Patient Resources at www.thyroid.org.

thyroid hormone that is stored in the gland leaks out, increasing thyroid hormone levels in the blood, and produces symptoms of thyrotoxicosis, which are similar to hyperthyroidism. These symptoms often include anxiety, insomnia, palpitations (fast heart rate) fatigue, weight loss, and irritability. This is seen in patients with the toxic phase of subacute, painless, and postpartum thyroiditis. The symptoms of thyrotoxicosis and hyperthyroidism are identical, as elevated levels of thyroid hormone in the blood cause both conditions. Thyrotoxicosis is the term used with thyroiditis since the gland is not overactive. In subacute, painless and postpartum thyroiditis, the thyroid gland often becomes depleted of thyroid hormone as the course of inflammation continues, leading to a fall in thyroid hormone levels in the blood and symptoms of hypothyroidism. Pain in the thyroid can be seen in patients with subacute thyroiditis.

Causes

What causes thyroiditis?

Thyroiditis is caused by an attack on the thyroid, causing inflammation and damage to the thyroid cells. Antibodies that attack the thyroid cause most types of thyroiditis. As such, thyroiditis is often an autoimmune disease, like juvenile diabetes and rheumatoid arthritis. No one knows why certain people make thyroid antibodies, although this tends to run in families. Thyroiditis can also be caused by an infection, such as a virus or bacteria, which work in the same way as the antibodies to cause inflammation in the gland. Finally, drugs such as interferon and amiodarone, can also damage thyroid cells and cause thyroiditis.

What is the clinical course of thyroiditis?

The course of thyroiditis depends on the type of thyroiditis.

Hashimoto thyroiditis: Patients usually present with hypothyroidism, which is usually permanent.

Painless and postpartum thyroiditis: These disorders are similar and follow the same general clinical course of thyrotoxicosis followed by hypothyroidism. The only real difference between them is that postpartum thyroiditis occurs after the delivery of a baby while painless thyroiditis occurs in men and in women not related to a pregnancy. Not all patients demonstrate evidence of going through both phases; approximately one-third of patients will manifest both phases, while one-third of patients will have only a thyrotoxic or hypothyroid phase. The thyrotoxic phase lasts for 1–3 months and is associated with symptoms including anxiety, insomnia, palpitations (fast heart rate) fatigue, weight loss, and irritability. The hypothyroid phase typically occurs 1–3 months after the thyrotoxic phase and may last up to 9–12 months. Typical symptoms include fatigue, weight gain, constipation, dry skin, depression and poor exercise tolerance. Most patients (approximately 80%) will have a return of their thyroid function to normal within 12–18 months of the onset of symptoms.

Subacute thyroiditis: Subacute thyroiditis follows the same clinical course as painless and postpartum thyroiditis, with the exception of the symptoms of thyroidal pain. The thyroidal pain in patients with subacute thyroiditis usually follows the same time-frame of the thyrotoxic phase (1–3 months). However, not all patients with thyroidal pain necessarily have thyrotoxicosis. As noted with painless and postpartum thyroiditis, resolution of all thyroidal abnormalities after 12–18 months is seen in most patients (approximately 95%). Recurrence of subacute thyroiditis is rare.

Drug-induced and radiation thyroiditis: Both thyrotoxicosis and hypothyroidism may be seen in these disorders. The thyrotoxicosis is usually short-lived. Drug-induced hypothyroidism often resolves with the cessation of the drug, while the hypothyroidism related to radiation thyroiditis is usually permanent.

Acute or infectious thyroiditis: Symptoms range from thyroidal pain, systemic illness, painless enlargement of the thyroid, and hypothyroidism. The symptoms usually resolve once the infection resolves.

Types

What are the types of thyroiditis?

There are many types of thyroiditis, which are summarized in Table 23.1.

Treatment

How is thyroiditis treated?

Treatment depends on the type of thyroiditis and the clinical presentation.

Table 23.1. Types of Thyroiditis

TYPE	CAUSE	CLINICAL FEATURES	DIAGNOSIS (NOT ALL TESTS MAY BE NEEDED)	DURATION AND RESOLUTION
Hashimoto's thyroiditis	Anti-thyroid antibodies, autoimmune disease	Hypothyroidism, rare cases of transient thyrotoxicosis	Thyroid function tests, thyroid antibody tests	Hypothyroidism is usually permanent
Subacute thyroiditis (de Quervain's thyroiditis)	Possible viral cause	Painful thyroid, thyrotoxicosis followed by hypothyroidism	Thyroid function tests, sedimentation rate, radioactive iodine uptake	Resolves to normal thyroid function within 12-18 months, 5% possibility of permanent hypothyroidism.
Silent thyroiditis, Painless thyroiditis	Anti-thyroid antibodies, autoimmune disease	Thyrotoxicosis followed by hypothyroidism.	Thyroid function tests, thyroid antibody tests, radioactive iodine uptake	Resolves to normal thyroid function within 12-18 months, 20% possibility of permanent hypothyroidism.
Post partum thyroiditis	Anti-thyroid antibodies, autoimmune disease	Thyrotoxicosis followed by hypothyroidism.	Thyroid function tests, thyroid antibody tests, radioactive iodine uptake (contraindicated if the women is breast-feeding)	Resolves to normal thyroid function within 12-18 months, 20% possibility of permanent hypothyroidism
Drug induced	Drugs include: amiodarone, lithium, interferons, cytokines	Either thyrotoxicosis or hypothyroidism.	Thyroid function tests, thyroid antibody tests	Often continues as long as the drug is taken
Radiation induced	Follows treatment with radioactive iodine for hyperthyroidism or external beam radiation therapy for certain cancers.	Occasionally thyrotoxicosis, more frequently hypothyroidism.	Thyroid function tests	Thyrotoxicosis is transient, hypothyroidism is usually permanent
Acute thyroiditis, Suppurative thyroiditis	Bacteria mainly, but any infectious organism	Occasionally painful thyroid, generalized illness, occasional mild hypothyroidism	Thyroid function tests, radioactive iodine uptake, fine needle aspiration biopsy	Resolves after treatment of infectious cause, may cause severe illness

Thyrotoxicosis: Beta blockers to decrease palpitations and reduce shakes and tremors may be helpful. As symptoms improve, the medication is tapered off since the thyrotoxic phase is transient. Antithyroid medications are not used for the thyrotoxic phase of thyroiditis of any kind since the thyroid is not overactive.

Hypothyroidism: Treatment is initiated with thyroid hormone replacement for hypothyroidism due to Hashimoto thyroiditis. In patients who are symptomatic with the hypothyroid phase of subacute, painless, and postpartum thyroiditis, thyroid hormone therapy is also indicated. If the hypothyroidism in these latter disorders is mild and the patient has few, if any, symptoms, then no therapy may be necessary. If thyroid hormone therapy is begun in patients with subacute, painless, and postpartum thyroiditis, treatment should be continued for approximately 6–12 months and then tapered to see if thyroid hormone is required permanently.

Thyroidal pain: The pain associated with subacute thyroiditis usually can be managed with mild anti-inflammatory medications such as aspirin or ibuprofen. Occasionally, the pain can be severe and require steroid therapy with prednisone.

Chapter 24

Hashimoto Thyroiditis

Hashimoto thyroiditis is a type of autoimmune thyroid disease in which the immune system attacks and destroys the thyroid gland. The thyroid helps set the rate of metabolism, which is the rate at which the body uses energy. Hashimoto stops the gland from making enough thyroid hormones for the body to work the way it should. It is the most common thyroid disease in the U.S.

An autoimmune disease occurs when the body's immune system becomes misdirected and attacks the organs, cells, or tissues that it was designed to protect. About 75% of autoimmune diseases occur in women, most often during their childbearing years.

There is some evidence that Hashimoto thyroiditis can have a hereditary link. If autoimmune diseases in general run in your family, you are at a higher risk of developing one yourself.

Symptoms of Hashimoto Thyroiditis

Some patients with Hashimoto thyroiditis may have no symptoms. However, the common symptoms are fatigue, depression, sensitivity to cold, weight gain, forgetfulness, muscle weakness, puffy face, dry skin and hair, constipation, muscle cramps, and increased menstrual flow. Some patients have major swelling of the thyroid gland in the front of the neck called goiter.

National Women's Health Information Center, January 2006.

Diagnosis

Your doctor will perform a simple blood test that will be able to tell if your body has the right amount of thyroid hormones. This test measures the TSH (thyroid stimulating hormone) to find out if the levels are in the normal range. The range is set by your doctor and should be discussed with you. Work with your doctor to figure out what level is right for you. There are other available tests that your doctor may choose to do if need be, such as a blood test to measure the level of active thyroid hormone or Free T_4 and a scan (picture) to look at the thyroid.

Treatment

Hypothyroidism caused by Hashimoto thyroiditis is treated with thyroid hormone replacement. A small pill taken once a day should be able to keep the thyroid hormone levels normal. This medicine will, in most cases, need to be taken for the rest of the patient's life. When trying to figure out the amount of hormone you need, you may have to return to your doctor several times for blood tests to guide adjustments in the medicine dose. It is important that the dose be right for you. A yearly visit to your doctor will help keep your levels normal and help you stay healthy overall. Be aware of the symptoms. If you note any changes or the return of symptoms, return to your doctor to see if you need to have your medicine dosage adjusted.

What would happen without medication to regulate my thyroid function?

If left untreated, hypothyroidism can cause further problems, including changes in menstrual cycles, prevention of ovulation, and an increased risk of miscarriage. Symptoms such as fatigue, depression, and constipation may progress, and there can be other serious consequences, including heart failure. It is also important to know that too much thyroid replacement hormone can mimic the symptoms of hyperthyroidism. This is a condition that happens when there is too much thyroid hormone. These symptoms include insomnia, irritability, weight loss without dieting, heat sensitivity, increased perspiration, thinning of your skin, fine or brittle hair, muscular weakness, eye changes, lighter menstrual flow, rapid heart beat, and shaky hands.

What happens if I have this disease and I get pregnant?

It is important to get checked out by your doctor more often if you are pregnant. Inadequately treated thyroid problems can affect a growing baby, and the thyroid replacement needs of pregnant women often change. A doctor can help you figure out your changing medicine needs.

Additional Information

American Thyroid Association
6066 Leesburg Pike, Suite 550
Falls Church, VA 22041
Toll-Free: 800-THYROID (849-7643)
Phone: 703-998-8890
Fax: 703-998-8893
Website: http://www.thyroid.org
E-mail: thyroid@thyroid.org

Thyroid Foundation of America
One Longfellow Place, Suite 1518
Boston, MA 02114
Toll-Free: 800-832-8321
Fax: 617-534-1515
Website: http://www.tsh.org
E-mail: info@allthyroid.org

Chapter 25

Hypothyroidism

Primary hypothyroidism is a condition of decreased hormone production by the thyroid gland.

Causes, Incidence, and Risk Factors

The thyroid gland is an important organ that regulates metabolism. It is located in the front of the neck just below the voice box (larynx). The thyroid gland secretes two forms of thyroid hormone—thyroxine (T_4) and triiodothyronine (T_3). The secretion of T_3 and T_4 by the thyroid is controlled by a feedback system involving the pituitary gland, a small organ at the base of the brain, and the hypothalamus, a structure in the brain.

Hypothyroidism caused by the inability of the thyroid gland to make T_3 and T_4 is called primary hypothyroidism. Worldwide, the most common cause of primary hypothyroidism is deficiency of the element iodine. In the U.S., the most common cause is destruction of the thyroid gland by the immune system, a condition called Hashimoto thyroiditis.

Other causes of primary hypothyroidism include surgical removal of part or all of the thyroid gland, radioactive iodine used for treatment of hyperthyroidism (overactive thyroid), radiation exposure to the neck, special x-ray dyes, and certain drugs such as lithium. Approximately 5–10% of women develop hypothyroidism after pregnancy (often referred to as postpartum thyroiditis). Some cases of hypothyroidism may be caused by a lack of enzymes that convert T_3 and T_4 for use in the body. In other cases, the cause of hypothyroidism is unknown.

Since the thyroid gland is regulated by the pituitary gland and hypothalamus, disorders of these organs can cause the thyroid gland to produce too little thyroid hormone as well. This condition is called secondary hypothyroidism.

Primary hypothyroidism affects the whole body and may cause a variety of symptoms. The body's normal rate of functioning slows, causing mental and physical sluggishness. Symptoms may vary from mild to severe. The most severe form is called myxedema coma and is a medical emergency. Risk factors for hypothyroidism include age (older than age 50), female gender, obesity, thyroid surgery, and x-ray or radiation treatments to the neck.

Symptoms

Early Symptoms

- weakness
- fatigue
- cold intolerance
- constipation
- weight gain
- depression
- muscle or joint pain
- thin, brittle fingernails
- thin, brittle hair
- paleness

Late Symptoms

- slow speech
- dry flaky skin
- thickening of the skin
- puffy face, hands, and feet
- decreased sense of taste and smell
- thinning of eyebrows
- hoarseness
- menstrual disorders

Signs and Tests

Physical examination may reveal a smaller than normal gland, though sometimes the gland is normal in size or even enlarged (goiter). Other physical findings include pale, yellow, and dry skin; thin, brittle hair; loss of the edges of the eyebrows; coarse facial features; firm swelling of the arms and legs; and slow muscle relaxation when reflexes are tested. Vital signs may reveal a slow heart rate, low blood pressure, and low temperature. A chest x-ray sometimes reveals an enlarged heart.

Laboratory tests to determine thyroid function include:

- free T_4 test (low)
- total T_3 or free T_3 (low)
- serum TSH (high)

Additional laboratory abnormalities may include:

- increased cholesterol levels
- increased liver enzymes
- increased serum prolactin
- low serum sodium
- a complete blood count (CBC) shows anemia

Treatment

The purpose of treatment is to replace the deficient thyroid hormone. Levothyroxine (T_4) is the most commonly used medication, but a preparation of T_3 is also available. Most people feel their best when TSH is brought into the 1 to 2 millicurie international unit per milliliter (mc IU/mL) range. People get the lowest dose that is effective in relieving symptoms and normalizing blood tests.

Life-long therapy is needed. Relapses will occur if therapy is interrupted. Medication must be continued even when symptoms go away.

After replacement therapy has begun, report any symptoms of increased thyroid activity (hyperthyroidism), such as restlessness, rapid weight loss, heat intolerance, and sweating.

Myxedema coma is treated by intravenous thyroid replacement and steroid therapy. Supportive therapy (oxygen, assisted ventilation, and fluid replacement) and intensive care nursing may be indicated.

Expectations (Prognosis)

With early treatment, the condition can be completely controlled. However, relapses will occur if the medication is not continued. Myxedema coma can result in death.

Complications

Myxedema coma, the most severe form of hypothyroidism, is rare. It may be caused by an infection, illness, exposure to cold, or certain medications. Symptoms and signs of myxedema coma include:

- unresponsiveness
- decreased breathing
- low blood pressure
- low blood sugar
- below-normal temperature

Other complications include:

- heart disease
- increased risk of infection
- infertility
- miscarriage
- pituitary tumors

Calling Your Health Care Provider

Call your health care provider if signs or symptoms of hypothyroidism or myxedema are present.

Call your health care provider if restlessness, rapid weight loss, heat intolerance, rapid heart rate, excessive sweating, or symptoms of hyperthyroidism occur after beginning thyroid replacement.

Prevention

Primary hypothyroidism is preventable by supplemental iodine in areas where iodine in the food supply is low. Otherwise, the condition is not preventable. Awareness of risk may allow early diagnosis and treatment. Some experts advocate screening TSH testing in certain high-risk groups (for example, women older than 50 years).

Chapter 26

Congenital Hypothyroidism

Babies who are born with underactive thyroid function have a disorder known as congenital hypothyroidism. The usual cause of this condition is the failure of the thyroid gland to develop during pregnancy. At birth the infants look normal and then slowly over a period of weeks the clinical features of hypothyroidism appear. Because there are no conspicuous signs or symptoms, the diagnosis of congenital hypothyroidism is seldom made at birth by the examining physician. If the condition goes unrecognized, which is usually the case, then signs and symptoms such as constipation, dry skin, hoarse cry, large tongue, swelling around the eyes, failure to suckle well, and prolonged periods of sleep will appear within a few weeks.

Accompanying these overt clinical changes in the infant is the less obvious damage to the brain resulting in mental retardation. Although treatment at this juncture will reverse the clinical signs and symptoms, the damage to the baby's brain is irreversible. The longer the disorder goes unrecognized (and thus untreated) the greater the insult to the brain.

Fortunately, in recent years the burden of diagnosing congenital hypothyroidism in the newborn period has been shifted from the physician to the laboratory. In the early nineteen-seventies a French-Canadian physician, Jean Dussault, found a way to measure thyroid hormone (T_4) in a tiny amount of dried blood in filter paper. The filter paper was the same type that had been used for years to collect blood from newborns before discharge from the hospital. The dried blood specimens were sent to public health laboratories where tests were done for phenylketonuria (PKU) and other metabolic diseases. Thus, this pre-existing network for collecting newborn blood specimens provided the framework upon which the same public health laboratories could not only screen for metabolic diseases but could screen for congenital hypothyroidism as well. It was not long before most industrialized nations had established newborn screening programs to identify infants born with hypothyroidism. Without question, the screening process has revolutionized the diagnosis and early treatment of congenital hypothyroidism, and thereby, prevented countless number of children from becoming mentally retarded.

The Screening Process

Every child born in North America has blood collected on filter paper by heel stick before discharge from the hospital or birthing center. The dried blood specimens are forwarded to a central laboratory where a one-eighth inch paper blood spot is tested for the amount of T_4 and/ or thyroid stimulating hormone (TSH). A low T_4 and elevated TSH indicate that an infant lacks normal thyroid function. Although an elevated TSH is a more sensitive and specific marker of hypothyroidism, the majority of North American screening programs use T_4 as the initial test and confirm the diagnosis with the measurement of TSH.

Incidence and Types

Approximately one baby with congenital hypothyroidism is born out of 3,500 births. However, it is estimated that 15–20% of hypothyroid infants have a temporary form of the disorder and will only require treatment for a limited number of years. When there is a question of permanence of the disorder, the physician should discontinue treatment after three years of age and repeat the blood tests for TSH and T_4 in a few weeks to be sure they are now normal.

There are three different types of thyroid abnormalities that are associated with congenital hypothyroidism. Approximately 40% of infants have underdeveloped or absent thyroid glands; 40% have thyroid glands that are in the wrong place, such as under the tongue or at the far side of the neck; and the remaining 20% are unable to manufacture thyroid hormone because of defects within the thyroid gland. The latter condition is usually familial in nature.

216

Low T_4 Values

Only a tiny number of infants with low T_4 levels actually have congenital hypothyroidism. More than 90% of low T_4 values (not accompanied by elevated TSH levels) in neonates are associated with other conditions such as prematurity, low birth weight, illness, a deficiency in the protein that carries T_4 to various body tissues, or pituitary failure. The latter is a rare disorder in which the pituitary gland is unable to secrete TSH. This condition should be considered in an infant whose growth rate falls off its expected growth curve and has a low T_4 and a low or normal TSH.

Treatment

The infant with suspected hypothyroidism should be seen without delay by a physician, preferably by a pediatric endocrinologist. Blood should be obtained to confirm the diagnosis, and treatment with thyroxine should begin before the confirmatory T_4 and TSH values are available. Measurements of T_4 and TSH should be made two and four weeks after starting the thyroxine, two weeks after a dosage change, and every one to two months during the first year of life. Optimal intellectual outcome depends on maintaining the circulating level of T_4 in the upper half of the normal range (10–16 micrograms per deciliter [mcg/dl]) during the first year of life.

If the T_4 value is not above 10 mcg/dl and the TSH is below 20 milliunits per liter (mU/l) within two to four weeks after starting therapy, the physician should consider the possibility that the baby has not been receiving the medication or that there is a problem with absorption of T_4 (soy-based formula or iron supplement will interfere with absorption of T_4).

Outcome

After recovering from the emotional shock of learning that their baby has congenital hypothyroidism, the first question invariably asked by the parents is, "Will our baby be normal?" Many parents confuse congenital hypothyroidism with cretinism and harbor the vision of their child becoming dwarfed and mentally retarded.

It is gratifying to be able to reassure parents that their children will not be deficient in brain power and that the children are not cretins. Severe iodine deficiency, the cause of cretinism in many parts of the world, has not been a problem in the United States since the introduction of iodized salt in the 1920s. Unfortunately, mild degrees of iodine deficiency are now beginning to reappear in the United States.

When treatment is initiated before the appearance of clinical signs and symptoms of hypothyroidism, the intellectual outcome of the child is the same as that of children with normal thyroid function. This was shown by a group of New England hypothyroid children whose results in intelligence tests and in school performance were the same as those of their unaffected classmates.

It is prudent to remember that as children grow older they have a tendency to neglect their medication. This is especially true for adolescents. A recent study in teenagers found a significant decline in intelligence quotient (IQ) that returned to normal after the appropriate blood levels of T_4 were restored. Consider non-compliance with medication when school performance undergoes a change for the worse in your adolescent child who is on treatment for hypothyroidism.

Conclusion

There are few instances in the practice of medicine where the health and welfare of future generations can be positively affected; early treatment of congenital hypothyroidism through newborn screening is one of those instances.

Chapter 27

Hyperthyroidism

Alternative names: Thyrotoxicosis; overactive thyroid

Definition: Hyperthyroidism is a condition caused by an overactive thyroid gland. The gland makes too much T_4 and T_3 hormones. Hormones are substances that affect and control many important functions in the body.

Causes, Incidence, and Risk Factors

The thyroid gland is located in the neck. It produces several hormones which control the way that every cell in the body uses energy (metabolism). The thyroid is part of the endocrine system. Hyperthyroidism or thyrotoxicosis occurs when the thyroid releases too many of its hormones over a short (acute) or long (chronic) period of time. Many diseases and conditions can cause this problem, including:

- Graves disease
- non-cancerous growths of the thyroid gland or pituitary gland
- tumors of the testes or ovaries
- inflammation (irritation and swelling) of the thyroid due to viral infections or other causes

- ingestion (taking in through the mouth, such as in eating) of large amounts of thyroid hormone
- ingestion of excessive iodine

Graves disease accounts for 85% of all cases of hyperthyroidism.

Symptoms

- weight loss
- increased appetite
- nervousness
- restlessness
- heat intolerance
- increased sweating
- fatigue
- frequent bowel movements
- menstrual irregularities in women
- goiter (visibly enlarged thyroid) may be present

Additional symptoms that may be associated with this disease:

- weakness
- sleeping difficulty
- clammy skin
- skin blushing or flushing
- bounding pulse
- nausea and vomiting
- lack of menstruation
- itching - overall
- heartbeat sensations
- hand tremor
- hair loss
- diarrhea
- breast development in men
- high blood pressure
- protruding eyes (exophthalmos)

Signs and Tests

Physical examination may reveal thyroid enlargement or goiter. Vital signs (temperature, pulse, rate of breathing, blood pressure) show increased heart rate. Systolic blood pressure (the first number in a blood pressure reading) may be high.

Laboratory tests that evaluate thyroid function:

- serum TSH is usually low
- T_3 and free T_4 are usually high

This disease may also alter the results of the following tests:

- vitamin B_{12}
- thyroid-stimulating immunoglobulins (TSI)
- triglycerides
- thyroid hormone-binding ratio (RT3U)
- radioactive iodine uptake
- glucose test
- cholesterol test
- antithyroglobulin antibody

Treatment

Treatment varies depending on the cause of the condition and the severity of symptoms. Hyperthyroidism is usually treated with anti-thyroid medications, radioactive iodine (which destroys the thyroid and stops the excess production of hormones), or surgery to remove the thyroid.

If the thyroid must be removed with radiation or surgery, replacement thyroid hormones must be taken for the rest of the person's life.

Beta-blockers like propranolol are used to treat some of the symptoms including rapid heart rate, sweating, and anxiety until the hyperthyroidism can be controlled.

Expectations (Prognosis)

Hyperthyroidism caused by Graves disease is usually progressive and has many associated complications, some of which are severe and affect quality of life. These include complications caused by treatment such as use of radioactive iodine, surgery, and medications to replace thyroid hormones. However, hyperthyroidism is generally treatable and rarely fatal.

Complications

- Heart-related complications include rapid heart rate, congestive heart failure, and atrial fibrillation.

- Thyroid crisis or storm is an acute worsening of the symptoms of hyperthyroidism that may occur with infection or stress. Fever, decreased mental alertness, and abdominal pain may occur, and immediate hospitalization is needed.

- Hyperthyroidism increases the risk for osteoporosis.

- There may be complications related to surgery, including visible scarring of the neck, hoarseness due to nerve damage to the voice box, and a low calcium level because of damage to the parathyroid glands.

- Complications may be related to replacement of thyroid hormones. If too little hormone is given, symptoms of underactive thyroid can occur including fatigue, increased cholesterol levels, mild weight gain, depression, and slowing of mental and physical activity. If too much hormone is given, the symptoms of hyperthyroidism will come back.

Calling Your Health Care Provider

Call your health care provider if you have symptoms which could be caused by excessive thyroid hormone production. If the symptoms are associated with a rapid, irregular heartbeat, dizziness, or change in consciousness, go to the emergency room or call the local emergency number (such as 911).

Call your health care provider if treatment for hyperthyroidism induces symptoms of under-active thyroid, including mental and physical sluggishness, weight gain, and depression.

Prevention

There are no general prevention measures to prevent hyperthyroidism.

Chapter 28

Graves Disease

Graves disease, a type of hyperthyroidism, is caused by a generalized overactivity of the entire thyroid gland. It is named for Robert Graves, an Irish physician, who was the first to describe this form of hyperthyroidism about 150 years ago.

Symptoms of Graves Disease

Hyperthyroidism

The hyperthyroid symptoms of Graves disease are often the same as those caused by other types of hyperthyroidism.

Eye Disease

Graves disease is the only kind of hyperthyroidism that has inflammation of the eyes, swelling of the tissues around the eyes, and bulging of the eyes (called Graves ophthalmopathy). The cause of these problems is unknown. Although many patients with Graves disease have redness and irritation of the eyes at some time, less than 1% ever develop enough inflammation of the eye tissues to cause serious or permanent trouble. Patients who have severe eye symptoms may benefit from visiting an eye doctor (an ophthalmologist).

Eye symptoms generally begin about six months before or after the diagnosis of Graves disease has been made. Seldom do eye problems

Reprinted with permission from The American Thyroid Association, Inc., © 2005 Online Patient Resources at www.thyroid.org.

occur long after the disease has been treated. In some patients with eye symptoms, hyperthyroidism never develops. The severity of the eye problems is not related to the severity of the hyperthyroidism. Early signs of trouble might be red or inflamed eyes or a bulging of the eyes due to inflammation of the tissues behind the eyeball. Diminished or double vision are rare problems that usually occur later. We do not know why, but problems with the eyes occur much more often in people with Graves disease who smoke cigarettes than in those who don't smoke.

Skin Disease

Rarely, patients with Graves disease develop a lumpy reddish thickening of the skin in front of the shins known as pretibial myxedema. This skin condition is usually painless and is not serious. Like the eye trouble of Graves disease, the skin problem does not necessarily begin precisely when the hyperthyroidism starts. Its severity is not related to the level of thyroid hormone. We don't know why this problem is usually limited to the lower leg or why so few people have it.

Causes of Graves Disease

Graves disease is triggered by some process in the body's immune system, which normally protects us from foreign invaders such as bacteria and viruses. The immune system destroys foreign invaders with substances called antibodies produced by blood cells known as lymphocytes. Many people inherit an immune system that can cause problems. Their lymphocytes make antibodies against their own tissues that stimulate or damage them. In Graves disease, antibodies bind to the surface of thyroid cells and stimulate those cells to overproduce thyroid hormones. This results in an overactive thyroid. Physicians have long suspected that severe emotional stress, such as the death of a loved one, can set off Graves disease in some patients. Dr. Graves himself commented on stressful events in his patients' lives that came several months before the development of hyperthyroidism. However, many patients who develop Graves disease report no stress in their lives.

Diagnosis of Graves Disease

The diagnosis of hyperthyroidism is made on the basis of findings during a physical exam and confirmed by laboratory tests that measure the amount of thyroid hormone (thyroxine, or T_4, and triiodothyronine, or T_3) and thyroid-stimulating hormone (TSH) in your blood. Sometimes your doctor may want you to have a radioactive image, or scan, of the thyroid to see whether the entire thyroid gland is overactive. Your doctor may also wish to do a blood test to confirm the presence of thyroid-stimulating antibodies (TSAb) that cause Graves disease, but this test is not usually necessary.

Clues that your hyperthyroidism is caused by Graves disease are the presence of Graves eye disease, an enlarged thyroid, and a history of other family members with thyroid problems. Some relatives may have had hyperthyroidism or an underactive thyroid; others may have acquired gray hair prematurely (beginning in their 20s). Similarly, there may be a history of related immune problems in the family, including juvenile diabetes, pernicious anemia (due to lack of vitamin B_{12}), or painless white patches on the skin known as vitiligo.

Treatment of Graves Disease

Treatment includes antithyroid drugs (methimazole [Tapazole®]) or propylthiouracil [PTU]), radioiodine, and surgery. Although each treatment has its advantages and disadvantages, most patients will find one that is just right for them. Hyperthyroidism due to Graves disease is, in general, easily controlled and safely treated, and treatment is almost always successful.

What will be the outcome of treatment?

No matter how your hyperthyroidism is controlled, you probably will have hypothyroidism someday. Hyperthyroidism tends to lead towards hypothyroidism, probably because of low-grade inflammation within your thyroid gland. Hypothyroidism will occur sooner if your thyroid has been damaged by radioactive iodine or removed in an operation. Even if you are treated with antithyroid drugs alone, hypothyroidism still can occur.

Because of this natural tendency to progress toward hypothyroidism sometime after you have been hyperthyroid, every patient who has ever had hyperthyroidism due to Graves disease should have blood tests at least once a year to measure thyroid function. Low thyroid hormone levels cause your pituitary gland to produce increased amounts of thyroid-stimulating hormone (TSH). A high TSH blood level is the most sensitive indicator of hypothyroidism, and so your annual thyroid evaluation should always include a TSH test. When hypothyroidism occurs, a thyroid hormone tablet taken once a day can treat it simply and safely.

Are other family members at risk?

Because Graves disease is an inherited condition, examinations of the members of your family may reveal other individuals with thyroid problems.

Additional Information

American Thyroid Association
6066 Leesburg Pike, Suite 550
Falls Church, VA 22041
Phone: 703-998-8890
Fax: 703-998-8893
Website: http://www.thyroid.org
E-mail: admin@thyroid.org

Chapter 29

Thyroid Nodule

What is a thyroid nodule?

The thyroid gland is located in the lower front of the neck, below the larynx (Adam's apple) and above the collarbone. A thyroid nodule is a lump in or on the thyroid gland. Thyroid nodules are common and detected in about 6.4% of women and 1.5% of men; they are less common in younger patients and occur 10 times as often in older individuals, but are usually not diagnosed. Sometimes several nodules will develop in the same person. Any time a lump is discovered in thyroid tissue, the possibility of malignancy (cancer) must be considered. Fortunately, the vast majority of thyroid nodules are benign (not cancerous).

Many patients with thyroid nodules have no symptoms whatsoever, and are found by chance to have a lump in the thyroid gland on a routine physical exam or an imaging study of the neck done for unrelated reasons (computed tomography (CT) or magnetic resonance imaging (MRI) scan of spine or chest, carotid ultrasound, etc.) However, a minority of patients may become aware of a gradually enlarging lump in the front portion of the neck, and/or may experience a vague pressure sensation or discomfort when swallowing. Obviously, finding a lump in the neck should be brought to the attention of your physician, even in the absence of symptoms.

Nodules can be caused by a simple overgrowth of normal thyroid tissue, fluid-filled cysts, inflammation (thyroiditis), or a tumor (either benign or cancerous). Most nodules were surgically removed until the 1980s. In retrospect, this approach led to many unnecessary operations, since fewer than 10% of the removed nodules proved to be cancer. Most removed nodules could have simply been observed or treated medically.

It is not usually possible for a physician to determine whether a thyroid nodule is cancerous on the basis of a physical examination or blood tests. Endocrinologists rely heavily on three specialized tests for help in deciding which nodules should be treated surgically:

- thyroid fine needle biopsy
- thyroid scan
- thyroid ultrasonography

What is a thyroid needle biopsy?

A thyroid fine needle biopsy is a simple procedure that can be performed in the physician's office. Many physicians numb the skin over the nodule prior to the biopsy, but it is not necessary to be put to sleep, and patients can usually return to work or home afterward with no ill effects. This test provides specific information about a particular patient's nodule, information that no other test can offer short of surgery. Although the test is not perfect, a thyroid needle biopsy will provide sufficient information on which to base a treatment decision more than 75% of the time, eliminating the need for additional diagnostic studies.

Use of fine needle biopsy has drastically reduced the number of patients who have undergone unnecessary operations for benign nodules. However, about 10–20% of biopsy specimens are interpreted as inconclusive or inadequate, that is, the pathologist cannot be certain whether the nodule is cancerous or benign. This situation is particularly common with cystic (fluid-filled) nodules, which contain very few thyroid cells to examine, and with those nodules composed of a particular cell type called follicular. In such cases, a physician who is experienced with thyroid disease can use other criteria to make a decision about whether or not to operate. The fine needle biopsy can be repeated in those patients whose initial attempt failed to yield enough material to make a diagnosis. Many physicians use thyroid ultrasonography to guide the needle's placement.

What is a thyroid scan?

A thyroid scan is a picture of the thyroid gland taken after a small dose of a radioactive isotope, normally concentrated by thyroid cells, has been injected or swallowed. The scan tells whether the nodule is hyperfunctioning (a hot nodule), or taking up more radioactivity than normal thyroid tissue does, taking up the same amount as normal tissue (a warm nodule), or taking up less (a cold nodule). Because cancer is rarely found in hot nodules, a scan showing a hot nodule eliminates the need for fine needle biopsy. If a hot nodule causes hyperthyroidism, it can be treated with radioiodine or surgery.

Fortunately, the vast majority (90–95%) of thyroid nodules are benign. Unfortunately, thyroid scans show that most thyroid nodules, both benign and malignant, are cold or nonfunctioning. Therefore, although almost all thyroid cancers are nonfunctional on scan, the majority of nonfunctional nodules are benign. For this reason, thyroid scans are of relatively little value in most patients unless hyperthyroidism exists along with the nodule.

What is thyroid ultrasonography?

Thyroid ultrasonography is a procedure for obtaining pictures of the thyroid gland by using high frequency sound waves that pass through the skin, bounce off the inner structures of the neck, and are converted into a live image by a computer. It can visualize nodules as small as 2 to 3 millimeters (mm). Ultrasound studies were first used to distinguish thyroid cysts (fluid-filled nodules) from solid nodules. Cysts are usually benign, and solid nodules are potentially cancerous. Most nodules, however, have both solid and cystic components, and very few purely cystic nodules occur. Therefore, ultrasonography alone is rarely able to distinguish between a benign (non-cancerous) nodule and a malignant (cancerous) one.

A more important use of thyroid ultrasonography is in guiding the placement of a biopsy needle to decrease the frequency of inadequate specimens. Such guidance allows the biopsy sample to be obtained from the solid portion of those nodules that are both solid and cystic, and it avoids getting a specimen from the surrounding normal thyroid tissue if the nodule is small.

Even when a thyroid biopsy sample is reported as benign, the size of the nodule should be monitored. A thyroid ultrasound examination provides an objective and precise method for detection of a change in the size of the nodule. A nodule with a benign biopsy that is stable or decreasing in size is unlikely to be malignant or require surgical treatment.

How are thyroid nodules treated?

Your endocrinologist will use the mentioned tests to arrive at a recommendation for optimal management of your nodule. Most patients who appear to have benign nodules require no specific treatment, and can simply be followed expectantly. Some physicians prescribe levothyroxine with hopes of preventing nodule growth or reducing the size of cold nodules, while radioiodine may be used to treat hot nodules.

If cancer is suspected, surgical treatment will be recommended. The primary goal of therapy is to remove all thyroid nodules that are cancerous (and, if malignancy is confirmed, remove the rest of the thyroid gland along with any abnormal lymph glands). If surgery is not recommended, it is important to have regular follow-up of the nodule by a physician experienced in such an evaluation.

Additional Information

American Association of Clinical Endocrinologists (AACE)
245 Riverside Ave., Suite 200
Jacksonville, FL 32202
Phone: 904-353-7878
Fax: 904-353-8185
Website: http://www.aace.com
E-mail: info@aace.com

The AACE also offers an interactive thyroid health awareness tool and other resources for patients and physicians on their Thyroid Awareness website at http://www.thyroidawareness.com.

Chapter 30

Thyroid Cancer

Thyroid cancer is a disease in which cancer (malignant) cells are found in the tissues of the thyroid gland. The thyroid gland is at the base of the throat. It has two lobes, one on the right side and one on the left. The thyroid gland makes important hormones that help the body function normally. Certain factors may increase the risk of developing thyroid cancer.

* Thyroid cancer occurs more often in people between the ages of 25 and 65 years.

* People who have been exposed to radiation or received radiation treatments to the head and neck during infancy or childhood have a greater chance of developing thyroid cancer. The cancer may occur as early as five years after exposure or may occur twenty or more years later.

* People who have had goiter (enlarged thyroid) or a family history of thyroid disease have an increased risk of developing thyroid cancer.

* Thyroid cancer is more common in women than in men.

* Asian people have an increased risk of developing thyroid cancer.

PDQ® Cancer Information Summary. National Cancer Institute, Bethesda, MD. Thyroid Cancer (PDQ®) Treatment–Patient. Updated 07/2005. Available at http://cancer.gov. Accessed 02/07/2007.

A doctor should be seen if there is a lump or swelling in the front of the neck or in other parts of the neck. If there are symptoms, a doctor will feel the patient's thyroid and check for lumps in the neck. The doctor may order blood tests and special scans to see whether a lump in the thyroid is making too many hormones. The doctor may want to take a small amount of tissue from the thyroid. This is called a biopsy. To do this, a small needle is inserted into the thyroid at the base of the throat and some tissue is drawn out. The tissue is then looked at under a microscope to see whether it contains cancer.

There are four main types of thyroid cancer (based on how the cancer cells look under a microscope):

- papillary
- follicular
- medullary
- anaplastic

Some types of thyroid cancer grow faster than others. The chance of recovery (prognosis) depends on the type of thyroid cancer, whether it is in the thyroid only or has spread to other parts of the body (stage), and the patient's age and overall health. The prognosis is better for patients younger than forty years who have cancer that has not spread beyond the thyroid.

The genes in our cells carry the hereditary information from our parents. An abnormal gene has been found in patients with some forms of thyroid cancer. If medullary thyroid cancer is found, the patient may have been born with a certain abnormal gene which may have led to the cancer. Family members may have also inherited this abnormal gene. Tests have been developed to determine who has the genetic defect long before any cancer appears. It is important that the patient and his or her family members (children, grandchildren, parents, brothers, sisters, nieces, and nephews) see a doctor about tests that will show if the abnormal gene is present. These tests are confidential and can help the doctor help patients. Family members, including young children, who don't have cancer, but do have this abnormal gene, may reduce the chance of developing medullary thyroid cancer by having surgery to safely remove the thyroid gland (thyroidectomy).

Stage Explanation

Once thyroid cancer is found (diagnosed), more tests will be done to find out if cancer cells have spread to other parts of the body. This is called staging. A doctor needs to know the stage of the disease to plan treatment.

Papillary and Follicular Thyroid Cancer

Stage I

- In patients younger than 45 years, cancer may have spread within the neck or upper chest and/or to nearby lymph nodes but not to other parts of the body.

- In patients aged 45 years and older, the tumor is two centimeters (about ¾ inch) or smaller and in the thyroid only.

Stage II

- In patients younger than 45 years, the cancer has spread to distant parts of the body, such as the lung or bone, and may have spread to nearby lymph nodes.

- In patients aged 45 years and older, the tumor is larger than two centimeters but not larger than four centimeters (between ¾ and 1½ inches) in the thyroid only.

Stage III

The cancer is found in patients aged 45 years or older. The tumor either:

- is larger than four centimeters; or
- may be any size and has spread just outside the thyroid and/or to lymph nodes in the neck.

Stage IVA

The cancer is found in patients aged 45 years or older. The tumor may be any size and has spread within the neck and/or to lymph nodes in the neck or upper chest.

Stage IVB

The cancer is found in patients aged 45 years or older. The tumor may be any size and has spread to neck tissues near the backbone or around blood vessels in the neck or upper chest. Cancer may have spread to lymph nodes.

Stage IVC

The cancer has spread to other parts of the body, such as the lung or bone, and may have spread to nearby lymph nodes.

Medullary Thyroid Cancer

Stage 0

No tumor is found in the thyroid, but the cancer is detected by screening tests. Stage 0 is also called carcinoma in situ.

Stage I

The tumor is two centimeters or smaller and in the thyroid only.

Stage II

The tumor is larger than two centimeters but not larger than four centimeters and is in the thyroid only.

Stage III

The tumor either:

- is larger than four centimeters; or
- may be any size and has spread just outside the thyroid and/or to lymph nodes in the neck.

Stage IVA

The tumor may be any size and has spread within the neck and/or to lymph nodes in the neck or upper chest.

Stage IVB

The tumor may be any size and has spread to neck tissues near the backbone or around blood vessels in the neck or upper chest. Cancer may have spread to lymph nodes.

Stage IVC

Cancer has spread to other parts of the body, such as the lung or bone, and may have spread to nearby lymph nodes.

Anaplastic Thyroid Cancer

Anaplastic thyroid cancer is considered to be stage IV thyroid cancer. It grows quickly and has usually spread within the neck when it is found. Anaplastic thyroid cancer develops most often in older people.

Recurrent Thyroid Cancer

Recurrent disease means that the cancer has come back (recurred) after it has been treated. It may come back in the thyroid or in other parts of the body.

Treatment Option Overview

There are treatments for all patients with thyroid cancer. Four types of treatment are used:

- surgery (taking out the cancer)
- radiation therapy (using high-dose x-rays or other high-energy rays to kill cancer cells)
- hormone therapy (using hormones to stop cancer cells from growing)
- chemotherapy (using drugs to kill cancer cells)

Surgery is the most common treatment of thyroid cancer. A doctor may remove the cancer using one of the following operations:

- Lobectomy removes only the side of the thyroid where the cancer is found. Lymph nodes in the area may be taken out (biopsied) to see if they contain cancer.
- Near-total thyroidectomy removes all of the thyroid except for a small part.
- Total thyroidectomy removes the entire thyroid.
- Lymph node dissection removes lymph nodes in the neck that contain cancer.

Radiation therapy uses high-energy x-rays to kill cancer cells and shrink tumors. Radiation for thyroid cancer may come from a machine outside the body (external radiation therapy) or from drinking a liquid that contains radioactive iodine. Because the thyroid takes up iodine, the radioactive iodine collects in any thyroid tissue remaining in the body and kills the cancer cells.

Hormone therapy uses hormones to stop cancer cells from growing. In treating thyroid cancer, hormones can be used to stop the body from making other hormones that might make cancer cells grow. Hormones are usually given as pills. Chemotherapy uses drugs to kill cancer cells.

Chemotherapy may be taken by pill, or it may be put into the body by a needle in the vein or muscle. Chemotherapy is called a systemic treatment because the drug enters the bloodstream, travels through the body, and can kill cancer cells outside the thyroid.

Treatment by Stage

Treatment of thyroid cancer depends on the type and stage of the disease, and the patient's age and overall health.

Standard treatment may be considered because of its effectiveness in patients in past studies, or participation in a clinical trial may be considered. Not all patients are cured with standard therapy and some standard treatments may have more side effects than are desired. For these reasons, clinical trials are designed to find better ways to treat cancer patients and are based on the most up-to-date information. Clinical trials are ongoing in many parts of the country for some patients with thyroid cancer.

Stage I and II Papillary and Follicular Thyroid Cancer

Treatment may be one of the following:

1. Surgery to remove the thyroid (total thyroidectomy). This may be followed by hormone therapy and radioactive iodine.

2. Surgery to remove one lobe of the thyroid (lobectomy), followed by hormone therapy. Radioactive iodine also may be given following surgery.

Stage III Papillary and Follicular Thyroid Cancer

Treatment may be one of the following:

1. Surgery to removes the entire thyroid gland (total thyroidectomy) and lymph nodes where cancer has spread.

2. Total thyroidectomy followed by radiation therapy with radio-active iodine or external-beam radiation therapy.

Stage IV Papillary and Follicular Thyroid Cancer

Treatment may be one of the following:

1. Radioactive iodine.
2. External-beam radiation therapy.
3. Surgery to remove the cancer from places where it has spread.
4. Hormone therapy.
5. A clinical trial of new treatments, including chemotherapy.

Medullary Thyroid Cancer

Treatment may be one of the following:

1. Total thyroidectomy for tumors in the thyroid only. Lymph nodes in the neck may also be removed.
2. Radiation therapy for tumors that come back in the thyroid as palliative treatment to relieve symptoms and improve the patient's quality of life.
3. Chemotherapy for cancer that has spread to other parts of the body, as palliative treatment to relieve symptoms and improve the patient's quality of life.

Anaplastic Thyroid Cancer

Treatment may be one of the following:

1. Surgery to create an opening in the windpipe, for tumors that block the airway. This is called a tracheostomy.
2. Total thyroidectomy to reduce symptoms if the tumor is in the area of the thyroid only.
3. External-beam radiation therapy.
4. Chemotherapy.
5. Clinical trials of chemotherapy and radiation therapy following thyroidectomy.
6. Clinical trials studying new methods of treatment of thyroid cancer.

Recurrent Thyroid Cancer

The choice of treatment depends on the type of thyroid cancer the patient has, the kind of treatment the patient had before, and where the cancer comes back. Treatment may be one of the following:

1. Surgery with or without radioactive iodine. A second surgery may be done to remove tumor that remains.

2. Radioactive iodine.

3. External-beam radiation therapy or radiation therapy given during surgery to relieve symptoms caused by the cancer.

4. Chemotherapy.

5. Clinical trials of new treatments.

Additional Information

National Cancer Institute
Cancer Information Service
6116 Executive Blvd., Room 3036A
Bethesda, MD 20892-8322
Toll-Free: 800-4-CANCER (422-6237)
Toll-Free TTY: 800-332-8615
Website: http://www.cancer.gov
E-mail: cancergovstaff@mail.nih.gov

Chapter 31

Hypoparathyroidism

Hypoparathyroidism is a condition in which the body produces too little parathyroid hormone.

Causes, Incidence, and Risk Factors

Calcium and phosphorus are important body minerals. They form the mineral component of bones, and they exist as charged particles called ions in the blood and inside cells.

Parathyroid hormone (PTH) regulates the amount of calcium and phosphorus in bone and blood. PTH is made by four small parathyroid glands located in the neck behind the thyroid gland. Hypoparathyroidism occurs when there is too little PTH. Blood calcium levels fall, and phosphorus levels rise.

The most common cause of hypoparathyroidism is injury to the parathyroid glands during head and neck surgery. Rarely, hypoparathyroidism is a side effect of radioactive iodine treatment for hyperthyroidism. PTH secretion also may be impaired when blood levels of magnesium are low, or when blood pH is too high, a condition called metabolic alkalosis.

DiGeorge syndrome is a childhood disease in which hypoparathyroidism occurs due to a total absence of the parathyroid glands at birth. Familial hypoparathyroidism occurs with other endocrine diseases, such as adrenal insufficiency, in a syndrome called type I polyglandular autoimmune syndrome (PGA I).

The risk factors for hypoparathyroidism include recent thyroid or neck surgery, a family history of parathyroid disorder, or certain autoimmune endocrine diseases, such as Addison disease.

Symptoms

- tingling lips, fingers, and toes
- muscle cramps
- pain in the face, legs, and feet
- abdominal pain
- dry hair
- brittle nails
- dry, scaly skin
- cataracts
- weakened tooth enamel (in children)
- muscle spasms called tetany (can lead to spasms of the larynx, causing breathing difficulties)
- convulsions (seizures)

Additional symptoms that may be associated with this disease include:

- painful menstruation
- hand or foot spasms
- decreased consciousness
- delayed or absent tooth formation

Signs and Tests

This disease may produce the following test results:

- low serum calcium level
- high serum phosphorus level
- low serum parathyroid hormone level
- low serum magnesium level (possible)
- abnormal heart rhythms on electrocardiogram (ECG)

This disease may also alter the results of the following tests:

- urine calcium
- ionized calcium in the blood

Treatment

The goal of treatment is to restore the calcium and mineral balance in the body. Oral calcium carbonate and vitamin D supplements are usually lifelong therapy. Blood levels are measured regularly to make sure that the dose is correct. A high-calcium, low-phosphorous diet is recommended.

In the event of a life-threatening attack of low calcium levels or tetany (prolonged muscle contractions), calcium is administered by intravenous (IV) infusion. Precautions are taken to prevent seizures or larynx spasms. The heart is monitored for abnormal rhythms until the person is stable. When the life-threatening attack has been controlled, treatment continues with medicine taken by mouth.

Expectations (Prognosis)

The outcome is likely to be good if the diagnosis is made early. However, changes in the teeth, the development of cataracts, and brain calcifications are irreversible.

Complications

- Tetany can lead to a blocked airway, requiring a tracheostomy.
- Stunted growth, malformed teeth, and slow mental development can occur if hypoparathyroidism develops in childhood.
- Over-treatment with vitamin D and calcium can cause hypercalcemia (high blood calcium) and sometimes interfere with kidney function.
- There is an increased risk of pernicious anemia, Addison disease, cataract development, and Parkinson disease.

Calling Your Health Care Provider

Call your health care provider if you develop any symptoms of hypoparathyroidism.

Seizures or difficulty breathing are an emergency. Call 911 immediately.

Prevention

If you undergo thyroid or neck surgery, watch for early signs of hypoparathyroidism and inform your health care provider promptly. This will enable treatment with calcium and vitamin D supplements to be started as quickly as possible.

Chapter 32

Hyperparathyroidism

Primary hyperparathyroidism is a disorder of the parathyroid glands, also called parathyroids. Primary means this disorder originates in the parathyroids: One or more enlarged, overactive parathyroid glands secretes too much parathyroid hormone (PTH). In secondary hyperparathyroidism, a problem such as kidney failure causes the parathyroids to be overactive. This chapter focuses on primary hyperparathyroidism.

What are the parathyroid glands?

The parathyroid glands are four pea-sized glands located on the thyroid gland in the neck. Occasionally, a person is born with one or more of the parathyroid glands embedded in the thyroid, in the thymus, or located elsewhere around this area. In most such cases, however, the glands function normally.

Though their names are similar, the thyroid and parathyroid glands are entirely different glands, each producing distinct hormones with specific functions. The parathyroid glands secrete PTH, a substance that helps maintain the correct balance of calcium and phosphorous in the body. PTH regulates the level of calcium in the blood, release of calcium from bone, absorption of calcium in the intestine, and excretion of calcium in the urine.

National Institute of Diabetes and Digestive and Kidney Diseases (NIDDK), NIH Publication No. 06-3425, May 2006.

When the level of calcium in the blood falls too low, the parathyroid glands secrete just enough PTH to restore the blood calcium level.

What is hyperparathyroidism?

If the parathyroid glands secrete too much hormone, as happens in primary hyperparathyroidism, the balance is disrupted: Blood calcium rises. This condition of excessive calcium in the blood, called hypercalcemia, is what usually signals the doctor that something may be wrong with the parathyroid glands. In 85 percent of people with primary hyperparathyroidism, a benign tumor called an adenoma has formed on one of the parathyroid glands, causing it to become overactive. Benign tumors are noncancerous. In most other cases, the excess hormone comes from two or more enlarged parathyroid glands, a condition called hyperplasia. Very rarely, hyperparathyroidism is caused by cancer of a parathyroid gland.

This excess PTH triggers the release of too much calcium into the bloodstream. The bones may lose calcium, and too much calcium may be absorbed from food. The levels of calcium may increase in the urine, causing kidney stones. PTH also lowers blood phosphorous levels by increasing excretion of phosphorus in the urine.

Why are calcium and phosphorous so important?

Calcium is essential for good health. It plays an important role in bone and tooth development and in maintaining bone strength. Calcium is also important in nerve transmission and muscle contraction. Phosphorous is found in all bodily tissue. It is a main part of every cell with many roles in each. Combined with calcium, phosphorous gives strength and rigidity to your bones and teeth.

What causes hyperparathyroidism?

In most cases doctors don't know the cause. The vast majority of cases occur in people with no family history of the disorder. Only about five percent of cases can be linked to an inherited problem.

Familial multiple endocrine neoplasia type 1 (MEN-1) is a rare, inherited syndrome that affects the parathyroids as well as the pancreas and the pituitary gland. Another rare genetic disorder, familial hypocalciuric hypercalcemia, is sometimes confused with typical hyperparathyroidism. Each accounts for about two percent of primary hyperparathyroidism cases.

How common is hyperparathyroidism?

In the United States, about 100,000 people develop the disorder each year. Women outnumber men two to one, and risk increases with age. In women 60 years and older, two out of 1,000 will develop hyperparathyroidism each year.

What are the symptoms of hyperparathyroidism?

A person with hyperparathyroidism may have severe symptoms, subtle ones, or none at all. Increasingly, routine blood tests that screen for a wide range of conditions, including high calcium levels, are alerting doctors to people who have mild forms of the disorder even though they are symptom-free.

When symptoms do appear, they are often mild and nonspecific, such as a feeling of weakness and fatigue, depression, or aches and pains. With more severe disease, a person may have a loss of appetite, nausea, vomiting, constipation, confusion or impaired thinking and memory, and increased thirst and urination. Patients may have thinning of the bones without symptoms, but with risk of fractures. Increased calcium and phosphorous excretion in the urine may cause kidney stones.

How is hyperparathyroidism diagnosed?

Hyperparathyroidism is diagnosed when tests show that blood levels of calcium and parathyroid hormone are too high. Other diseases can cause high blood calcium levels, but only in hyperparathyroidism is the elevated calcium the result of too much parathyroid hormone. A blood test that accurately measures the amount of parathyroid hormone has simplified the diagnosis of hyperparathyroidism.

Once the diagnosis is established, other tests may be done to assess complications. Because high PTH levels can cause bones to weaken from calcium loss, a measurement of bone density can help assess bone loss and the risk of fractures. Abdominal images may reveal the presence of kidney stones and a 24-hour urine collection may provide information on kidney damage, the risk of stone formation, and the risk of familial hypocalciuric hypercalcemia.

How is hyperparathyroidism treated?

Surgery to remove the enlarged gland (or glands) is the main treatment for the disorder and cures it in 95 percent of operations.

Calcimimetic agents are a new class of drugs that turn off secretion of PTH. They have been approved by the Food and Drug Administration for the treatment of hyperparathyroidism secondary to kidney failure with dialysis, and primary hyperparathyroidism caused by parathyroid cancer. They have not been approved for primary hyperparathyroidism, but some physicians have begun prescribing calcimimetic for some patients with this condition. Patients can discuss this class of drug in more detail with their physicians.

Some patients who have mild disease may not need immediate treatment, according to panels convened by the National Institutes of Health (NIH) in 2002. Patients who are symptom-free, whose blood calcium is only slightly elevated, and whose kidneys and bones are normal may wish to talk with their physicians about long-term monitoring. In the 2002 recommendation, periodic monitoring would consist of clinical evaluation, measurement of serum calcium levels, and bone mass measurement. If the patient and physician choose long-term follow-up, the patient should try to drink lots of water, get plenty of exercise, and avoid certain diuretics, such as the thiazides. Immobilization (unable to move) and gastrointestinal illness with vomiting or diarrhea can cause calcium levels to rise. Patients with hyperparathyroidism should seek medical attention if they find themselves immobilized, vomiting, or having diarrhea.

Are there any complications associated with parathyroid surgery?

Surgery for hyperparathyroidism is highly successful with a low complication rate when performed by surgeons experienced with this condition. About one percent of patients undergoing surgery experience damage to the nerves controlling the vocal cords, which can affect speech. One to five percent of patients lose all their parathyroid tissue and thus develop chronic low calcium levels, which may require treatment with calcium or vitamin D. The complication rate is slightly higher for hyperplasia than it is for adenoma since more extensive surgery is needed.

Are parathyroid imaging tests needed before surgery?

The NIH panels recommended against the use of expensive imaging tests to locate benign tumors before initial surgery. Such tests are not likely to improve the success rate of surgery, which is about 95 percent when performed by experienced surgeons. Simple imaging tests before surgery are preferred by some surgeons. Localization tests are useful in patients having a second operation for recurrent or persistent hyperparathyroidism.

Which doctors specialize in treating hyperparathyroidism?

Endocrinologists are doctors who specialize in hormonal problems. Nephrologists are doctors who specialize in kidney and mineral disorders. Along with surgeons who are experienced in endocrine surgery, endocrinologists and nephrologists are best qualified to treat people with hyperparathyroidism. Organizations that help people with hyperparathyroidism may have additional information to assist in finding a qualified health professional nearby.

Additional Information

American Association of Clinical Endocrinologists (AACE)
245 Riverside Ave., Suite 200
Jacksonville, FL 32202
Phone: 904-353-7878
Fax: 904-353-8185
Website: http://www.aace.com
E-mail: info@aace.com

Endocrine and Metabolic Diseases Information Service
6 Information Way
Bethesda, MD 20892-3569
Toll-Free: 888-828-0904
Fax: 703-738-4929
Website: http://www.endocrine.niddk.nih.gov
E-mail: endoandmeta@info.niddk.nih.gov

Hormone Foundation
8401 Connecticut Ave., Suite 900
Chevy Chase, MD 20815
Toll-Free: 800-HORMONE (467-6663)
Fax: 301-941-0259
Website: http://www.hormone.org
E-mail: hormone@endo-society.org

Chapter 33

Parathyroid Cancer

Key Points about Parathyroid Cancer

- Parathyroid cancer is a rare disease in which malignant (cancer) cells form in the tissues of a parathyroid gland.
- Having certain inherited disorders can increase the risk of developing parathyroid cancer.
- Possible signs of parathyroid cancer include weakness, feeling tired, and a lump in the neck.
- Tests that examine the neck and blood are used to detect (find) and diagnose parathyroid cancer.
- Certain factors affect prognosis (chance of recovery) and treatment options.

The parathyroid glands are four pea-sized organs found in the neck near the thyroid gland. The parathyroid glands make parathyroid hormone (PTH or parathormone). PTH helps the body use and store calcium to keep the calcium in the blood at normal levels.

A parathyroid gland may become overactive and make too much PTH, a condition called hyperparathyroidism. Hyperparathyroidism can occur when a benign tumor (noncancer), called an adenoma, forms

PDQ® Cancer Information Summary. National Cancer Institute; Bethesda, MD. Parathyroid Cancer (PDQ®): Treatment–Patient. Updated 10/13/2006. Available at http://cancer.gov. Accessed 02/07/2007.

on one of the parathyroid glands, and causes it to grow and become overactive. Sometimes hyperparathyroidism can be caused by parathyroid cancer, but this is very rare.

The extra PTH causes:

• the calcium stored in the bones to move into the blood; and

• the intestines to absorb more calcium from the food we eat.

This condition is called hypercalcemia (too much calcium in the blood). The hypercalcemia caused by hyperparathyroidism is more serious and life-threatening than parathyroid cancer itself and treating hypercalcemia is as important as treating the cancer.

Risk Factors

Having certain inherited disorders can increase the risk of developing parathyroid cancer. Anything that increases the chance of getting a disease is called a risk factor. Risk factors for parathyroid cancer include the following rare disorders that are inherited (passed down from parent to child):

• familial isolated hyperparathyroidism (FIHP)

• multiple endocrine neoplasia type 1 (MEN1) syndrome

Treatment with radiation therapy may increase the risk of developing a parathyroid adenoma.

Symptoms

Possible signs of parathyroid cancer include weakness, feeling tired, and a lump in the neck. Most parathyroid cancer symptoms are caused by the hypercalcemia that develops. Symptoms of hypercalcemia include:

• weakness

• feeling very tired

• nausea and vomiting

• loss of appetite

• weight loss for no known reason

• being much more thirsty than usual

• urinating much more than usual

- constipation
- trouble thinking clearly

Other symptoms of parathyroid cancer include:

- pain in the abdomen, side, or back that doesn't go away
- pain in the bones
- a broken bone
- a lump in the neck
- change in voice such as hoarseness
- trouble swallowing

Other conditions may cause the same symptoms as parathyroid cancer. A doctor should be consulted if any of these problems occur.

Diagnosis

Tests that examine the neck and blood are used to detect (find) and diagnose parathyroid cancer. Once blood tests are done and hyperparathyroidism is diagnosed, imaging tests may be done to help find which of the parathyroid glands is overactive. Sometimes the parathyroid glands are hard to find and imaging tests are done to find exactly where they are.

Parathyroid cancer may be hard to diagnose because the cells of a benign parathyroid adenoma and a malignant parathyroid cancer look alike. The patient's symptoms, blood levels of calcium and parathyroid hormone, and characteristics of the tumor are also used to make a diagnosis.

The following tests and procedures may be used:

- Physical exam and history: An exam of the body to check general signs of health, including checking for signs of disease, such as lumps or anything else that seems unusual. A history of the patient's health habits and past illnesses and treatments will also be taken.

- Blood chemistry studies: A procedure in which a blood sample is checked to measure the amounts of certain substances released into the blood by organs and tissues in the body. An unusual (higher or lower than normal) amount of a substance can be a sign of disease in the organ or tissue that makes it. To diagnose parathyroid cancer, the sample of blood is checked for its calcium level.

- Parathyroid hormone test: A procedure in which a blood sample is checked to measure the amount of parathyroid hormone released into the blood by the parathyroid glands. A higher than normal amount of parathyroid hormone can be a sign of disease.

- Sestamibi scan: A type of radionuclide scan used to find an overactive parathyroid gland. A small amount of a radioactive substance called technetium 99 is injected into a vein and travels through the bloodstream to the parathyroid gland. The radioactive substance will collect in the overactive gland and show up brightly on a special camera that detects radioactivity.

- Computed tomography scan (CT scan): A procedure that makes a series of detailed pictures of areas inside the body, taken from different angles. The pictures are made by a computer linked to an x-ray machine. A dye may be injected into a vein or swallowed to help the organs or tissues show up more clearly. This procedure is also called computerized tomography, or computerized axial tomography.

- Ultrasound exam: A procedure in which high-energy sound waves (ultrasound) are bounced off internal tissues or organs and make echoes. The echoes form a picture of body tissues called a sonogram.

- Angiogram: A procedure to look at blood vessels and the flow of blood. A contrast dye is injected into the blood vessel. As the contrast dye moves through the blood vessel, x-rays are taken to see if there are any blockages.

- Venous sampling: A procedure in which a sample of blood is taken from specific veins and checked to measure the amounts of certain substances released into the blood by nearby organs and tissues. If imaging tests do not show which parathyroid gland is overactive, blood samples may be taken from veins near each parathyroid gland to find which one is making too much PTH.

Prognosis

Certain factors affect prognosis (chance of recovery) and treatment options. The prognosis (chance of recovery) and treatment options depend on:

- whether the calcium level in the blood can be controlled;

- the stage of the cancer;

- whether the tumor and the capsule around the tumor can be completely removed by surgery; and

- the patient's general health.

Stages of Parathyroid Cancer

Staging is the process used to find out how far the cancer has spread. The following imaging tests may be used to determine if cancer has spread to other parts of the body such as the lungs, liver, bone, heart, pancreas, or lymph nodes:

- CT scan (CAT scan)

- MRI (magnetic resonance imaging): A procedure that uses a magnet, radio waves, and a computer to make a series of detailed pictures of areas inside the body. This procedure is also called nuclear magnetic resonance imaging (NMRI).

There is no standard staging process for parathyroid cancer. The disease is described as either localized or metastatic.

- Localized parathyroid cancer is found in a parathyroid gland and may have spread to nearby tissues.

- Metastatic parathyroid cancer has spread to other parts of the body, such as the lungs, liver, bone, sac around the heart, pancreas, or lymph nodes.

Recurrent Parathyroid Cancer

Recurrent parathyroid cancer is cancer that has recurred (come back) after it has been treated. More than half of patients have a recurrence. The parathyroid cancer usually recurs between two and five years after the first surgery, but can recur up to 20 years later. It usually comes back in the tissues or lymph nodes of the neck. High blood calcium levels that appear after treatment may be the first sign of recurrence.

Treatment Option Overview

Key Points

- There are different types of treatment for patients with parathyroid cancer.

- Treatment includes control of hypercalcemia (too much calcium in the blood) in patients who have an overactive parathyroid gland.

- Four types of standard treatment are used:

  - surgery

  - radiation therapy

  - chemotherapy

  - supportive care

- New types of treatment are being tested in clinical trials.

- Lifelong follow-up is important.

Types of Treatment

Different types of treatment are available for patients with parathyroid cancer. Some treatments are standard (the currently used treatment), and some are being tested in clinical trials. Before starting treatment, patients may want to think about taking part in a clinical trial. A treatment clinical trial is a research study meant to help improve current treatments or obtain information on new treatments for patients with cancer. When clinical trials show that a new treatment is better than the standard treatment, the new treatment may become the standard treatment.

Clinical trials are taking place in many parts of the country. Information about ongoing clinical trials is available from the National Cancer Institute website. Choosing the most appropriate cancer treatment is a decision that ideally involves the patient, family, and health care team.

Control of Hypercalcemia

Treatment includes control of hypercalcemia (too much calcium in the blood) in patients who have an overactive parathyroid gland. In order to reduce the amount of parathyroid hormone that is being made and control the level of calcium in the blood, as much of the tumor as possible is removed in surgery. For patients who cannot have surgery, medication may be used.

Four Types of Standard Treatment

Surgery: Surgery (removing the cancer in an operation) is the most common treatment for parathyroid cancer that is in the parathyroid glands or has spread to other parts of the body. Because parathyroid cancer grows very slowly, cancer that has spread to other parts of the body may be removed by surgery in order to cure the patient or control the effects of the disease for a long time. Before surgery, treatment is given to control hypercalcemia.

The following surgical procedures may be used:

- En bloc resection: Surgery to remove the entire parathyroid gland and the capsule around it. Sometimes lymph nodes, half of the thyroid gland on the same side of the body as the cancer, and muscles, tissues, and a nerve in the neck are also removed.

- Tumor debulking: Surgery to remove as much of the tumor as possible. Sometimes, not all of the tumor can be removed.

- Metastasectomy: Surgery to remove any cancer that has spread to distant organs such as the lung.

Surgery for parathyroid cancer sometimes damages nerves of the vocal cords. There are treatments to help with speech problems caused by this nerve damage.

Radiation Therapy: Radiation therapy is a cancer treatment that uses high-energy x-rays or other types of radiation to kill cancer cells or stop them from growing. There are two types of radiation therapy. External radiation therapy uses a machine outside the body to send radiation toward the cancer. Internal radiation therapy uses a radioactive substance sealed in needles, seeds, wires, or catheters that are placed directly into or near the cancer. The way the radiation therapy is given depends on the type and stage of the cancer being treated.

Chemotherapy: Chemotherapy is a cancer treatment that uses drugs to stop the growth of cancer cells, either by killing the cells or by stopping them from dividing. When chemotherapy is taken by mouth or injected into a vein or muscle, the drugs enter the bloodstream and can reach cancer cells throughout the body (systemic chemotherapy). When chemotherapy is placed directly into the spinal column, an organ, or a body cavity such as the abdomen, the drugs mainly affect cancer cells in those areas (regional chemotherapy). The way the chemotherapy is given depends on the type and stage of the cancer being treated.

Supportive Care: Supportive care is given to lessen the problems caused by the disease or its treatment. Supportive care for hypercalcemia caused by parathyroid cancer may include:

- intravenous (IV) fluids;

- drugs that increase how much urine the body makes;

- drugs that stop the body from absorbing calcium from the food we eat; or

- drugs that stop the parathyroid gland from making parathyroid hormone.

Clinical Trials

New types of treatment are being tested in clinical trials. Information about ongoing clinical trials is available from the National Cancer Institute website.

Follow-Up

Lifelong follow-up is important. Parathyroid cancer often recurs. Patients should have regular check-ups for the rest of their lives, to find and treat recurrences early.

Treatment Options for Parathyroid Cancer

Localized Parathyroid Cancer

Treatment of localized parathyroid cancer may include:

- surgery (en bloc resection);

- surgery followed by radiation therapy;

- radiation therapy; and

- supportive care to treat hypercalcemia (too much calcium in the blood).

Metastatic Parathyroid Cancer

Treatment of metastatic parathyroid cancer may include:

- surgery (metastasectomy) to remove cancer from the places where it has spread;

- surgery followed by radiation therapy;

- radiation therapy;

- chemotherapy; and

- supportive care to treat hypercalcemia (too much calcium in the blood).

Recurrent Parathyroid Cancer

Treatment of recurrent parathyroid cancer may include:

- surgery (metastasectomy) to remove cancer from the places where it has recurred;

- surgery (tumor debulking);

- surgery followed by radiation therapy;

- radiation therapy;

- chemotherapy; and

- supportive care to treat hypercalcemia (too much calcium in the blood).

Additional Information

National Cancer Institute
6116 Executive Blvd., Room 3036A
Bethesda, MD 20892-8322
Toll-Free: 800-4-Cancer (422-6237)
Toll-Free TTY: 800-332-8615
Website: http://www.cancer.gov
E-mail: cancergovstaff@mail.nih.gov

Part Four

Adrenal Gland Disorders

Chapter 34

Addison Disease

Addison disease is an endocrine or hormonal disorder that occurs in all age groups and afflicts men and women equally. The disease is characterized by weight loss, muscle weakness, fatigue, low blood pressure, and sometimes darkening of the skin in both exposed and unexposed parts of the body. Addison disease occurs when the adrenal glands do not produce enough of the hormone cortisol and, in some cases, the hormone aldosterone. The disease is also called adrenal insufficiency, or hypocorticoidism.

Cortisol

Cortisol is normally produced by the adrenal glands, located just above the kidneys. It belongs to a class of hormones called glucocorticoids, which affect almost every organ and tissue in the body. Scientists think that cortisol has possibly hundreds of effects in the body, but its most important job is to help the body respond to stress. Among its other vital tasks, cortisol helps to:

- maintain blood pressure and cardiovascular function;
- slow the immune system's inflammatory response;
- balance the effects of insulin in breaking down sugar for energy;

National Institute of Diabetes and Digestive and Kidney Diseases (NIDDK), NIH Publication No. 04-3054, June 2004.

- regulate the metabolism of proteins, carbohydrates, and fats; and

- maintain proper arousal and sense of well-being.

Because cortisol is so vital to health, the amount of cortisol produced by the adrenals is precisely balanced. Like many other hormones, cortisol is regulated by the brain's hypothalamus and the pituitary gland, a bean-sized organ at the base of the brain. First, the hypothalamus sends releasing hormones to the pituitary gland. The pituitary responds by secreting hormones that regulate growth and thyroid and adrenal function, and sex hormones such as estrogen and testosterone. One of the pituitary's main functions is to secrete adrenocorticotropic hormone (ACTH), a hormone that stimulates the adrenal glands. When the adrenals receive the pituitary's signal in the form of ACTH, they respond by producing cortisol. Completing the cycle, cortisol then signals the pituitary to lower secretion of ACTH.

Aldosterone

Aldosterone belongs to a class of hormones called mineralocorticoids, also produced by the adrenal glands. It helps maintain blood pressure and water and salt balance in the body by helping the kidney retain sodium and excrete potassium. When aldosterone production falls too low, the kidneys are not able to regulate salt and water balance, causing blood volume and blood pressure to drop.

Causes

Failure to produce adequate levels of cortisol can occur for different reasons. The problem may be due to a disorder of the adrenal glands themselves (primary adrenal insufficiency) or to inadequate secretion of ACTH by the pituitary gland (secondary adrenal insufficiency).

Primary Adrenal Insufficiency

Addison disease affects about one in 100,000 people. Most cases are caused by the gradual destruction of the adrenal cortex, the outer layer of the adrenal glands, by the body's own immune system. About 70 percent of reported cases of Addison disease are caused by autoimmune disorders, in which the immune system makes antibodies that attack the body's own tissues or organs and slowly destroy them. Adrenal insufficiency occurs when at least 90 percent of the adrenal cortex has been destroyed. As a result, often both glucocorticoid (cortisol) and mineralocorticoid (aldosterone) hormones are lacking. Sometimes only the adrenal gland is affected, as in idiopathic adrenal insufficiency; sometimes other glands also are affected, as in the polyendocrine deficiency syndrome.

Polyendocrine Deficiency Syndrome

The polyendocrine deficiency syndrome is classified into two separate forms, referred to as type I and type II.

Type I occurs in children, and adrenal insufficiency may be accompanied by:

- underactive parathyroid glands,
- slow sexual development,
- pernicious anemia,
- chronic candida infections,
- chronic active hepatitis, or
- hair loss (in very rare cases).

Type II, often called Schmidt syndrome, usually afflicts young adults. Features of type II may include:

- an underactive thyroid gland,
- slow sexual development,
- diabetes,
- vitiligo, or
- loss of pigment on areas of the skin.

Scientists think that the polyendocrine deficiency syndrome is inherited because frequently more than one family member tends to have one or more endocrine deficiencies.

Tuberculosis

Tuberculosis (TB), an infection which can destroy the adrenal glands, accounts for about 20 percent of cases of primary adrenal insufficiency in developed countries. When adrenal insufficiency was first identified by Dr. Thomas Addison in 1849, TB was found at autopsy in 70 to 90 percent of cases. As the treatment for TB improved, however, the incidence of adrenal insufficiency due to TB of the adrenal glands has greatly decreased.

Other Causes

Less common causes of primary adrenal insufficiency include:

* chronic infection, mainly fungal infections;
* cancer cells spreading from other parts of the body to the adrenal glands;
* amyloidosis; and
* surgical removal of the adrenal glands.

Secondary Adrenal Insufficiency

This form of adrenal insufficiency is much more common than primary adrenal insufficiency and can be traced to a lack of ACTH. Without ACTH to stimulate the adrenals, the adrenal glands' production of cortisol drops, but not aldosterone. A temporary form of secondary adrenal insufficiency may occur when a person who has been receiving a glucocorticoid hormone such as prednisone for a long time abruptly stops or interrupts taking the medication. Glucocorticoid hormones, which are often used to treat inflammatory illnesses like rheumatoid arthritis, asthma, or ulcerative colitis, block the release of both corticotropin-releasing hormone (CRH) and ACTH. Normally, CRH instructs the pituitary gland to release ACTH. If CRH levels drop, the pituitary is not stimulated to release ACTH, and the adrenals then fail to secrete sufficient levels of cortisol.

Another cause of secondary adrenal insufficiency is the surgical removal of benign, or noncancerous, ACTH-producing tumors of the pituitary gland (Cushing disease). In this case, the source of ACTH is suddenly removed, and replacement hormone must be taken until normal ACTH and cortisol production resumes.

Less commonly, adrenal insufficiency occurs when the pituitary gland either decreases in size or stops producing ACTH. These events can result from:

* tumors or infections of the area;
* loss of blood flow to the pituitary;
* radiation for the treatment of pituitary tumors;
* surgical removal of parts of the hypothalamus; or
* surgical removal of the pituitary gland.

Symptoms

The symptoms of adrenal insufficiency usually begin gradually. Characteristics of the disease are:

- chronic, worsening fatigue;
- muscle weakness;
- loss of appetite; and/or
- weight loss.

Other symptoms include:

- nausea, vomiting, and diarrhea (about 50 percent of the time);
- low blood pressure that falls further when standing, causing dizziness or fainting; or
- skin changes in Addison disease, with areas of hyperpigmentation, or dark tanning, covering exposed and unexposed parts of the body; this darkening of the skin is most visible on scars; skin folds; pressure points such as the elbows, knees, knuckles, and toes; lips; and mucous membranes.

Addison disease can cause irritability and depression. Because of salt loss, a craving for salty foods also is common. Hypoglycemia, or low blood glucose, is more severe in children than in adults. In women, menstrual periods may become irregular or stop.

Because the symptoms progress slowly, they are usually ignored until a stressful event like an illness or an accident causes them to become worse. This is called an addisonian crisis, or acute adrenal insufficiency. In most cases, symptoms are severe enough that patients seek medical treatment before a crisis occurs. However, in about 25 percent of patients, symptoms first appear during an addisonian crisis.

Symptoms of an addisonian crisis include:

- sudden penetrating pain in the lower back, abdomen, or legs;
- severe vomiting and diarrhea;
- dehydration;
- low blood pressure; and
- loss of consciousness.

Left untreated, an addisonian crisis can be fatal.

Diagnosis

In its early stages, adrenal insufficiency can be difficult to diagnose. A review of a patient's medical history based on the symptoms, especially the dark tanning of the skin, will lead a doctor to suspect Addison disease. A diagnosis of Addison disease is made by laboratory tests. The aim of these tests is first to determine whether levels of cortisol are insufficient and then to establish the cause. X-ray exams of the adrenal and pituitary glands also are useful in helping to establish the cause.

ACTH Stimulation Test

This is the most specific test for diagnosing Addison disease. In this test, blood cortisol, urine cortisol, or both are measured before and after a synthetic form of ACTH is given by injection. In the so-called short, or rapid, ACTH test, measurement of cortisol in blood is repeated 30 to 60 minutes after an intravenous ACTH injection. The normal response after an injection of ACTH is a rise in blood and urine cortisol levels. Patients with either form of adrenal insufficiency respond poorly, or do not respond at all.

Corticotropin-Releasing Hormone (CRH) Stimulation Test

When the response to the short ACTH test is abnormal, a long CRH stimulation test is required to determine the cause of adrenal insufficiency. In this test, synthetic CRH is injected intravenously and blood cortisol is measured before and 30, 60, 90, and 120 minutes after the injection. Patients with primary adrenal insufficiency have high ACTH but do not produce cortisol. Patients with secondary adrenal insufficiency have deficient cortisol responses but absent or delayed ACTH responses. Absent ACTH response points to the pituitary as the cause; a delayed ACTH response points to the hypothalamus as the cause.

In patients suspected of having an Addisonian crisis, the doctor must begin treatment with injections of salt, fluids, and glucocorticoid hormones immediately. Although a reliable diagnosis is not possible while the patient is being treated for the crisis, measurement of blood ACTH and cortisol during the crisis and before glucocorticoids are given, is enough to make the diagnosis. Once the crisis is controlled and medication has been stopped, the doctor will delay further testing for up to one month to obtain an accurate diagnosis.

Other Tests

Once a diagnosis of primary adrenal insufficiency has been made, x-ray exams of the abdomen may be taken to see if the adrenals have any signs of calcium deposits. Calcium deposits may indicate TB. A tuberculin skin test also may be used.

If secondary adrenal insufficiency is the cause, doctors may use different imaging tools to reveal the size and shape of the pituitary gland. The most common is the computed tomography (CT) scan, which produces a series of x-ray pictures giving a cross-sectional image of a body part. The function of the pituitary and its ability to produce other hormones also are tested.

Treatment

Treatment of Addison disease involves replacing, or substituting, the hormones that the adrenal glands are not making. Cortisol is replaced orally with hydrocortisone tablets, a synthetic glucocorticoid, taken once or twice a day. If aldosterone is also deficient, it is replaced with oral doses of a mineralocorticoid called fludrocortisone acetate (Florinef), which is taken once a day. Patients receiving aldosterone replacement therapy are usually advised by a doctor to increase their salt intake. Because patients with secondary adrenal insufficiency normally maintain aldosterone production, they do not require aldosterone replacement therapy. The doses of each of these medications are adjusted to meet the needs of individual patients.

During an addisonian crisis, low blood pressure, low blood glucose, and high levels of potassium can be life threatening. Standard therapy involves intravenous injections of hydrocortisone, saline (salt water), and dextrose (sugar). This treatment usually brings rapid improvement. When the patient can take fluids and medications by mouth, the amount of hydrocortisone is decreased until a maintenance dose is achieved. If aldosterone is deficient, maintenance therapy also includes oral doses of fludrocortisone acetate.

Special Problems

Surgery

Patients with chronic adrenal insufficiency who need surgery with general anesthesia are treated with injections of hydrocortisone and saline. Injections begin on the evening before surgery and continue until the patient is fully awake and able to take medication by mouth.

The dosage is adjusted until the maintenance dosage given before surgery is reached.

Pregnancy

Women with primary adrenal insufficiency who become pregnant are treated with standard replacement therapy. If nausea and vomiting in early pregnancy interfere with oral medication, injections of the hormone may be necessary. During delivery, treatment is similar to that of patients needing surgery; following delivery, the dose is gradually tapered and the usual maintenance doses of hydrocortisone and fludrocortisone acetate by mouth are reached by about ten days after childbirth.

Patient Education

A person who has adrenal insufficiency should always carry identification stating his or her condition in case of an emergency. The card should alert emergency personnel about the need to inject 100 milligrams (mg) of cortisol if its bearer is found severely injured or unable to answer questions. The card should also include the doctor's name and telephone number and the name and telephone number of the nearest relative to be notified. When traveling, a needle, syringe, and an injectable form of cortisol should be carried for emergencies. A person with Addison disease also should know how to increase medication during periods of stress or mild upper respiratory infections. Immediate medical attention is needed when severe infections, vomiting, or diarrhea occur. These conditions can precipitate an addisonian crisis. A patient who is vomiting may require injections of hydrocortisone.

People with medical problems may wish to wear a descriptive warning bracelet or neck chain to alert emergency personnel. A number of companies manufacture medical identification products.

Additional Information

American Autoimmune Related Diseases Association
National Office
22100 Gratiot Ave.
East Detroit, MI 48021
Phone: 586-776-3900
Website: http://www.aarda.org
E-mail: aarda@aarda.org

Endocrine and Metabolic Diseases Information Service
6 Information Way
Bethesda, MD 20892-3569
Toll-Free: 888-828-0904
Fax: 703-738-4929
Website: http://www.endocrine.niddk.nih.gov
E-mail: endoandmeta@info.niddk.nih.gov

National Adrenal Diseases Foundation (NADF)
505 Northern Blvd.
Great Neck, NY 11021
Phone: 516-487-4992
Fax: 516-829-5710
Website: http://www.nadf.us
E-mail: nadfmail@aol.com

Chapter 35

Conn Syndrome (Hyperaldosteronism)

What Is It?

Conn syndrome is another name for primary hyperaldosteronism which is the most common cause of secondary hypertension and may also be referred to as aldosteronism. It is a condition characterized by the excess secretion of aldosterone from the cortex—the outer layer—of the adrenal glands. The adrenal glands are small triangular organs located on the top of the kidneys. They are part of the endocrine system, a group of glands that produce and secrete hormones that act on and regulate many systems throughout the body. Aldosterone is a hormone that plays an important role in maintaining blood volume, pressure, and electrolyte balance. Its production is normally regulated by renin, an enzyme produced in the kidneys. When renin increases—due to low blood pressure, decreased blood flow to the kidneys, or to a sodium deficiency—aldosterone increases; when renin decreases, aldosterone decreases.

With Conn syndrome, excessive amounts of aldosterone are produced by one or more adrenal tumors (usually benign), by hyperplasia (an increased number of aldosterone-producing cells), for unknown reasons (idiopathic), or rarely, due to a cancerous adrenal tumor. Regardless of the cause, increased aldosterone can most commonly lead

"Conn's Syndrome: What is it?, Tests, and Treatments," © 2006 American Association for Clinical Chemistry. Reprinted with permission. For additional information about clinical lab testing, visit the Lab Tests Online website at www.labtestsonline.org.

to hypokalemia (decreased potassium), increased blood pH (alkalosis), and hypertension.

Somewhat less frequently, increased aldosterone will lead to polyuria (frequent urination), increased thirst, weakness, temporary paralysis, headaches, muscle cramps, and tingling.

Very rarely, increased aldosterone will lead to hypernatremia (increased sodium).

The presence of hypokalemia (low potassium) in a person with hypertension suggests the need to look for primary hyperaldosteronism.

Diagnosing Conn syndrome is important because it represents one of the few causes of hypertension that is potentially curable. Although anyone can get primary hyperaldosteronism, it commonly occurs in adults between the ages of 30 and 50 and is more common in women than men. It can sometimes be difficult to diagnose as patients may have variable symptoms or no symptoms at all. Suspicion of Conn syndrome may be raised in patients who are resistant to standard hypertension therapies.

Secondary aldosteronism, which is not considered Conn syndrome, can occur as a result of anything that increases renin levels, such as decreased blood flow to the kidneys, low blood pressure, or low sodium levels in the urine. The most important cause is narrowing of the blood vessels that supply the kidney, termed renal artery stenosis. Other causes of secondary hyperaldosteronism include congestive heart failure, cirrhosis, kidney disease, and toxemia of pregnancy.

Tests

The goal with testing for Conn syndrome is to identify primary hyperaldosteronism, distinguish between primary and secondary types, and distinguish between those types of primary hyperaldosteronism that may benefit from surgical intervention, and those that will usually not.

Laboratory Tests

Doctors will frequently order blood renin tests along with blood and/or 24-hour urine aldosterone tests to help diagnose primary hyperaldosteronism and to monitor the effectiveness of treatment. The ratio of aldosterone to renin is used to screen for primary hyperaldosteronism. If renin levels are low and aldosterone high, then the ratio will be significantly increased and primary hyperaldosteronism is likely to be present. Based on the results of these tests, a doctor

272

may do a suppression test, using sodium chloride or captopril administration, to see if aldosterone secretion decreases.

Electrolytes may be measured to look for an electrolyte imbalance—primarily decreased potassium and chloride but increased carbon dioxide. If they are present, then the doctor may give the patient spironolactone, a drug that blocks the action of aldosterone, to see if balance is restored.

These tests may be followed by a computed tomography (CT) scan of the adrenal glands to look for a tumor. This process can be complicated as benign adrenal tumors are relatively common, especially as people get older. Many of them do not secrete aldosterone and are found during procedures for other reasons. Determining hyperplasia can also be tricky because the size of normal adrenal glands may vary significantly from one person to the next.

If hyperplasia or an aldosterone-producing tumor is suspected, but not easily locatable, then a doctor may order adrenal venous sampling. In this procedure, blood is collected from the vein that carries blood away from each adrenal gland. These blood samples are tested for aldosterone (sometimes cortisol is also measured and an aldosterone to cortisol ratio calculated) and then the results from the two adrenal glands compared. If they are significantly different, then it is likely that an adenoma is occurring in the gland with the highest aldosterone concentration.

Non-Laboratory Tests

- Blood pressure measurement is often the first indicator of possible primary hyperaldosteronism.

- CT scan or magnetic resonance imaging (MRI) is used to locate adrenal tumors.

Treatments

The goal with treatment of Conn syndrome is to lower blood pressure to normal or near normal levels, decrease blood aldosterone levels, and resolve any electrolyte imbalance. The type(s) of treatment depend on the cause of the excess aldosterone secretion. If it is due to a single benign adrenal tumor, then the affected gland may be surgically removed. In many cases, this will completely resolve hypertension and other associated symptoms, but in others some treatment will still be necessary to control blood pressure. If the primary hyperaldosteronism is due to a cancerous tumor (rare), then organs located next to the affected adrenal gland will need to be evaluated during surgery, and more than the adrenal gland may need to be removed.

If the cause of the primary hyperaldosteronism cannot be determined (idiopathic) or appears to be due to hyperplasia in both adrenals, then surgery is usually not recommended. The patient's condition will be treated with spironolactone (which blocks the action of aldosterone) and one or more blood pressure drug therapies.

Patients should consult with their doctors and, when indicated, with an endocrinologist (a specialist in the endocrine system). Treatment for primary hyperaldosteronism must often be adjusted to accommodate underlying hypertension, kidney disease, congestive heart failure, and a variety of other disorders.

Chapter 36

Cushing Syndrome

Cushing syndrome is a hormonal disorder caused by prolonged exposure of the body's tissues to high levels of the hormone cortisol. Sometimes called hypercortisolism, it is relatively rare and most commonly affects adults aged 20 to 50. An estimated 10 to 15 of every million people are affected each year.

Symptoms

Symptoms vary, but most people have upper body obesity, rounded face, increased fat around the neck, and thinning arms and legs. Children tend to be obese with slowed growth rates.

Other symptoms appear in the skin, which becomes fragile and thin. It bruises easily and heals poorly. Purplish pink stretch marks may appear on the abdomen, thighs, buttocks, arms, and breasts. The bones are weakened, and routine activities such as bending, lifting, or rising from a chair may lead to backaches, rib, and spinal column fractures.

Most people have severe fatigue, weak muscles, high blood pressure, and high blood sugar. Irritability, anxiety, and depression are common.

Women usually have excess hair growth on their faces, necks, chests, abdomens, and thighs. Their menstrual periods may become

National Institute of Diabetes and Digestive and Kidney Diseases (NIDDK), NIH Publication No. 02–3007, June 2002. Reviewed in February 2007 by Dr. David A. Cooke, M.D., Diplomate, American Board of Internal Medicine.

irregular or stop. Men have decreased fertility with diminished or absent desire for sex.

Causes of Cushing Syndrome

Cushing syndrome occurs when the body's tissues are exposed to excessive levels of cortisol for long periods of time. Many people suffer the symptoms of Cushing syndrome because they take glucocorticoid hormones such as prednisone for asthma, rheumatoid arthritis, lupus, and other inflammatory diseases, or for immunosuppression after transplantation.

Others develop Cushing syndrome because of overproduction of cortisol by the body. Normally, the production of cortisol follows a precise chain of events. First, the hypothalamus, a part of the brain which is about the size of a small sugar cube, sends corticotropin releasing hormone (CRH) to the pituitary gland. CRH causes the pituitary to secrete adrenocorticotropic hormone (ACTH), a hormone that stimulates the adrenal glands. When the adrenals, which are located just above the kidneys, receive the ACTH, they respond by releasing cortisol into the bloodstream.

Cortisol performs vital tasks in the body. It helps maintain blood pressure and cardiovascular function, reduces the immune system's inflammatory response, balances the effects of insulin in breaking down sugar for energy, and regulates the metabolism of proteins, carbohydrates, and fats. One of its most important jobs is to help the body respond to stress. For this reason, women in their last three months of pregnancy and highly trained athletes normally have high levels of cortisol. People suffering from depression, alcoholism, malnutrition, and panic disorders also have increased cortisol levels.

When the amount of cortisol in the blood is adequate, the hypothalamus and pituitary release less CRH and ACTH. This ensures that the amount of cortisol released by the adrenal glands is precisely balanced to meet the body's daily needs. However, if something goes wrong with the adrenals, or their regulating switches in the pituitary gland or the hypothalamus, cortisol production can go awry.

Pituitary Adenomas

Pituitary adenomas cause most cases of Cushing syndrome. They are benign, or non-cancerous, tumors of the pituitary gland which secrete increased amounts of ACTH. Most patients have a single adenoma. This form of the syndrome, known as Cushing disease, affects women five times more frequently than men.

Ectopic Adrenocorticotropic Hormone (ACTH) Syndrome

Some benign or malignant (cancerous) tumors that arise outside the pituitary can produce ACTH. This condition is known as ectopic ACTH syndrome. Lung tumors cause over 50 percent of these cases. Men are affected three times more frequently than women. The most common forms of ACTH-producing tumors are oat cell, or small cell lung cancer, which accounts for about 25 percent of all lung cancer cases, and carcinoid tumors. Other less common types of tumors that can produce ACTH are thymomas, pancreatic islet cell tumors, and medullary carcinomas of the thyroid.

Adrenal Tumors

Sometimes, an abnormality of the adrenal glands, most often an adrenal tumor, causes Cushing syndrome. The average age of onset is about 40 years. Most of these cases involve non-cancerous tumors of adrenal tissue, called adrenal adenomas, which release excess cortisol into the blood.

Adrenocortical carcinomas, or adrenal cancers, are the least common cause of Cushing syndrome. Cancer cells secrete excess levels of several adrenal cortical hormones, including cortisol and adrenal androgens. Adrenocortical carcinomas usually cause very high hormone levels and rapid development of symptoms.

Familial Cushing Syndrome

Most cases of Cushing syndrome are not inherited. Rarely, however, some individuals have special causes of Cushing syndrome due to an inherited tendency to develop tumors of one or more endocrine glands. In primary pigmented micronodular adrenal disease, children or young adults develop small cortisol-producing tumors of the adrenal glands. In multiple endocrine neoplasia type I (MEN I), hormone secreting tumors of the parathyroid glands, pancreas, and pituitary occur. Cushing syndrome in MEN I may be due to pituitary, ectopic, or adrenal tumors.

Diagnosing Cushing Syndrome

Diagnosis is based on a review of the patient's medical history, physical examination, and laboratory tests. Often x-ray exams of the adrenal or pituitary glands are useful for locating tumors. These tests help to determine if excess levels of cortisol are present and why.

Twenty-Four Hour Urinary Free Cortisol Level

This is the most specific diagnostic test. The patient's urine is collected over a 24-hour period and tested for the amount of cortisol. Levels higher than 50–100 micrograms a day for an adult suggest Cushing syndrome. The normal upper limit varies in different laboratories, depending on which measurement technique is used.

Once Cushing syndrome has been diagnosed, other tests are used to find the exact location of the abnormality that leads to excess cortisol production. The choice of test depends, in part, on the preference of the endocrinologist or the center where the test is performed.

Dexamethasone Suppression Test

This test helps to distinguish patients with excess production of ACTH due to pituitary adenomas from those with ectopic ACTH-producing tumors. Patients are given dexamethasone, a synthetic glucocorticoid, by mouth every six hours for four days. For the first two days, low doses of dexamethasone are given, and for the last two days, higher doses are given. Twenty-four hour urine collections are made before dexamethasone is administered and on each day of the test. Since cortisol and other glucocorticoids signal the pituitary to lower secretion of ACTH, the normal response after taking dexamethasone is a drop in blood and urine cortisol levels. Different responses of cortisol to dexamethasone are obtained depending on whether the cause of Cushing syndrome is a pituitary adenoma or an ectopic ACTH-producing tumor.

The dexamethasone suppression test can produce false-positive results in patients with depression, alcohol abuse, high estrogen levels, acute illness, and stress. Conversely, drugs such as phenytoin and phenobarbital may cause false-negative results in response to dexamethasone suppression. For this reason, patients are usually advised by their physicians to stop taking these drugs at least one week before the test.

Corticotropin-Releasing Hormone (CRH) Stimulation Test

This test helps to distinguish between patients with pituitary adenomas and those with ectopic ACTH syndrome or cortisol-secreting adrenal tumors. Patients are given an injection of CRH, the corticotropin-releasing hormone which causes the pituitary to secrete ACTH. Patients with pituitary adenomas usually experience a rise in blood levels of ACTH and cortisol. This response is rarely seen in patients with ectopic ACTH syndrome, and practically never in patients with cortisol-secreting adrenal tumors.

Direct Visualization of the Endocrine Glands (Radiologic Imaging)

Imaging tests reveal the size and shape of the pituitary and adrenal glands and help determine if a tumor is present. The most common are the computed tomography (CT) scan and magnetic resonance imaging (MRI). A CT scan produces a series of x-ray pictures giving a cross-sectional image of a body part. MRI also produces images of the internal organs of the body but without exposing the patient to ionizing radiation.

Imaging procedures are used to find a tumor after a diagnosis has been established. Imaging is not used to make the diagnosis of Cushing syndrome because a mass lesion, sometimes called incidentaloma, is commonly found in the pituitary and adrenal glands. These tumors do not produce hormones detrimental to health and are not removed unless blood tests show they are a cause of symptoms or they are unusually large. Conversely, pituitary tumors are not detected by imaging in almost 50 percent of patients who ultimately require pituitary surgery for Cushing syndrome.

Petrosal Sinus Sampling

This test is not always required, but in many cases, it is the best way to separate pituitary from ectopic causes of Cushing syndrome. Samples of blood are drawn from the petrosal sinuses, veins which drain the pituitary, by introducing catheters through a vein in the upper thigh (groin) region, with local anesthesia and mild sedation. X-rays are used to confirm the correct position of the catheters. Often CRH, the hormone which causes the pituitary to secrete ACTH, is given during this test to improve diagnostic accuracy. Levels of ACTH in the petrosal sinuses are measured and compared with ACTH levels in a forearm vein. ACTH levels higher in the petrosal sinuses than in the forearm vein indicate the presence of a pituitary adenoma; similar levels suggest ectopic ACTH syndrome.

The Dexamethasone-Corticotropin-Releasing Hormone (CRH) Test

Some individuals have high cortisol levels, but do not develop the progressive effects of Cushing syndrome, such as muscle weakness, fractures and thinning of the skin. These individuals may have pseudo-Cushing syndrome, which was originally described in people who were depressed or drank excess alcohol, but is now known to be more common. Pseudo-Cushing does not have the same long-term effects on health as Cushing syndrome and does not require treatment directed at the endocrine glands. Although observation over months to years will distinguish pseudo-Cushing from Cushing, the dexamethasone-CRH test was developed to distinguish between the conditions rapidly, so that Cushing patients can receive prompt treatment. This test combines the dexamethasone suppression and the CRH stimulation tests. Elevations of cortisol during this test suggest Cushing syndrome.

Some patients may have sustained high cortisol levels without the effects of Cushing syndrome. These high cortisol levels may be compensating for the body's resistance to cortisol effects. This rare syndrome of cortisol resistance is a genetic condition that causes hypertension and chronic androgen excess.

Sometimes other conditions may be associated with many of the symptoms of Cushing syndrome. These include polycystic ovarian syndrome, which may cause menstrual disturbances, weight gain from adolescence, excess hair growth, and sometimes impaired insulin action and diabetes. Commonly, weight gain, high blood pressure, and abnormal levels of cholesterol and triglycerides in the blood are associated with resistance to insulin action and diabetes; this has been described as the metabolic syndrome-X. Patients with these disorders do not have abnormally elevated cortisol levels.

Treatment

Treatment depends on the specific reason for cortisol excess and may include surgery, radiation, chemotherapy, or the use of cortisol-inhibiting drugs. If the cause is long-term use of glucocorticoid hormones to treat another disorder, the doctor will gradually reduce the dosage to the lowest dose adequate for control of that disorder. Once control is established, the daily dose of glucocorticoid hormones may be doubled and given on alternate days to lessen side effects.

Pituitary Adenomas

Several therapies are available to treat the ACTH-secreting pituitary adenomas of Cushing disease. The most widely used treatment is surgical removal of the tumor, known as transsphenoidal adenomectomy. Using a special microscope and very fine instruments, the surgeon approaches the pituitary gland through a nostril or an opening made below the upper lip. Because this is an extremely delicate procedure, patients are often referred to centers specializing in this type of surgery. The success, or cure, rate of this procedure is over 80 percent when performed by a surgeon with extensive experience. If surgery fails, or only produces a temporary cure, surgery can be repeated, often with good results. After curative pituitary surgery, the production of ACTH drops two levels below normal. This is a natural, but temporary, drop in ACTH production, and patients are given a synthetic form of cortisol (such as hydrocortisone or prednisone). Most patients can stop this replacement therapy in less than a year.

For patients in whom transsphenoidal surgery has failed or who are not suitable candidates for surgery, radiotherapy is another possible treatment. Radiation to the pituitary gland is given over a six-week period, with improvement occurring in 40 to 50 percent of adults and up to 80 percent of children. It may take several months or years before patients feel better from radiation treatment alone. However, the combination of radiation and the drug mitotane (Lysodren®) can help speed recovery. Mitotane suppresses cortisol production and lowers plasma and urine hormone levels. Treatment with mitotane alone can be successful in 30 to 40 percent of patients. Other drugs used alone or in combination to control the production of excess cortisol are aminoglutethimide, metyrapone, trilostane, and ketoconazole. Each has its own side effects that doctors consider when prescribing therapy for individual patients.

Ectopic Adrenocorticotropic Hormone (ACTH) Syndrome

To cure the overproduction of cortisol caused by ectopic ACTH syndrome, it is necessary to eliminate all of the cancerous tissue that is secreting ACTH. The choice of cancer treatment—surgery, radiotherapy, chemotherapy, immunotherapy, or a combination of these treatments—depends on the type of cancer and how far it has spread. Since ACTH-secreting tumors (for example, small cell lung cancer) may be very small or widespread at the time of diagnosis, cortisol-inhibiting drugs, like mitotane, are an important part of treatment. In some cases, if pituitary surgery is not successful, surgical removal of the adrenal glands (bilateral adrenalectomy) may take the place of drug therapy.

Adrenal Tumors

Surgery is the mainstay of treatment for benign as well as cancerous tumors of the adrenal glands. In primary pigmented micronodular adrenal disease and the familial Carney complex, surgical removal of the adrenal glands is required.

Additional Information

Cushing's Support and Research Foundation, Inc.
65 East India Row, Suite 22B
Boston, MA 02110
Phone/Fax: 617-723-3674
Website: http://www.CSRF.net
E-mail: cushinfo@csrf.net

Pituitary Network Association
P.O. Box 1958
Thousand Oaks, CA 91358
Phone: 805-499-9973
Fax: 805-480-0633
Website: http://www.pituitary.org
E-mail: pna@pituitary.org

Endocrine and Metabolic Diseases Information Service
6 Information Way
Bethesda, MD 20892-3569
Toll-Free: 888-828-0904
Fax: 703-738-4929
Website: http://www.endocrine.niddk.nih.gov
E-mail: endoandmeta@info.niddk.nih.gov

Chapter 37

Pheochromocytoma

Pheochromocytoma, a rare cancer, is a disease in which cancer (malignant) cells are found in special cells in the body called chromaffin cells. Most pheochromocytomas start inside the adrenal gland (the adrenal medulla) where most chromaffin cells are located. There are two adrenal glands, one above each kidney in the back of the upper abdomen. Cells in the adrenal glands make important hormones that help the body work properly. Usually pheochromocytoma affects only one adrenal gland. Pheochromocytoma may also start in other parts of the body, such as the area around the heart or bladder.

Most tumors that start in the chromaffin cells do not spread to other parts of the body and are not cancer. These are called benign tumors. If a tumor is found, the doctor will need to determine whether it is cancer or benign.

Pheochromocytomas often cause the adrenal glands to make too many hormones called catecholamines. The extra catecholamines cause high blood pressure (hypertension), which can cause headaches, sweating, pounding of the heart, pain in the chest, and a feeling of anxiety. High blood pressure that goes on for a long time without treatment can lead to heart disease, stroke, and other major health problems.

If there are symptoms, a doctor may order blood and urine tests to see if there are extra hormones in the body. A patient may also have

PDQ® Cancer Information Summary. National Cancer Institute, Bethesda, MD. Pheochromocytoma (PDQ®): Treatment–Patient. Updated 6/2003. Available at: http://cancer.gov. Accessed 02/12/2007.

a special nuclear medicine scan. A computed tomography (CT) scan, an x-ray that uses a computer to make a picture of the inside of a part of the body, or a magnetic resonance imaging (MRI) scan, which uses magnetic waves to make a picture of the abdomen, may also be done.

Pheochromocytoma is sometimes part of a condition called multiple endocrine neoplasia syndrome (MEN). People with MEN often have other cancers (such as thyroid cancer) and other hormonal problems.

The chance of recovery (prognosis) depends on how far the cancer has spread, and the patient's age and general health.

Stage Explanation

Once pheochromocytoma is found, more tests will be done to see how far the cancer has spread. This is called staging. A doctor needs to know the stage of the disease to plan treatment. The following stages are used for pheochromocytoma.

Localized benign pheochromocytoma: Tumor is found in only one area and has not spread to other tissues. Most pheochromocytomas do not spread to other parts of the body and are not cancer.

Regional pheochromocytoma: Cancer has spread to lymph nodes in the area or to other tissues around the original cancer. (Lymph nodes are small bean-shaped structures that are found throughout the body. They produce and store infection-fighting cells.)

Metastatic pheochromocytoma: The cancer has spread to other parts of the body.

Recurrent pheochromocytoma: Recurrent disease means that the cancer has come back (recurred) after it has been treated. It may come back in the area where it started or in another part of the body.

Treatment Option Overview

There are treatments for all patients with pheochromocytoma. Three kinds of treatment are used:

- surgery (taking out the cancer)
- radiation therapy (using high-dose x-rays or other high-energy rays to kill cancer cells)
- chemotherapy (using drugs to kill cancer cells)

Surgery is the most common treatment of pheochromocytoma. A doctor may remove one or both adrenal glands in an operation called adrenalectomy. The doctor will look inside the abdomen to make sure all the cancer is removed. If the cancer has spread, lymph nodes or other tissues may also be taken out.

Chemotherapy uses drugs to kill cancer cells. Chemotherapy may be taken by pill, or it may be put into the body by a needle in the vein or muscle. Chemotherapy is called a systemic treatment because the drug enters the bloodstream, travels through the body, and can kill cancer cells throughout the body.

Radiation therapy uses high energy x-rays to kill cancer cells and shrink tumors. Radiation comes from a machine outside the body (external radiation therapy).

Treatment by Stage

Treatments for pheochromocytoma depend on the stage of the disease, and the patient's age and overall health.

Localized benign pheochromocytoma: Treatment will probably be surgery to remove one or both adrenal glands (adrenalectomy). After surgery the doctor will order blood and urine tests to make sure hormone levels return to normal.

Regional pheochromocytoma: Treatment may be one of the following:

1. Surgery to remove one or both adrenal glands (adrenalectomy) and as much of the cancer as possible. If cancer remains after surgery, drugs will be given to control high blood pressure.

2. External radiation therapy to relieve symptoms (in rare cases).

3. Chemotherapy.

Metastatic pheochromocytoma: Treatment may be one of the following:

1. Surgery to remove as much of the cancer as possible. If cancer remains after surgery, drugs will be given to control high blood pressure.

2. External radiation therapy to relieve symptoms.

3. Chemotherapy.

Recurrent pheochromocytoma: Treatment may be one of the following:

1. Surgery to remove as much of the cancer as possible. If cancer remains after surgery, drugs will be given to control high blood pressure.

2. External radiation therapy to relieve symptoms.

3. Chemotherapy.

Additional Information

National Cancer Institute (NCI)
Cancer Information Service
6116 Executive Blvd., Room 3036A
Bethesda, MD 20892-8322
Toll-Free: 800-4-CANCER (422-6237)
Toll-Free TTY: 800-332-8615
Website: http://www.cancer.gov
E-mail: cancergovstaff@mail.nih.gov

Chapter 38

Adrenal Gland Cancer

Cancer of the adrenal cortex, a rare cancer, is a disease in which cancer (malignant) cells are found in the adrenal cortex, which is the outside layer of the adrenal gland. Cancer of the adrenal cortex is also called adrenocortical carcinoma. There are two adrenal glands, one above each kidney in the back of the upper abdomen. The adrenal glands are also called the suprarenal glands. The inside layer of the adrenal gland is called the adrenal medulla. Cancer that starts in the adrenal medulla is called pheochromocytoma.

The cells in the adrenal cortex make important hormones that help the body work properly. When cells in the adrenal cortex become cancerous, they may make too much of one or more hormones, which can cause symptoms such as high blood pressure, weakening of the bones, or diabetes. If male or female hormones are affected, the body may go through changes such as a deepening of the voice, growing hair on the face, swelling of the sex organs, or swelling of the breasts. Cancers that make hormones are called functioning tumors. Many cancers of the adrenal cortex do not make extra hormones and are called nonfunctioning tumors.

A doctor should be seen if the following symptoms appear and won't go away—pain in the abdomen, loss of weight without dieting, or weakness.

PDQ® Cancer Information Summary. National Cancer Institute, Bethesda, MD. Adrenocortical Carcinoma (PDQ®): Treatment–Patient. Updated 7/2005. Available at http://cancer.gov. Accessed 02/12/2007.

If there is a functioning tumor, there may be symptoms or signs caused by too many hormones. If there are symptoms, a doctor will order blood and urine tests to see whether the amounts of hormones in the body are normal. A doctor may also order a computed tomography (CT) scan of the abdomen, a special x-ray that uses a computer to make a picture of the inside of the abdomen. Other special x-rays may also be done to tell what kind of tumor is present.

The chance of recovery (prognosis) depends on how far the cancer has spread (stage) and on whether a doctor was able to surgically remove all of the cancer.

Stages of Cancer of the Adrenal Cortex

Once cancer of the adrenal cortex has been found, more tests will be done to see how far the cancer has spread. This is called staging. A doctor needs to know the stage of the cancer to plan treatment. The following stages are used for cancer of the adrenal cortex.

Stage I: The cancer is less than five centimeters (less than two inches) and has not spread into tissues around the adrenal gland.

Stage II: The cancer is more than five centimeters (greater than two inches) and has not spread into tissues around the adrenal gland.

Stage III: The cancer has spread into tissues around the adrenal gland or has spread to the lymph nodes around the adrenal gland. Lymph nodes are part of the lymph system and are small, bean shaped organs that make and store infection-fighting cells.

Stage IV: The cancer has spread to tissues or organs in the area and to lymph nodes around the adrenal cortex, or the cancer has spread to other parts of the body.

Recurrent: The cancer has come back (recurred) after it has been treated. It may come back in the adrenal cortex or in another part of the body.

Treatment Option Overview

There are treatments for all patients with cancer of the adrenal cortex. Three kinds of treatment are used:

- surgery (taking out the cancer),

- chemotherapy (using drugs to kill cancer cells), and

- radiation therapy (using high-dose x-rays or other high-energy rays to kill cancer cells).

A doctor may take out the adrenal gland in an operation called an adrenalectomy. Tissues around the adrenal glands that contain cancer may be removed. Lymph nodes in the area may also be removed (lymph node dissection).

Chemotherapy uses drugs to kill cancer cells. Chemotherapy may be taken by pill, or it may be put into the body by a needle in a vein or muscle. Chemotherapy is called a systemic treatment because the drug enters the bloodstream, travels through the body, and kills cancer cells throughout the body.

Radiation therapy uses high-energy x-rays to kill cancer cells and shrink tumors. Radiation for cancer of the adrenal cortex usually comes from a machine outside the body (external radiation therapy).

Besides treatment for cancer (chemotherapy, radiation therapy, or surgery), a patient may also receive therapy to prevent or treat symptoms caused by the extra hormones that are made by the cancer.

Treatment by Stage

Treatment depends on how far the cancer has spread, and a patient's age and overall health. Standard treatment may be considered because of its effectiveness in past studies, or participation in a clinical trial may be considered. Not all patients are cured with standard therapy, and some standard treatments may have more side effects than are desired. For these reasons, clinical trials are designed to find better ways to treat cancer patients and are based on the most up-to-date information. Clinical trials are ongoing in some parts of the country for patients with cancer of the adrenal cortex.

Stage I: Treatment will probably be surgery to remove the cancer.

Stage II: Treatment will probably be surgery to remove the cancer. Clinical trials are testing new treatments.

Stage III: Treatment may be one of the following:

1. Surgery to remove the cancer. Lymph nodes in the area may also be removed (lymph node dissection).

2. A clinical trial of radiation therapy.

3. A clinical trial of chemotherapy if the size of the tumor can be measured with x-rays and/or if the tumor is making hormones.

Stage IV: Treatment may be one of the following:

1. Chemotherapy. Clinical trials are testing new drugs.

2. Radiation therapy to bones where the cancer has spread.

3. Surgery to remove the cancer in places where it has spread.

Recurrent: Treatment depends on many factors, including where the cancer came back and what treatment has already been received. In some cases, surgery can be effective in decreasing the symptoms of the disease by removing some of the tumor. Clinical trials are testing new treatments.

Additional Information

National Cancer Institute (NCI)
Cancer Information Service
6116 Executive Blvd., Room 3036A
Bethesda, MD 20892-8322
Toll-Free: 800-4-CANCER (422-6237)
Toll-Free TTY: 800-332-8615
Website: http://www.cancer.gov
E-mail: cancergovstaff@mail.nih.gov

Chapter 39

X-Linked Adrenal Hypoplasia Congenita (AHC)

X-linked adrenal hypoplasia congenita is a disorder that mainly affects males. It involves many hormone-producing (endocrine) tissues in the body, especially the adrenal glands (small glands on top of the kidneys). One of the main characteristics of this disorder is adrenal insufficiency, a reduction in adrenal gland function that results from incomplete development of the gland's outer layer (the adrenal cortex). Adrenal insufficiency typically begins in infancy or in childhood and can cause vomiting, difficulty with feeding, dehydration, extremely low blood sugar (hypoglycemia), and shock.

Affected males may also lack male sex hormones, which leads to underdeveloped reproductive tissues, undescended testicles (cryptorchidism), delayed puberty, and an inability to father children (infertility). These characteristics are known as hypogonadotropic hypogonadism.

Females are rarely affected by this disorder, but a few cases have been reported of adrenal insufficiency or a lack of female sex hormones, resulting in underdeveloped reproductive tissues, delayed puberty, and an absence of menstruation (hypogonadotropic hypogonadism).

How common is X-linked adrenal hypoplasia congenita?

X-linked adrenal hypoplasia congenita is estimated to affect one in 12,500 newborns.

Genetics Home Reference, National Library of Medicine, June 2006.

What genes are related to X-linked adrenal hypoplasia congenita?

Mutations in the NR0B1 gene cause X-linked adrenal hypoplasia congenita. The NR0B1 gene provides instructions to make a protein called DAX1 that helps control the activity of certain genes. Proteins that control the activity of other genes are known as transcription factors. When the NR0B1 gene is deleted or mutated, the activity of certain genes is not properly controlled. This leads to problems with the development of the adrenal glands, two structures in the brain (the hypothalamus and pituitary gland), and reproductive tissues (the ovaries or testes). These tissues are important for the production of many hormones that control various functions in the body. When these hormones are not present in the correct amounts, the signs and symptoms of adrenal insufficiency and hypogonadotropic hypogonadism can result.

How do people inherit X-linked adrenal hypoplasia congenita?

This condition is inherited in an X-linked recessive pattern. A condition is considered X-linked if the mutated gene that causes the disorder is located on the X chromosome, one of the two sex chromosomes. Males are affected by X-linked recessive disorders much more frequently than females. A striking characteristic of X-linked inheritance is that fathers cannot pass X-linked traits to their sons.

What other names do people use for X-linked adrenal hypoplasia congenita?

- adrenal hypoplasia congenita
- congenital adrenal hypoplasia
- X-linked AHC

Chapter 40

Congenital Adrenal Hyperplasia (CAH)

Congenital adrenal hyperplasia (CAH), also termed adrenogenital syndrome in older literature, is a common inherited form of adrenal insufficiency. This group of diseases is due to mutations (genetic defects) in the gene coding for several enzymes needed to produce vital adrenal cortex hormones.

About 95% of cases of CAH are caused because of lack of the enzyme 21-hydroxylase. When this enzyme is missing, or functioning at low levels, the body cannot make adequate amounts of two vital adrenal steroid hormones: cortisol and aldosterone. This causes disruption in the delicate balance of hormones. Sensing low levels of cortisol, the adrenal, directed by the master hypothalamus and pituitary glands, goes into high gear. Because cortisol production is impeded, the adrenal cortex instead manufactures androgens, or male steroid hormones, an undesired by-product.

In short, while one part of the adrenal functions poorly, making inadequate amounts of cortisol and aldosterone, another portion of the gland overproduces androgens. This last feature distinguishes CAH-21-hydroxylase deficiency from another form of adrenal insufficiency, Addison disease, since in Addisonian patients the adrenals are most often completely non-functional.

"Congenital Adrenal Hyperplasia: The Facts You Need to Know," © 2004 National Adrenal Diseases Foundation. Reprinted with permission.

Classical CAH-21-hydroxylase Deficiency

Lack of both cortisol and aldosterone predispose three-quarters of severely affected individuals with CAH to adrenal crises with dehydration and shock, or even death, if not properly diagnosed and treated. Excess adrenal androgen production begins in early fetal life in classical CAH-21 affected infants, and causes abnormal growth of the clitoris in girls and masculinization of other genital-urinary structures. Severely affected girls may be mistaken for boys at birth. Affected boys have no genital malformations at birth, but continued androgen excess causes unusually fast body growth.

Inappropriately early puberty leads to premature completion of growth and short adult height. Proper medical treatment with the class of medications called glucocorticoids resets the abnormal balance of hormones, permits near-normal growth, and puberty. Another type of medication, mineralocorticoids, preserve salt balance and help prevent adrenal crisis.

Proper surgical treatment by an experienced pediatric urologist reconstructs near-normal female genitals. Some surgeons are now able to reconstruct the vagina at the same time as they reduce the size of the clitoris in early infancy, whereas in the past surgery was at least a two-step process, finished in late adolescence. Some families may opt to defer genital surgery.

Nonclassical CAH-21-hydroxylase Deficiency

A milder, non-life-threatening form of CAH becomes manifest in later childhood or even young adult life, and is not characterized by ambiguous genitalia in girls. Rather, these individuals have a partial enzyme deficiency, and thus have better cortisol production, normal aldosterone production, and lower levels of adrenal androgens. They do not suffer adrenal crisis.

Generally, such individuals seek medical attention because of premature development of pubic hair, irregular menstrual periods, hirsutism (unwanted body hair), or severe acne. About 10–15% of these young women may suffer from fertility problems. Some people affected with nonclassical CAH are not at all symptomatic, and are identified only because of an affected relative.

Nonclassical CAH is among the most common genetic disorders, with Ashkenazi Jews having the highest prevalence. In the general population, depending on the ethnic breakdown of a given community, 1–5% may be affected with non-classical CAH. Nonclassical CAH does not progress to classical CAH in affected individuals. The symptoms of non-classical CAH are treatable with very low dose glucocorticoids. This type of treatment may be optional and need not be lifelong.

Diagnosis of CAH

The diagnosis of CAH has traditionally rested on hormone measurements combined with clinical evaluation, including history and physical examination. Most states in the U.S. as well as several foreign countries now perform a hormonal test for CAH within the first few days of life. These heel-prick blood specimens are obtained at the time when blood is drawn for thyroid tests and a number of other inherited diseases.

The rationale for newborn screening is that mainly in boys, who have no outward sign of the disease, the mortality from adrenal crisis is high, and this could be entirely prevented by early diagnosis and medical treatment. Since the incidence of classical CAH worldwide is about one in 5,000 male births (or one in 15,000 total births), this amounts to a substantial number of potentially preventable infant deaths. These screening programs have achieved their goals. Diagnostic methods are continually being refined, both for the hormonal methods, and for the newer genetic typing discussed later.

Since the advent of molecular genetic technology, we can now examine the genes of CAH patients and family members. This type of study has application for prenatal testing, neonatal screening, and genetic counseling, as well as confirming diagnosis in questionable cases. Molecular diagnosis is available in several specialized laboratories. Families should receive genetic counseling in conjunction with genetic testing, if they choose this procedure.

Just as there are potential inaccuracies in hormonal testing, there are pitfalls in genetic testing. In most cases, except in prenatal diagnosis, people affected with classical and nonclassical forms of CAH can be detected with hormone measurements alone, without genetic testing.

Standard CAH Treatment

Currently, standard medical treatment consists of giving a glucocorticoid (a cortisol-like steroid medication; for example, oral hydrocortisone in children, or prednisone or dexamethasone in older patients). In addition, those classical patients who have aldosterone deficiency (salt-wasters) need another drug, fludrocortisone (Florinef, which acts like the missing hormone, aldosterone) to be able to retain salt. Infants also receive supplemental salt (as crushed tablets or solutions), whereas older patients with classical forms of CAH eat salty foods.

Although many patients are well-managed on these types of medical regimens, it is very difficult to precisely mimic the native adrenal hormone rhythms and achieve perfect hormonal balance. Thus, most CAH patients have intermittent periods of fluctuating control with peaks and valleys in the hormones doctors use to monitor the effectiveness of treatment (specifically, 17-hydroxyprogesterone and androgens). This leads to increases in the steroid medication doses, and sometimes these become excessive. A known complication of high dose glucocorticoids is growth inhibition.

Individuals with classical CAH are about one to two standard deviations below the adult population average in height, meaning they are "short normal." A particularly important factor in determining final height in CAH patients is the amount of steroids given as treatment in the first two years of life. To preserve height potential, children with CAH should be seen frequently by a pediatric endocrinologist who not only measures blood hormone levels, but also carefully assesses height, weight, blood pressure, and an annual x-ray of the wrist (bone age x-ray).

Nonclassical CAH patients, if they require medical therapy, are usually effectively treated with low dose hydrocortisone (children), prednisone, or dexamethasone (the latter two drugs should mainly be used in older adolescents or adults). Excessive dosing with these medications may inhibit growth in young children, and may cause weight gain and/or hypertension. Girls with nonclassical CAH do not require genital surgery.

Newer Treatment Modalities

Because of these difficulties in fine-tuning medical treatment of classical, severe CAH with standard therapy, some research centers have designed experimental types of drug therapy. One such example consists of a four drug combination, with an androgen blocking agent (flutamide), an inhibitor of aromatase, an enzyme responsible for estrogen formation from androgens (testolactone), low dose hydrocortisone and fludrocortisone. Preliminary results after two years in a small group of patients are encouraging with respect to more age appropriate growth and less rapid bone fusion in the experimental group. A longer trial is in progress. Other experimental therapies involve the use of growth hormone with or without depot leuprolide (Lupron) to delay puberty.

It will take many years and many more patients in clinical trials to fully understand the safety and effectiveness of experimental therapies, since a large number of patients will have to reach final height to determine whether the short-term benefits are sustained.

A more radical suggestion for alternative CAH therapy is a surgical one: adrenalectomy. This therapy was in common use in the days before physicians had access to steroid medications. It is now suggested again for selected patients, particularly females with little- to-no enzyme activity and severe virilization that cannot readily be controlled with medications. Adrenalectomy can help avoid high dose glucocorticoids needed to control persistently high adrenal androgens.

A major motivation for considering adrenalectomy is that it can now be accomplished by laparoscopy. Laparoscopy is surgery done through one or more 1-inch incisions, with insertion of a fiberoptic light containing a tube with openings for surgical instruments. Laparoscopic appendectomy, for instance, has minimal morbidity and low potential for operative complications. Obviously, removing both adrenals leaves the patient in a vulnerable Addisonian state, and one would still have to supplement both cortisol and aldosterone equivalents.

Advocates of adrenalectomy point out that replacement hormone doses in Addisonian patients are lower than in CAH patients, and Addisonian children do not suffer from short stature, overweight, masculinization, and ill-timed puberty. However, if the patient is unwilling or unable to take his or her medications, it should be understood that there are potential dire, life-threatening consequences.

Prenatal Therapy

Prenatal therapy for CAH has been practiced since 1984. It is still considered somewhat experimental, as dexamethasone is not approved by the U.S. Food and Drug Administration (FDA), or by the European regulatory agencies, for this use. In families where one child already has CAH, parents can benefit from genetic counseling explaining how the disease is inherited, and what their options are during subsequent pregnancies.

The aim of giving dexamethasone to the pregnant woman at risk for a second CAH-affected child is to reduce secretion of androgens from the female fetus' adrenal gland, and thus reduce the chance that the baby will be born with male-like genitals. Because adrenal production of androgen begins in the mid-to-late first trimester before prenatal diagnosis is done, the treatment is begun before it is known whether the fetus is male or female, and before it is known whether the child has CAH.

Since CAH is a recessive disease, one has a 50% chance of inheriting a mutant gene from each carrier parent. The risk of an affected child is thus 25% (or 50% multiplied by 50%) in each pregnancy. Since only half of the children are female, only one in eight fetuses may benefit from prenatal treatment. Thus, seven of eight fetuses would be exposed unnecessarily to steroid treatment via placental passage of the drug given to their mothers.

Several hundred children have undergone such prenatal treatment, and cursory surveys show no major ill effects. An expert international panel urges caution in the use of prenatal dexamethasone therapy and strict monitoring of its application by hospital institutional review boards and ethics committees. It is always prudent to consider the long-term potential for unrecognized complications when experimental therapies are used.

Present and Future Directions

For the present, most patients with CAH can be reasonably well-managed with the standard diagnostic and therapeutic approaches. Molecular diagnosis does not directly add to patient well-being, but is of use in prenatal diagnosis and other genetic counseling.

Looking toward the future, important diagnostic issues are demonstrating the cost-effectiveness of newer methods of newborn screening, including molecular genetic testing. Treatment questions to be resolved will include whether either the newer experimental drug therapies or adrenalectomy improve patient outcome substantially, or whether enzyme replacement by gene therapy is a possible research breakthrough. Much work also remains in assessing outcomes among young women with respect to psychosexual development with and without surgical intervention.

Quick Facts about CAH

- CAH is an inherited disorder that affects the adrenal gland. In its classical form, this disease appears in approximately one in 15,000 births.

- CAH is caused by a deficiency of an enzyme (adrenal steroid 21-hydroxylase) necessary for the synthesis of two vital hormones, cortisol and aldosterone, by the human body. In its severest form, classical CAH results in the uncontrolled loss of salt and fluids from the body, a condition which, if undetected, can lead to adrenal crisis and death.

- One must inherit a defective enzyme trait from each parent to become affected with CAH. This is termed an autosomal recessive disease. CAH affects males and females in equal numbers.

- For parents who have had an affected child with CAH, there is a 25% (1 in 4) chance of producing a second affected child. Prenatal diagnosis, and prenatal treatment of a potentially affected fetus, are available.

- Classical CAH can be detected through newborn screening. Newborn screening for CAH saves lives.

- CAH is treatable with medications. In its classical form, CAH requires lifelong medical management.

- Classical, severe CAH can cause genital anomalies in affected females, with baby girls occasionally misidentified as boys. Whether and when to consider genital surgery for females with CAH is a question to be decided on an individual basis in conjunction with experienced health professionals.

- The non-classical form of CAH (also known as late-onset or mild CAH) presents with milder symptoms, which may appear at any time from infancy through adulthood.

- Non-classical CAH is not life-threatening, but can present serious quality of life issues for the individual affected.

- The non-classical form of CAH can result in rapid growth and premature puberty in early childhood, but in some cases shorter than expected height, hirsutism (excessive hair growth), irregular menstrual periods, acne, and more rarely, infertility in either males or females. In young women, these features may be confused with a polycystic ovary syndrome.

- The symptoms of non-classical CAH are treatable with a type of steroid hormone, glucocorticoids, in very low doses. This type of treatment may be optional and need not be life-long.

- Non-classical CAH is among the most common genetic disorders, with Ashkenazi Jews having the highest prevalence. In the general population depending on the ethnic breakdown of a given community, 1–5% may be affected with non-classical CAH.

- Non-classical CAH does not progress to classical CAH in affected individuals.

- Since marriage between two individuals with non-classical CAH may, in a minority of cases, result in the birth of a child with classical CAH, those affected by any form of CAH, or with a close family member affected by the condition, should consider undergoing genetic counseling.

- Doctors, legislators, and members of those populations most often affected by CAH, as well as the general public, need to be educated about the disease and its symptoms, and newborn screening for CAH will eventually become mandatory.

Additional Information

CARES Foundation, Inc.
Congenital Adrenal Hyperplasia Support
2414 Morris Ave., Suite 110
Union, NJ 07083
Toll-Free: 866-227-3737
Phone: 973-912-3895
Fax: 973-912-8990
Website: http://www.caresfoundation.org

National Adrenal Diseases Foundation (NADF)
505 Northern Blvd.
Great Neck, NY 11021
Phone: 516-487-4992
Fax: 516-829-5710
Website: http://www.nadf.us
E-mail: nadfmail@aol.com

Chapter 41

Exogenous Adrenal Insufficiency

Alternative name: Drug-induced adrenal insufficiency

Definition

Exogenous adrenal insufficiency is a condition of low levels of hormones released by the adrenal glands, caused by factors other than problems with the glands themselves. See Addison disease for information on adrenal deficiency caused by problems within these glands.

Causes, Incidence, and Risk Factors

Glucocorticoid medications such as prednisone, hydrocortisone, and dexamethasone are similar to natural hormones produced by the adrenal glands. They are used to treat a variety of conditions, including many inflammatory diseases such as asthma and some forms of arthritis.

Treatment with glucocorticoids can slow down the production of adrenal hormones, because of the effect the medicine has on the pituitary gland, the master gland that controls the adrenal glands.

If glucocorticoids are stopped or decreased too quickly, the adrenal glands may not begin making their own hormones again fast enough to meet the body's needs, and symptoms of adrenal insufficiency result. This condition usually occurs when these drugs are given by pills or injections, rather than on the skin, or when they are given in inhaled forms. Higher doses and longer treatments increase the risk of adrenal insufficiency.

Abruptly stopping treatment with glucocorticoids is the most common cause of adrenal insufficiency.

Other drugs that may cause adrenal insufficiency include the following:

- megestrol
- ketoconazole
- metyrapone
- aminoglutethimide
- mitotane

These drugs have direct effects on the adrenal glands, decreasing glucocorticoid production.

Symptoms

Symptoms may include:

- weakness
- fatigue
- nausea and vomiting
- arthralgias (joint pains), myalgias (muscle pains)
- low blood pressure (hypotension), which may cause light-headedness or fainting when the affected person stands after sitting or lying down
- shock

Signs and Tests

Typically, a patient who has been taking steroids and has developed this condition will have physical characteristics similar to a person with Cushing syndrome (round face, obesity around the waist, streaks on the stomach area), while having symptoms of adrenal insufficiency.

Tests will look for:

- low cortisol level

- low sodium
- hypoglycemia (low sugar)
- depressed response to adrenocorticotropic hormone (ACTH)

Treatment

Treatment consists of giving additional glucocorticoids. Higher doses are needed in stressful situations (such as during infections, or prior to and after surgery).

Expectations (Prognosis)

Patients usually get better with treatments of glucocorticoids. The long-term outlook depends on the degree of dependence on these drugs, and any resulting complications. If glucocorticoids treatment is no longer needed for the original condition, the drugs can be very slowly tapered (dosage decreased gradually, over time), under the supervision of a physician.

The length of the taper can extend over many months, and some level of withdrawal symptoms is likely.

Complications

Complications include ongoing steroid dependence, and need for stress-situation steroids treatments for an unknown length of time. Complications related to steroid use, such as diabetes, high blood pressure, and osteoporosis, may also occur.

Serious complications include adrenal crisis, which requires immediate treatment with glucocorticoids. Symptoms include dizziness, nausea and vomiting, and extreme fatigue, which usually follow a stress on the body such as dehydration, infection, or another illness or injury. Adrenal crisis can generally be prevented by increasing (doubling or tripling) the steroid dose during illness or other physical stress.

Calling Your Health Care Provider

Call your health care provider if you are taking glucocorticoid drugs and experience any of the symptoms of adrenal insufficiency. If the symptoms are severe, go to the emergency room or call 911.

People with adrenal insufficiency should wear a Medic-Alert tag to alert health care professionals to this condition in case of emergency.

Prevention

Using glucocorticoids for the shortest time possible, in the smallest dose possible, using alternate-day steroids (taking steroids every other day, instead of daily), and use of steroid-sparing agents (for treatment of asthma or arthritis, for example) may help minimize development of exogenous adrenal insufficiency. Persons using inhaled steroids can lessen their exposure to these steroids by using a spacer, and by rinsing their mouths out after the inhalation.

Chapter 42

Managing Adrenal Insufficiency

This information was developed by the patient care staff of the National Institutes of Health (NIH) Clinical Center to help patients with adrenal insufficiency (AI) understand their condition and how to take care of it. It explains what causes adrenal insufficiency and how it can be controlled. If left untreated, adrenal insufficiency can cause serious illness or death. But by working with their doctors and nurses, patients can learn how to manage this condition.

What are the adrenal glands?

Your body has two adrenal glands. Each gland is located above a kidney. The adrenal glands secrete many hormones needed for the body's normal functioning.

Cortisol helps the body use sugar and protein for energy and enables the body to recover from infections and stresses (for example, surgery, illness). Aldosterone maintains the right amount of salt, potassium, and water in the body.

What is adrenal insufficiency?

Adrenal insufficiency means that there are not enough adrenal hormones. Without the right levels of these hormones, your body cannot maintain essential life functions. Adrenal insufficiency can occur

National Institutes of Health (NIH) Clinical Center, March 30, 2005.

because of a problem with the adrenal glands, themselves. In this case, there is not enough cortisol or aldosterone.

Adrenal insufficiency can also occur when the pituitary gland does not make enough adrenocorticotropic hormone (ACTH). ACTH stimulates cortisol production. In this case, there is enough aldosterone but not enough cortisol.

Adrenal insufficiency may be permanent or temporary. When AI is permanent, medication must be taken daily for the rest of the patient's life. Causes of permanent AI include the following:

- Addison disease
- CAH (congenital adrenal hyperplasia)
- complete surgical removal of the pituitary gland
- surgical removal of the adrenals

Temporary adrenal insufficiency is brought on by physical stress, infection, surgery, or when the proper medication is not taken. Causes of temporary AI include:

- transsphenoidal surgery (for Cushing disease or for another reason) that removes a tumor from the pituitary gland;
- removal of a tumor that has been causing the adrenal glands to make too much cortisol; and
- medical treatment for Cushing syndrome with drugs that lower cortisol levels.

What are the signs and symptoms of adrenal insufficiency?

When your essential life functions are not being maintained because of a lack of adrenal hormones, you will not feel well. Your symptoms could include the following:

- unusual tiredness and weakness
- dizziness when standing up
- nausea, vomiting, diarrhea
- loss of appetite
- stomach ache

Other symptoms you may experience over time include these:

- weight loss

- darkened skin
- craving for salt

If any of these symptoms appear, and you know that you are at risk for AI, call your local doctor immediately.

What medication is used to treat AI?

To keep your AI under control, you must take medication daily. This medication is in pill form and must be taken in the amounts and at the times prescribed by your doctor. This medication is often referred to as your replacement dose. To replace the hormone cortisol, adults usually take hydrocortisone, prednisone, or dexamethasone. Children sometimes take liquid hydrocortisone.

You may be told to take your medication once a day or twice a day. Be sure to follow the instructions for taking your medication.

If your body cannot maintain the right levels of sodium (salt) and fluids, because of too little aldosterone, you will also be given a drug called fludrocortisone (Florinef). This drug replaces aldosterone, oral or injectable hydrocortisone.

Adults usually take tablets of Florinef. Children with AI who have trouble swallowing pills can take Florinef tablets dissolved in water or crushed.

What are the side effects of these drugs?

Replacement doses of hydrocortisone cause almost no side effects. Sometimes, however, an upset stomach may occur. If this happens, take your medication with meals. If you notice anything else out of the ordinary, call your local doctor.

What do I do when I do not feel well?

There may be times when you do not feel well. You may be working too hard (physical stress) or worried about something (psychological stress). Even though you may feel a little blue, be sure to take the right amount of medication at the right time of day.

There may also be times when you will need to take more than your normal replacement dose of hydrocortisone. Normally functioning adrenal glands produce more hydrocortisone when the body is under the physical stress of fever (over 100 degrees Fahrenheit), infection, surgery, vomiting, or diarrhea.

The fact that you have AI means that your body cannot deal with these stresses by making more hydrocortisone. Just as you must replace your basic hydrocortisone needs with your replacement dose, you must also replace your increased needs with an extra dose of oral or injectable hydrocortisone. If you are sick, call your local doctor right away. Ask if you should take extra hydrocortisone, and if so, how much to take.

What if I am so ill that I cannot take my medication?

If you are too ill to take your pills, or you cannot keep them down, you must take medicine by injection. You or someone who lives with you will need to learn how to give you this injection.

The shot will take the place of both hydrocortisone and Florinef pills. If you find it necessary to give yourself injectable medication, call your local doctor immediately or go to the nearest hospital emergency room.

How much medicine should I take once I feel better?

As soon as your illness is over and the symptoms are gone (for example, fever, vomiting, diarrhea), you can usually return to taking your usual amount of medication. But you should discuss this with your local doctor.

How do I give myself an injection?

Injectable hydrocortisone is given intramuscularly, which means that it is injected into a large muscle. When giving yourself an injection, the easiest and best place to give it is in the thigh on the same side as your dominant hand (for example, the right thigh if you are right handed). Adults should always carry injectable medication with them. If you have a child with AI, you or the child's caregiver must always carry the child's medication. If the child is in school, the school nurse must know about your child's condition and be able to provide such emergency care as giving an injection of hydrocortisone.

What else do I need to know about adrenal insufficiency?

You can control adrenal insufficiency by taking an active role in your care. Taking care of yourself involves:

• learning about your disease;

- taking your medication every day;
- recognizing stress in your life and taking special care of yourself during stressful times;
- getting regular medical check-ups; and
- wearing a Medic-Alert bracelet at all times.

If you follow the guidelines here and the instructions of your health care team, you will be able to lead a full and productive life. Only you can take care of yourself.

How to Give an Injection of Hydrocortisone

1. Wash your hands.

2. Assemble your equipment.

3. Mix the medication vial by pushing down on top of the vial to release the cork.

4. Shake the vial to mix the medication solution well.

5. Use alcohol to clean the rubber stopper on the vial.

6. Take the cap off the syringe needle and insert the needle into the vial.

7. Draw up the medication. Adults should use all the medication in the vial For a child, use the dose prescribed by the doctor.

8. Replace the needle cap.

9. Select the site for your injection. To inject yourself safely, become familiar with your body. Uncover your thigh and look at it. Now, draw an imaginary line in the middle of your thigh to divide it in half lengthwise. The outer part is where you will be injecting. Now, imagine your thigh divided into three equal parts, from the knee to the hip. The outer part of the inner third of your thigh is where you will do the injection.

10. Use alcohol to cleanse the injection site on your skin.

11. Remove the cap from the needle. Hold the syringe like a dart.

12. Using your thumb and first two fingers, spread your skin while pushing down lightly.

13. Dart the needle into the thigh injection site, going straight in at a 90-degree angle.

14. Hold the syringe in place. Pull back the plunger to make sure you are not injecting into a large blood vessel. If blood appears in the syringe, withdraw the syringe and discard it. (However, if this is the only dose of medication you have, inject the medication anyway.) If you have another dose, prepare another syringe with medication and inject yourself in a slightly different site.

15. After injecting the medication, place tissue or gauze near the needle, and pull the needle out quickly.

16. Massage the injection site gently.

17. Place the syringe and needle in a hard, unbreakable container (such as an empty coffee can with a lid) before disposing of it.

Chapter 43

Laparoscopic Adrenal Gland Removal

What are the adrenal glands?

The adrenal glands are two small organs, one located above each kidney. They are triangular in shape and about the size of a thumb. The adrenal glands are known as endocrine glands because they produce hormones. These hormones are involved in control of blood pressure, chemical levels in the blood, water use in the body, glucose usage, and the fight or flight reaction during times of stress. These adrenal-produced hormones include cortisol, aldosterone, the adrenaline hormones—epinephrine and norepinephrine—and a small fraction of the body's sex hormones (estrogen and androgens).

What causes adrenal gland problems?

Diseases of the adrenal gland are relatively rare. The most common reason that a patient may need to have the adrenal gland removed is excess hormone production by a tumor located within the adrenal. Most of these tumors are small and not cancers. They are known as benign growths that can usually be removed with laparoscopic techniques. Removal of the adrenal gland may also be required for certain tumors even if they aren't producing excess hormones, such as very large tumors, or if there is a suspicion that the tumor could be a cancer which is sometimes referred to as malignant. Fortunately, malignant adrenal tumors are rare. An adrenal mass or tumor is sometimes found by chance when a patient gets an x-ray study to evaluate another problem.

What are the symptoms of adrenal gland problems?

Patients with adrenal gland problems may have a variety of symptoms related to excess hormone production by the abnormal gland. Adrenal tumors associated with excess hormone production include pheochromocytomas, aldosterone-producing tumors, and cortisol-producing tumors. Some of these tumors and their typical features are listed.

- Pheochromocytomas produce excess hormones that can cause very high blood pressure and periodic spells characterized by severe headaches, excessive sweating, anxiety, palpitations, and rapid heart rate that may last from a few seconds to several minutes.

- Aldosterone producing tumors cause high blood pressure and low serum (blood) potassium levels. In some patients this may result in symptoms of weakness, fatigue, and frequent urination.

- Cortisol producing tumors cause a syndrome termed Cushing syndrome that can be characterized by obesity (especially of the face and trunk), high blood sugar, high blood pressure, menstrual irregularities, fragile skin, and prominent stretch marks. Most cases of Cushing syndrome, however, are caused by small pituitary tumors and are not treated by adrenal gland removal. Overall, adrenal tumors account for about 20% of cases of Cushing syndrome.

- An incidentally found mass in the adrenal may be any of the above types of tumors, or may produce no hormones at all. Most incidentally found adrenal masses do not make excess hormones, cause no symptoms, are benign, and do not need to be removed. Surgical removal of incidentally discovered adrenal tumors is indicated only if:
  - The tumor is found to make excess hormones.
  - The tumor is large in size (more than 4–5 centimeters or 2 inches in diameter).

- There is a suspicion that the tumor could be malignant.

- Adrenal gland cancers (adrenal cortical cancer) are rare tumors that are usually very large at the time of diagnosis. Removal of these tumors is usually done by open adrenal surgery.

If an adrenal tumor is suspected based on symptoms or has been identified by x-ray, the patient should undergo blood and urine tests to determine if the tumor is over-producing hormones. Special x-ray tests, such as a computed tomography (CT) scan, nuclear medicine scan, a magnetic resonance imaging (MRI) or selective venous sampling are commonly used to locate the suspected adrenal tumor.

Surgical removal of the adrenal gland is the preferred treatment for patients with adrenal tumors that secrete excess hormones and for primary adrenal tumors that appear malignant.

What are the advantages of laparoscopic adrenal gland removal?

In the past, making a large 6–12 inch incision in the abdomen, flank, or back was necessary for removal of an adrenal gland tumor. Today, with the technique known as minimally invasive surgery, removal of the adrenal gland (also known as laparoscopic adrenalectomy) can be performed through three or four, quarter- to half-inch incisions. Patients may leave the hospital in one or two days and return to work more quickly than patients recovering from open surgery.

Results of surgery may vary depending on the type of procedure and the patients overall condition. Common advantages are:

- less postoperative pain,

- shorter hospital stay,

- quicker return to normal activity,

- improved cosmetic result, and

- reduced risk of herniation or wound separation.

Are you a candidate for laparoscopic adrenal gland removal?

Although laparoscopic adrenal gland removal has many benefits, it may not be appropriate for some patients. Obtain a thorough medical evaluation by a surgeon qualified in laparoscopic adrenal gland

313

removal in consultation with your primary care physician or endocrinologist to find out if the technique is appropriate for you.

What preparation is required?

Prior to the operation, some patients may need medications to control the symptoms of the tumor, such as high blood pressure.

- Patients with a pheochromocytoma will need to be started on special medications several days prior to surgery to control their blood pressure and heart rate.

- Patients with an aldosterone-producing tumor may need to have their serum potassium checked and take extra potassium if the level is low.

- Patients with Cushing syndrome will need to receive extra doses of cortisone medication on the day of surgery and for a few months afterwards until the remaining adrenal gland has resumed normal function.

- Preoperative preparation includes blood work, medical evaluation, chest x-ray, and an EKG depending on your age and medical condition.

- After your surgeon reviews with you the potential risks and benefits of the operation, you will need to provide written consent for surgery.

- Blood transfusion and/or blood products may be needed depending on your condition.

- Your surgeon may request that you completely empty your colon and cleanse your intestines prior to surgery. You may be requested to drink clear liquids only, for one or several days prior to surgery.

- It is recommended that you shower the night before or morning of the operation.

- After midnight the night before the operation, you should not eat or drink anything except medications that your surgeon has told you are permissible to take with a sip of water the morning of surgery.

- Drugs such as aspirin, blood thinners, anti-inflammatory medications (arthritis medications), and large doses of vitamin E will need to be stopped temporarily for several days to a week prior to surgery.

- Diet medication or St. John's Wort should not be used for the two weeks prior to surgery.

- Quit smoking and arrange for any help you may need at home.

How is laparoscopic adrenal gland removal performed?

- The surgery is performed under a complete general anesthesia, so that the patient is asleep during the procedure.

- A cannula (a narrow tube-like instrument) is placed into the abdominal cavity in the upper abdomen or flank just below the ribs.

- A laparoscope (a tiny telescope) connected to a special camera is inserted through the cannula. This gives the surgeon a magnified view of the patient's internal organs on a television screen.

- Other cannulas are inserted which allow your surgeon to delicately separate the adrenal gland from its attachments. Once the adrenal gland has been dissected free, it is placed in a small bag and is then removed through one of the incisions. It is almost always necessary to remove the entire adrenal gland in order to safely remove the tumor.

- After the surgeon removes the adrenal gland, the small incisions are closed.

What happens if the procedure cannot be performed laparoscopically?

In a small number of patients the laparoscopic method cannot be performed. In that situation, the operation is converted to an open procedure. Factors that may increase the possibility of choosing or converting to the open procedure may include:

- obesity;

- a history of prior abdominal surgery causing dense scar tissue;

- inability to visualize the adrenal gland clearly;

- bleeding problems during the operation; or

- large tumor size (over 3 or 4 inches in diameter).

The decision to perform the open procedure is a judgment decision made by your surgeon either before or during the actual operation. When the surgeon feels that it is safest to convert the laparoscopic procedure to an open one, it is not a complication, but rather sound surgical judgment. The decision to convert to an open procedure is strictly based on patient safety.

What should I expect after surgery?

After the operation, it is important to follow your doctor's instructions. Although many people feel better in just a few days, remember that your body needs time to heal.

- After laparoscopic adrenal gland removal, most patients can be cared for on a regular surgical nursing unit. Occasionally, a patient with a pheochromocytoma may require admission to an intensive care unit after surgery to monitor their blood pressure. Most patients can be discharged from the hospital within one or two days after surgery.

- Patients with an aldosterone-producing tumor will need to have their serum potassium level checked after surgery and may need to continue to take medications to control their blood pressure.

- Patients with cortisol-producing tumors and Cushing syndrome will need to take prednisone or cortisol pills after surgery. The dose is then tapered over time as the remaining normal adrenal gland resumes adequate production of cortisol hormone.

- Patients are encouraged to engage in light activity while at home after surgery. Patients can remove any dressings and shower the day after the operation.

- Postoperative pain is generally mild and patients may require a pain pill or pain medication.

- Most patients can resume normal activities within one week, including driving, walking up stairs, light lifting, and work.

- You should call and schedule a follow-up appointment within two weeks after your operation.

What complications can occur?

As with any operation, there is a risk of a complication. Complications during the operation may include:

- adverse reaction to general anesthesia
- high blood pressure
- bleeding
- injury to other organs

Wound problems, blood clots, heart attacks, and other serious complications are uncommon after laparoscopic adrenalectomy.

When to Call Your Doctor

Be sure to call your physician or surgeon if you develop any of the following:

- persistent fever over 101° F (39° C)
- bleeding
- increasing abdominal swelling
- pain that is not relieved by your medications
- persistent nausea or vomiting
- chills
- persistent cough or shortness of breath
- purulent drainage (pus) from any incision
- redness surrounding any of your incisions that is worsening or getting bigger
- inability to eat or drink liquids

This information is not intended to take the place of your discussion with your surgeon about the need for adrenal gland surgery. If you have questions about your need for adrenal gland surgery, your alternatives billing or insurance coverage, or your surgeon's training and experience, do not hesitate to ask your surgeon or his or her office staff about it. If you have questions about the operation or subsequent follow-up, please discuss them with your surgeon before or after the operation.

Part Five

Pancreatic and Diabetic Disorders

Chapter 44

Pancreas Function Tests

Secretin Stimulation Test

The secretin stimulation test measures the ability of the pancreas to respond to the hormone secretin. The small intestines produce secretin in the presence of partially digested food. Normally, secretin stimulates the pancreas to secrete a fluid with a high concentration of bicarbonate. This fluid neutralizes stomach acid and is necessary for a number of enzymes to function in the breakdown and absorption of food. People with diseases involving the pancreas (for example, cystic fibrosis or pancreatic cancer) might have abnormal pancreatic function.

In performing a secretin stimulation test, a health care professional places a tube down the throat, into the stomach, then into the duodenum (upper section of small intestine). Secretin is administered and the contents of the duodenal secretions are aspirated (removed with suction) and analyzed over a period of about two hours.

Fecal Elastase Test

The fecal elastase test measures elastase, an enzyme found in fluids produced by the pancreas. Elastase digests and degrades various kinds of proteins. During this test, a patient's stool sample is analyzed for the presence of elastase.

Computed Tomography (CT) Scan with Contrast Dye

This scan can help rule out other causes of abdominal pain and also can determine whether tissue is dying (pancreatic necrosis). CT can identify complications such as fluid around the pancreas, a collection of pus (abscess), or a collection of tissue, fluid, and pancreatic enzymes (pseudocyst).

Abdominal Ultrasound

An abdominal ultrasound can detect gallstones and fluid from inflammation in the abdomen (ascites). It also can show an enlarged common bile duct, an abscess, or a pseudocyst.

Endoscopic Retrograde Cholangiopancreatography (ERCP)

During an ERCP, a health care professional places a tube down the throat, into the stomach, then into the small intestine. Dye is used to help the doctor see the structure of the common bile duct, other bile ducts, and the pancreatic duct on an x-ray.

Endoscopic Ultrasound

During this test, a probe attached to a lighted scope is placed down the throat and into the stomach. Sound waves show images of organs in the abdomen. Endoscopic ultrasound might reveal gallstones and can be helpful in diagnosing severe pancreatitis when an invasive test, such as ERCP, might make the condition worse.

Magnetic Resonance Cholangiopancreatography

This kind of magnetic resonance imaging (MRI) can be used to look at the bile ducts and the pancreatic duct.

Chapter 45

Pancreatitis

Pancreatitis is an inflammation of the pancreas. The pancreas is a large gland behind the stomach and close to the duodenum. The duodenum is the upper part of the small intestine. The pancreas secretes digestive enzymes into the small intestine through a tube called the pancreatic duct. These enzymes help digest fats, proteins, and carbohydrates in food. The pancreas also releases the hormones insulin and glucagon into the bloodstream. These hormones help the body use the glucose it takes from food for energy.

Normally, digestive enzymes do not become active until they reach the small intestine, where they begin digesting food. But if these enzymes become active inside the pancreas, they start "digesting" the pancreas itself.

Acute pancreatitis occurs suddenly and lasts for a short period of time and usually resolves itself. Chronic pancreatitis does not resolve itself and results in a slow destruction of the pancreas. Either form can cause serious complications. In severe cases, bleeding, tissue damage, and infection may occur. Pseudocysts, accumulations of fluid and tissue debris, may also develop. And enzymes and toxins may enter the bloodstream, injuring the heart, lungs, and kidneys, or other organs.

Acute Pancreatitis

Some people have more than one attack and recover completely after each, but acute pancreatitis can be a severe, life-threatening illness

National Institute of Diabetes and Digestive and Kidney Diseases (NIDDK), NIH Publication No. 04–1596, February 2004.

with many complications. About 80,000 cases occur in the United States each year; some 20 percent of them are severe. Acute pancreatitis occurs more often in men than women.

Acute pancreatitis is usually caused by gallstones or by drinking too much alcohol, but these are not the only causes. If alcohol use and gallstones are ruled out, other possible causes of pancreatitis should be carefully examined so that appropriate treatment, if available, can begin.

Symptoms

Acute pancreatitis usually begins with pain in the upper abdomen that may last for a few days. The pain may be severe and may become constant—just in the abdomen—or it may reach to the back and other areas. It may be sudden and intense or begin as a mild pain that gets worse when food is eaten. Someone with acute pancreatitis often looks and feels very sick. Other symptoms may include:

• swollen and tender abdomen

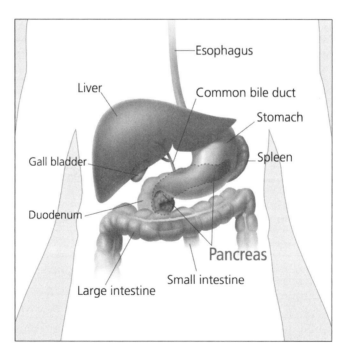

Figure 45.1. *The Pancreas and Nearby Organs (Source: National Cancer Institute, NIH Publication 01–1560, revised July 2001).*

- nausea
- vomiting
- fever
- rapid pulse

Severe cases may cause dehydration and low blood pressure. The heart, lungs, or kidneys may fail. If bleeding occurs in the pancreas, shock, and sometimes even death, follow.

Diagnosis

Besides asking about a person's medical history and doing a physical exam, a doctor will order a blood test to diagnose acute pancreatitis. During acute attacks, the blood contains at least three times more amylase and lipase than usual. Amylase and lipase are digestive enzymes formed in the pancreas. Changes may also occur in blood levels of glucose, calcium, magnesium, sodium, potassium, and bicarbonate. After the pancreas improves, these levels usually return to normal.

A doctor may also order an abdominal ultrasound to look for gallstones and a computerized axial tomography (CAT) scan to look for inflammation or destruction of the pancreas. CAT scans are also useful in locating pseudocysts.

Treatment

Treatment depends on the severity of the attack. If no kidney or lung complications occur, acute pancreatitis usually improves on its own. Treatment, in general, is designed to support vital bodily functions and prevent complications. A hospital stay will be necessary so that fluids can be replaced intravenously.

If pancreatic pseudocysts occur and are considered large enough to interfere with the pancreas's healing, your doctor may drain or surgically remove them.

Unless the pancreatic duct or bile duct is blocked by gallstones, an acute attack usually lasts only a few days. In severe cases, a person may require intravenous feeding for 3–6 weeks while the pancreas slowly heals. This process is called total parenteral nutrition. However, for mild cases of the disease, total parenteral nutrition offers no benefit.

Before leaving the hospital, a person will be advised not to drink alcohol and not to eat large meals. After all signs of acute pancreatitis are gone, the doctor will try to decide what caused it in order to prevent future attacks. In some people, the cause of the attack is clear, but in others, more tests are needed.

Complications

Acute pancreatitis can cause breathing problems. Many people develop hypoxia, which means that cells and tissues are not receiving enough oxygen. Doctors treat hypoxia by giving oxygen through a face mask. Despite receiving oxygen, some people still experience lung failure and require a ventilator.

Sometimes a person cannot stop vomiting and needs to have a tube placed in the stomach to remove fluid and air. In mild cases, a person may not eat for three or four days, and instead may receive fluids and pain relievers through an intravenous line.

If an infection develops, the doctor may prescribe antibiotics. Surgery may be needed for extensive infections. Surgery may also be necessary to find the source of bleeding, to rule out problems that resemble pancreatitis, or to remove severely damaged pancreatic tissue.

Acute pancreatitis can sometimes cause kidney failure. If your kidneys fail, you will need dialysis to help your kidneys remove wastes from your blood.

Gallstones and Pancreatitis

Gallstones can cause pancreatitis and they usually require surgical removal. Ultrasound or a CAT scan can detect gallstones and can sometimes give an idea of the severity of the pancreatitis. When gallstone surgery can be scheduled depends on how severe the pancreatitis is. If the pancreatitis is mild, gallstone surgery may proceed within about a week. More severe cases may mean gallstone surgery is delayed for a month or more. After the gallstones are removed and inflammation goes away, the pancreas usually returns to normal.

Chronic Pancreatitis

If injury to the pancreas continues, chronic pancreatitis may develop. Chronic pancreatitis occurs when digestive enzymes attack and destroy the pancreas and nearby tissues, causing scarring and pain. The usual cause of chronic pancreatitis is many years of alcohol abuse, but the chronic form may also be triggered by only one acute attack, especially if the pancreatic ducts are damaged. The damaged ducts cause the pancreas to become inflamed, tissue to be destroyed, and scar tissue to develop.

While common, alcoholism is not the only cause of chronic pancreatitis. The main causes of chronic pancreatitis are:

- alcoholism,
- blocked or narrowed pancreatic duct due to trauma or pseudocysts,
- heredity, or an
- unknown cause (idiopathic).

Damage from alcohol abuse may not appear for many years, and then a person may have a sudden attack of pancreatitis. In up to 70 percent of adult patients, chronic pancreatitis appears to be caused by alcoholism. This form is more common in men than in women and often develops between the ages of 30 and 40.

Hereditary pancreatitis usually begins in childhood but may not be diagnosed for several years. A person with hereditary pancreatitis usually has the typical symptoms that come and go over time. Episodes last from two days to two weeks. A determining factor in the diagnosis of hereditary pancreatitis is two or more family members with pancreatitis in more than one generation. Treatment for individual attacks is usually the same as it is for acute pancreatitis. Any pain or nutrition problems are treated just as they are for acute pancreatitis. Surgery can often ease pain and help manage complications.

Other causes of chronic pancreatitis are:

- congenital conditions such as pancreas divisum,
- cystic fibrosis,
- high levels of calcium in the blood (hypercalcemia),
- high levels of blood fats (hyperlipidemia or hypertriglyceridemia),
- some drugs, and
- certain autoimmune conditions.

Symptoms

Most people with chronic pancreatitis have abdominal pain, although some people have no pain at all. The pain may get worse when eating or drinking, spread to the back, or become constant and disabling.

In certain cases, abdominal pain goes away as the condition advances, probably because the pancreas is no longer making digestive enzymes. Other symptoms include nausea, vomiting, weight loss, and fatty stools.

People with chronic disease often lose weight, even when their appetite and eating habits are normal. The weight loss occurs because the body does not secrete enough pancreatic enzymes to break down food, so nutrients are not absorbed normally. Poor digestion leads to excretion of fat, protein, and sugar into the stool. If the insulin-producing cells of the pancreas (islet cells) have been damaged, diabetes may also develop at this stage.

Diagnosis

Diagnosis may be difficult, but new techniques can help. Pancreatic function tests help a doctor decide whether the pancreas is still making enough digestive enzymes. Using ultrasonic imaging, endoscopic retrograde cholangiopancreatography (ERCP), and CAT scans, a doctor can see problems indicating chronic pancreatitis. Such problems include calcification of the pancreas, in which tissue hardens from deposits of insoluble calcium salts. In more advanced stages of the disease, when diabetes and malabsorption occur, a doctor can use a number of blood, urine, and stool tests to help diagnose chronic pancreatitis and to monitor its progression.

Treatment

Relieving pain is the first step in treating chronic pancreatitis. The next step is to plan a diet that is high in carbohydrates and low in fat.

A doctor may prescribe pancreatic enzymes to take with meals if the pancreas does not secrete enough of its own. The enzymes should be taken with every meal to help the body digest food and regain some weight. Sometimes insulin or other drugs are needed to control blood glucose.

In some cases, surgery is needed to relieve pain. The surgery may involve draining an enlarged pancreatic duct or removing part of the pancreas. For fewer and milder attacks, people with pancreatitis must stop drinking alcohol, stick to their prescribed diet, and take the proper medications.

Pancreatitis in Children

Chronic pancreatitis is rare in children. Trauma to the pancreas and hereditary pancreatitis are two known causes of childhood pancreatitis.

Children with cystic fibrosis—a progressive, disabling, and incurable lung disease—may also have pancreatitis. But more often the cause is not known.

Points to Remember

- Pancreatitis begins when the digestive enzymes become active inside the pancreas and start "digesting" it.

- Pancreatitis has two forms—acute and chronic.

- Common causes of pancreatitis are gallstones or alcohol abuse.

- Sometimes no cause for pancreatitis can be found.

- Symptoms of acute pancreatitis include pain in the abdomen, nausea, vomiting, fever, and a rapid pulse.

- Treatment for acute pancreatitis can include intravenous fluids, oxygen, antibiotics, or surgery.

- Acute pancreatitis becomes chronic when pancreatic tissue is destroyed and scarring develops.

- Treatment for chronic pancreatitis includes easing the pain; eating a high-carbohydrate, low-fat diet; and taking enzyme supplements. Surgery is sometimes needed as well.

For More Information

American Gastroenterological Association
4930 Del Ray Avenue
Bethesda, MD 20814
Phone: 301-654-2055
Fax: 301-654-5920
Website: http://www.gastro.org
E-mail: member@gastro.org

National Digestive Diseases Information Clearinghouse
2 Information Way
Bethesda, MD 20892-3570
Toll-Free: 800-891-5389
Fax: 703-738-4929
Website: http://digestive.niddk.nih.gov
E-mail: nddic@info.niddk.nih.gov

Chapter 46

Insulin Resistance and Prediabetes

Insulin resistance is a silent condition that increases the chances of developing diabetes and heart disease. Learning about insulin resistance is the first step you can take toward making lifestyle changes that will help you prevent diabetes and other health problems.

What does insulin do?

After you eat, the food is broken down into glucose, the simple sugar that is the main source of energy for the body's cells. But your cells cannot use glucose without insulin, a hormone produced by the pancreas. Insulin helps the cells take in glucose and convert it to energy. When the pancreas does not make enough insulin or the body is unable to use the insulin that is present, the cells cannot use glucose. Excess glucose builds up in the bloodstream, setting the stage for diabetes.

Being obese or overweight affects the way insulin works in your body. Extra fat tissue can make your body resistant to the action of insulin, but exercise helps insulin work well.

How are insulin resistance, prediabetes, and type 2 diabetes linked?

If you have insulin resistance, your muscle, fat, and liver cells do not use insulin properly. The pancreas tries to keep up with the demand

National Institute of Diabetes and Digestive and Kidney Diseases (NIDDK), NIH Publication No. 06–4893, August 2006.

for insulin by producing more. Eventually, the pancreas cannot keep up with the body's need for insulin, and excess glucose builds up in the bloodstream. Many people with insulin resistance have high levels of blood glucose and high levels of insulin circulating in their blood at the same time.

People with blood glucose levels that are higher than normal, but not yet in the diabetic range, have prediabetes. Doctors sometimes call this condition impaired fasting glucose (IFG) or impaired glucose tolerance (IGT), depending on the test used to diagnose it. Prediabetes is becoming more common in the United States, according to new estimates provided by the U.S. Department of Health and Human Services. About 40 percent of U.S. adults ages 40 to 74—or 41 million people—had prediabetes in 2000. New data suggest that at least 54 million U.S. adults had prediabetes in 2002.

If you have prediabetes, you have a higher risk of developing type 2 diabetes, formerly called adult-onset diabetes or noninsulin-dependent diabetes. Studies have shown that most people with prediabetes go on to develop type 2 diabetes within ten years, unless they lose 5–7 percent of their body weight—which is about 10–15 pounds for someone who weighs 200 pounds—by making modest changes in their diet and level of physical activity. People with prediabetes also have a higher risk of heart disease.

Type 2 diabetes is sometimes defined as the form of diabetes that develops when the body does not respond properly to insulin, as opposed to type 1 diabetes, in which the pancreas makes no insulin at all. At first, the pancreas keeps up with the added demand by producing more insulin. In time, however, it loses the ability to secrete enough insulin in response to meals. Insulin resistance can also occur in people who have type 1 diabetes, especially if they are overweight.

What causes insulin resistance?

Because insulin resistance tends to run in families, we know that genes are partly responsible. Excess weight also contributes to insulin resistance because too much fat interferes with muscles' ability to use insulin. Lack of exercise further reduces muscles' ability to use insulin.

Many people with insulin resistance and high blood glucose have excess weight around the waist, high low density lipoprotein (LDL) or bad blood cholesterol levels, low high density lipoprotein (HDL) or good cholesterol levels, high levels of triglycerides (another fat in the blood), and high blood pressure—all conditions that also put the heart at risk.

This combination of problems is referred to as the metabolic syndrome, or the insulin resistance syndrome (formerly called syndrome X).

What are the symptoms of insulin resistance and prediabetes?

Insulin resistance and prediabetes usually have no symptoms. You may have one or both conditions for several years without noticing anything. If you have a severe form of insulin resistance, you may get dark patches of skin, usually on the back of your neck. Sometimes people get a dark ring around their neck. Other possible sites for these dark patches include elbows, knees, knuckles, and armpits. This condition is called acanthosis nigricans. If you have a mild or moderate form of insulin resistance, blood tests may show normal or high blood glucose and high levels of insulin at the same time.

Do you have insulin resistance or prediabetes?

Anyone 45 years or older should consider getting tested for diabetes. If you are overweight and aged 45 or older, it is strongly recommended that you get tested. You should consider getting tested if you are younger than 45, overweight, and have one or more of the following risk factors:

- family history of diabetes;
- low HDL cholesterol and high triglycerides;
- high blood pressure;
- history of gestational diabetes (diabetes during pregnancy) or gave birth to a baby weighing more than nine pounds; or
- minority group background (African American, American Indian, Hispanic American/Latino, or Asian American/Pacific Islander).

Diabetes and prediabetes can be detected with one of the following tests:

A fasting glucose test measures your blood glucose after you have gone overnight without eating. This test is most reliable when done in the morning. Fasting glucose levels of 100 to 125 milligram per deciliter (mg/dL) are above normal but not high enough to be called diabetes. This condition is called prediabetes or impaired fasting glucose, and it suggests that you have probably had insulin resistance for some time. IFG is considered a pre-diabetic state, meaning that you are more likely to develop diabetes, but do not have it yet.

A glucose tolerance test measures your blood glucose after an overnight fast and two hours after you drink a sweet liquid provided by the doctor or laboratory. If your blood glucose falls between 140 and 199 mg/dL two hours after drinking the liquid, your glucose tolerance is above normal but not high enough for diabetes. This condition, also a form of prediabetes, is called impaired glucose tolerance and, like IFG, it points toward a history of insulin resistance and a risk for developing diabetes.

These tests give only indirect evidence of insulin resistance. The test that most accurately measures insulin resistance is too complicated and expensive to use as a screening tool in most doctors' offices. The test, called the euglycemic clamp, is a research tool that helps scientists learn more about sugar metabolism problems. Insulin resistance can also be assessed with measurement of fasting insulin. If conventional tests show that you have IFG or IGT, your doctor may suggest changes in diet and exercise to reduce your risk of developing diabetes. If your blood glucose is higher than normal but lower than the diabetes range, have your blood glucose checked in 1–2 years.

Lab Tests and What They Show

* **Blood glucose:** High blood glucose may be a sign that your body does not have enough insulin or does not use it well. However, a fasting measurement or oral glucose tolerance test gives more precise information.

* **Insulin:** An insulin measurement helps determine whether a high blood glucose reading is the result of insufficient insulin or poor use of insulin.

* **Fasting glucose:** Your blood glucose level should be lower after several hours without eating. After an overnight fast, the normal level is below 100 mg/dL. If it is in the 100 to 125 mg/dL range, you have impaired fasting glucose or prediabetes. A result of 126 or higher, if confirmed on a repeat test, indicates diabetes.

* **Glucose tolerance:** Your blood glucose level will be higher after drinking a sugar solution, but it should still be below 140 mg/dL two hours after the drink. If it is higher than normal (in the 140 to 199 mg/dL range) two hours after drinking the solution, you have IGT or prediabetes, which is another strong indication that

your body has trouble using glucose. A level of 200 or higher, if confirmed, means diabetes is already present.

Can you reverse insulin resistance?

Yes. Physical activity and weight loss make the body respond better to insulin. By losing weight and being more physically active, you may avoid developing type 2 diabetes. In fact, a major study has verified the benefits of healthy lifestyle changes and weight loss. In 2001, the National Institutes of Health completed the Diabetes Prevention Program (DPP), a clinical trial designed to find the most effective ways of preventing type 2 diabetes in overweight people with prediabetes. The researchers found that lifestyle changes reduced the risk of diabetes by 58 percent. Also, many people with prediabetes returned to normal blood glucose levels. The main goal in treating insulin resistance and prediabetes is to help your body relearn to use insulin normally. You can do several things to help reach this goal.

Be Active and Eat Well

Physical activity helps your muscle cells use blood glucose because they need it for energy. Exercise makes those cells more sensitive to insulin. The DPP confirmed that people who follow a low-fat, low-calorie diet and who increase activities such as walking briskly or riding a bike for 30 minutes, five times a week, have a far smaller risk of developing diabetes than people who do not exercise regularly. The DPP also reinforced the importance of a low-calorie, low-fat diet. Following a low-calorie, low-fat diet can provide two benefits. If you are overweight, one benefit is that limiting your calorie and fat intake can help you lose weight. DPP participants who lost weight were far less likely to develop diabetes than others in the study who remained at an unhealthy weight. Increasing your activity and following a low-calorie, low-fat diet can also improve your blood pressure and cholesterol levels and has many other health benefits. Scientists have established some numbers to help people set goals that will reduce their risk of developing glucose metabolism problems.

Weight

Body mass index (BMI) is a measure used to evaluate body weight relative to height. You can use BMI to find out whether you are underweight, normal weight, overweight, or obese. Use Table 46.1 to find your BMI.

335

- Find your height in the left-hand column.

- Move across in the same row to the number closest to your weight.

- The number at the top of that column is your BMI. A BMI between 19 and 24 is considered normal, between 25 and 29 overweight, and 30 and more obese. If you are overweight or obese, talk with your doctor about ways to lose weight to reduce your risk of diabetes.

Blood Pressure

Blood pressure is expressed as two numbers that represent pressure in your blood vessels when your heart is beating (systolic pressure) and when it is resting (diastolic pressure). The numbers are usually written with a slash—for example, 140/90, which is expressed as "140 over 90." For the general population, blood pressure below 130/85 is considered normal, although people whose blood pressure is slightly elevated and who have no additional risk factors for heart disease may be advised to make lifestyle changes—that is, diet and exercise—rather than take blood pressure medicines. People who have diabetes, however, should take whatever steps necessary, including lifestyle changes and medicine, to reach a blood pressure goal of below 130/80.

Cholesterol

Your cholesterol is usually reported with three values: low density lipoprotein (LDL) cholesterol, high density lipoprotein (HDL) cholesterol, and total cholesterol. LDL cholesterol is sometimes called bad cholesterol, while HDL cholesterol is called good cholesterol. To lower your risk of cardiovascular problems if you have diabetes, you should try to keep your LDL cholesterol below 100 and your total cholesterol below 200. If you have metabolic syndrome, your doctor may recommend weight loss with diet and exercise, as well as medication to lower your cholesterol and blood pressure levels.

Stop Smoking

In addition to increasing your risk of cancer and cardiovascular disease, smoking contributes to insulin resistance. Quitting smoking is not easy, but it could be the single smartest thing you can do to improve your health. You will reduce your risk for respiratory problems, lung cancer, and diabetes.

Can Medicines Help?

Two classes of drugs can improve response to insulin and are used by prescription for type 2 diabetes—biguanides and thiazolidinediones. Other medicines used for diabetes act by other mechanisms. Alpha-glucosidase inhibitors restrict or delay the absorption of carbohydrates after eating, resulting in a slower rise of blood glucose levels. Sulfonylureas and meglitinides increase insulin production.

Table 46.1. *Body Mass Index Table (Source: Excerpted from "The Practical Guide: Identification, Evaluation, and Treatment of Overweight and Obesity in Adults," National Heart, Lung, and Blood Institute (NHLBI), NIH Publication Number 00-4084, October 2000).*

BMI	19	20	21	22	23	24	25	26	27	28	29	30	31	32	33	34	35
Height (inches)							Body Weight (pounds)										
58	91	96	100	105	110	115	119	124	129	134	138	143	148	153	158	162	167
59	94	99	104	109	114	119	124	128	133	138	143	148	153	158	163	168	173
60	97	102	107	112	118	123	128	133	138	143	148	153	158	163	168	174	179
61	100	106	111	116	122	127	132	137	143	148	153	158	164	169	174	180	185
62	104	109	115	120	126	131	136	142	147	153	158	164	169	175	180	186	191
63	107	113	118	124	130	135	141	146	152	158	163	169	175	180	186	191	197
64	110	116	122	128	134	140	145	151	157	163	169	174	180	186	192	197	204
65	114	120	126	132	138	144	150	156	162	168	174	180	186	192	198	204	210
66	118	124	130	136	142	148	155	161	167	173	179	186	192	198	204	210	216
67	121	127	134	140	146	153	159	166	172	178	185	191	198	204	211	217	223
68	125	131	138	144	151	158	164	171	177	184	190	197	203	210	216	223	230
69	128	135	142	149	155	162	169	176	182	189	196	203	209	216	223	230	236
70	132	139	146	153	160	167	174	181	188	195	202	209	216	222	229	236	243
71	136	143	150	157	165	172	179	186	193	200	208	215	222	229	236	243	250
72	140	147	154	162	169	177	184	191	199	206	213	221	228	235	242	250	258
73	144	151	159	166	174	182	189	197	204	212	219	227	235	242	250	257	265
74	148	155	163	171	179	186	194	202	210	218	225	233	241	249	256	264	272
75	152	160	168	176	184	192	200	208	216	224	232	240	248	256	264	272	279
76	156	164	172	180	189	197	205	213	221	230	238	246	254	263	271	279	287

BMI	36	37	38	39	40	41	42	43	44	45	46	47	48	49	50	51	52	53	54
58	172	177	181	186	191	196	201	205	210	215	220	224	229	234	239	244	248	253	258
59	178	183	188	193	198	203	208	212	217	222	227	232	237	242	247	252	257	262	267
60	184	189	194	199	204	209	215	220	225	230	235	240	245	250	255	261	266	271	276
61	190	195	201	206	211	217	222	227	232	238	243	248	254	259	264	269	275	280	285
62	196	202	207	213	218	224	229	235	240	246	251	256	262	267	273	278	284	289	295
63	203	208	214	220	225	231	237	242	248	254	259	265	270	278	282	287	293	299	304
64	209	215	221	227	232	238	244	250	256	262	267	273	279	285	291	296	302	308	314
65	216	222	228	234	240	246	252	258	264	270	276	282	288	294	300	306	312	318	324
66	223	229	235	241	247	253	260	266	272	278	284	291	297	303	309	315	322	328	334
67	230	236	242	249	255	261	268	274	280	287	293	299	306	312	319	325	331	338	344
68	236	243	249	256	262	269	276	282	289	295	302	308	315	322	328	335	341	348	354
69	243	250	257	263	270	277	284	291	297	304	311	318	324	331	338	345	351	358	365
70	250	257	264	271	278	285	292	299	306	313	320	327	334	341	348	355	362	369	376
71	257	265	272	279	286	293	301	308	315	322	329	338	343	351	358	365	372	379	386
72	265	272	279	287	294	302	309	316	324	331	338	346	353	361	368	375	383	390	397
73	272	280	288	295	302	310	318	325	333	340	348	355	363	371	378	386	393	401	408
74	280	287	295	303	311	319	326	334	342	350	358	365	373	381	389	396	404	412	420
75	287	295	303	311	319	327	335	343	351	359	367	375	383	391	399	407	415	423	431
76	295	304	312	320	328	336	344	353	361	369	377	385	394	402	410	418	426	435	443

The DPP showed that the diabetes drug metformin, a biguanide, reduced the risk of diabetes in those with prediabetes but was much less successful than losing weight and increasing activity. In another study, treatment with troglitazone, a thiazolidinedione later withdrawn from the market following reports of liver toxicity, delayed or prevented type 2 diabetes in Hispanic women with a history of gestational diabetes. Acarbose, an alpha-glucosidase inhibitor, has been effective in delaying development of type 2 diabetes. Additional studies using other diabetes medicines and some types of blood pressure medicines to prevent diabetes are underway. No drug has been approved by the Food and Drug Administration (FDA) specifically for insulin resistance or prediabetes.

Hope Through Research

Researchers sponsored by the National Institute of Diabetes and Digestive and Kidney Diseases conducted the DPP to find the most effective ways to prevent or delay the onset of type 2 diabetes. Volunteers were recruited from groups known to be at particularly high risk for IGT and type 2 diabetes. The study was designed to compare the effectiveness of lifestyle changes (weight loss through exercise and diet) with drug therapy (metformin). A control group received a placebo and information on diet and exercise. Participants assigned to the intensive lifestyle intervention reduced their risk of getting type 2 diabetes by 58 percent over three years. Participants treated with metformin reduced their risk by 31 percent. Metformin is not currently approved for use in preventing diabetes, but the FDA may determine whether to make diabetes prevention an added indication for this drug. In any event, the DPP demonstrates that a healthy diet and exercise are the most effective treatment for insulin resistance and the prediabetic states of IFG and IGT.

Points to Remember

- Glucose is the simple sugar that is the main source of energy for the body's cells.

- Insulin helps cells take in blood glucose and convert it to energy.

- If you have insulin resistance, your body's cells do not respond well to insulin.

- Insulin resistance is a stepping-stone to type 2 diabetes.

- Lack of exercise and excess weight contribute to insulin resistance.

- Engaging in moderate physical activity and maintaining proper weight can help prevent insulin resistance.

- Insulin resistance plays a role in the development of cardiovascular disease, which damages the heart and blood vessels.

- Controlling blood pressure and LDL cholesterol and not smoking can also help prevent cardiovascular problems.

- The Diabetes Prevention Program confirmed that exercise and a low-calorie, low-fat diet are the best ways to prevent type 2 diabetes.

Additional Information

American Diabetes Association
1701 N. Beauregard St.
Alexandria, VA 22311
Toll-Free: 800-DIABETES (342-2383)
Fax: 703-549-6995
Website: http://www.diabetes.org
E-mail: customerservice@diabetes.org

National Diabetes Information Clearinghouse
1 Information Way
Bethesda, MD 20892–3560
Toll-Free: 800-860-8747
Phone: 301-654-3327
Fax: 703-738-4929
Website: http://diabetes.niddk.nih.gov
E-mail: ndic@info.niddk.nih.gov

Additional information about the Diabetes Prevention Program (DPP) is available on the internet at http://diabetes.niddk.nih.gov/dm/pubs/preventionprogram/index.htm.

Chapter 47

Diabetes Mellitus

Diagnosis of Diabetes

Diabetes is a disease in which blood glucose levels are above normal. People with diabetes have problems converting food to energy. After a meal, food is broken down into a sugar called glucose, which is carried by the blood to cells throughout the body. Cells use insulin, a hormone made in the pancreas, to help them convert blood glucose into energy.

People develop diabetes because the pancreas does not make enough insulin or because the cells in the muscles, liver, and fat do not use insulin properly, or both. As a result, the amount of glucose in the blood increases while the cells are starved of energy. Over the years, high blood glucose, also called hyperglycemia, damages nerves and blood vessels, which can lead to complications such as heart disease and stroke, kidney disease, blindness, nerve problems, gum infections, and amputation.

Types of Diabetes

The three main types of diabetes are type 1, type 2, and gestational diabetes.

This chapter includes: "Diagnosis of Diabetes," National Institute of Diabetes and Digestive and Kidney Diseases (NIDDK), NIH Publication No. 05–4642, January 2005; and, "What I Need to Know about Physical Activity and Diabetes," NIDDK, NIH Publication No. 04–5180, June 2004.

- **Type 1 diabetes**, formerly called juvenile diabetes, is usually first diagnosed in children, teenagers, or young adults. In this form of diabetes, the beta cells of the pancreas no longer make insulin because the body's immune system has attacked and destroyed them.

- **Type 2 diabetes**, formerly called adult-onset diabetes, is the most common form. People can develop it at any age, even during childhood. This form of diabetes usually begins with insulin resistance, a condition in which muscle, liver, and fat cells do not use insulin properly. At first, the pancreas keeps up with the added demand by producing more insulin. In time, however, it loses the ability to secrete enough insulin in response to meals.

- **Gestational diabetes** develops in some women during the late stages of pregnancy. Although this form of diabetes usually goes away after the baby is born, a woman who has had it is more likely to develop type 2 diabetes later in life. Gestational diabetes is caused by the hormones of pregnancy or by a shortage of insulin.

To move away from basing the names of the two main types of diabetes on treatment or age at onset, an American Diabetes Association expert committee recommended in 1997 universal adoption of simplified terminology. The National Institute of Diabetes and Digestive and Kidney Diseases (NIDDK) agrees.

Table 47.1. Preferred Names for Diabetes

Former Names	Preferred Names
Type I	type 1 diabetes
juvenile diabetes	
insulin-dependent diabetes mellitus (IDDM)	
Type II	type 2 diabetes
adult-onset diabetes	
noninsulin-dependent diabetes mellitus (NIDDM)	

Prediabetes

In prediabetes, blood glucose levels are higher than normal but not high enough to be characterized as diabetes. However, many people with prediabetes develop type 2 diabetes within ten years. Prediabetes also increases the risk of heart disease and stroke. With modest weight loss and moderate physical activity, people with prediabetes can delay or prevent type 2 diabetes.

Diagnosing Diabetes and Prediabetes

The following tests are used for diagnosis:

- **A fasting plasma glucose test** measures your blood glucose after you have gone at least eight hours without eating. This test is used to detect diabetes or prediabetes.

- **An oral glucose tolerance test** measures your blood glucose after you have gone at least eight hours without eating and two hours after you drink a glucose-containing beverage. This test can be used to diagnose diabetes or prediabetes.

- **In a random plasma glucose test**, your doctor checks your blood glucose without regard to when you ate your last meal. This test, along with an assessment of symptoms, is used to diagnose diabetes but not prediabetes.

Positive test results should be confirmed by repeating the fasting plasma glucose test or the oral glucose tolerance test on a different day.

Fasting Plasma Glucose (FPG) Test

The FPG is the preferred test for diagnosing diabetes due to convenience and is most reliable when done in the morning. Results and their meaning are shown in Table 47.2. If your fasting glucose level is 100 to 125 milligrams per deciliter (mg/dL), you have a form of prediabetes called impaired fasting glucose (IFG), meaning that you are more likely to develop type 2 diabetes but do not have it yet. A

Table 47.2. Fasting Plasma Glucose Test

Plasma Glucose Result (mg/dL)	Diagnosis
99 and below	Normal
100 to 125	Prediabetes (impaired fasting glucose)
126 and above	Diabetes (Confirmed by repeating the test on a different day.)

level of 126 mg/dL or above, confirmed by repeating the test on another day, means that you have diabetes.

Oral Glucose Tolerance Test (OGTT)

Research has shown that the OGTT is more sensitive than the FPG test for diagnosing prediabetes, but it is less convenient to administer. The OGTT requires you to fast for at least eight hours before the test. Your plasma glucose is measured immediately before and two hours after you drink a liquid containing 75 grams of glucose dissolved in water. Results and what they mean are shown in Table 47.3. If your blood glucose level is between 140 and 199 mg/dL two hours after drinking the liquid, you have a form of prediabetes called impaired glucose tolerance or IGT, meaning that you are more likely to develop type 2 diabetes but do not have it yet. A 2-hour glucose level of 200 mg/dL or above, confirmed by repeating the test on another day, means that you have diabetes.

Table 47.3. Oral Glucose Tolerance Test

2-Hour Plasma Glucose Result (mg/dL)	Diagnosis
139 and below	Normal
140 to 199	Prediabetes (impaired glucose tolerance)
200 and above	Diabetes (Confirmed by repeating the test on a different day.)

Gestational diabetes is also diagnosed based on plasma glucose values measured during the OGTT. Blood glucose levels are checked four times during the test. If your blood glucose levels are above normal at least twice during the test, you have gestational diabetes. Table 47.4 shows the above-normal results for the OGTT for gestational diabetes.

Random Plasma Glucose Test

A random blood glucose level of 200 mg/dL or more, plus presence of the following symptoms, can mean that you have diabetes:

- increased urination
- increased thirst
- unexplained weight loss

Other symptoms include fatigue, blurred vision, increased hunger, and sores that do not heal. Your doctor will check your blood glucose level on another day using the FPG or the OGTT to confirm the diagnosis.

Factors that Increase Risk for Type 2 Diabetes

To find out your risk, note each item that applies to you.

- I am 45 or older.
- I am overweight or obese (see the body mass index [BMI] in Table 46.1).
- I have a parent, brother, or sister with diabetes.
- My family background is African American, American Indian, Asian American, Pacific Islander, or Hispanic American/Latino.
- I have had gestational diabetes, or I gave birth to at least one baby weighing more than nine pounds.
- My blood pressure is 140/90 or higher, or I have been told that I have high blood pressure.
- My cholesterol levels are not normal. My HDL cholesterol (good cholesterol) is 35 or lower, or my triglyceride level is 250 or higher.
- I am fairly inactive. I exercise fewer than three times a week.

If you are overweight, under 45 years of age, and have one or more of the risk factors, you should consider testing. If you are over 45, you should consider testing.

Table 47.4. Gestational Diabetes: Above-Norma Results for the Oral Glucose Tolerance Test

When	Plasma Glucose Result (mg/dL)
Fasting	95 or higher
At 1 hour	180 or higher
At 2 hours	155 or higher
At 3 hours	140 or higher

Note: Some laboratories use other numbers for this test.

Checking Your Weight

Body mass index (BMI) is a measure used to evaluate body weight relative to height. You can use BMI to find out whether you are underweight, normal weight, overweight, or obese. Use Table 46.1 [on page 337] to find your BMI. If you are overweight or obese, talk with your doctor about ways to lose weight to reduce your risk of diabetes or prediabetes.

Diabetes Testing

Anyone 45 years old or older should consider getting tested for diabetes. If you are 45 or older and your BMI indicates that you are overweight (see Table 46.1), it is strongly recommended that you get tested. If you are younger than 45, are overweight, and have one or more of the risk factors, you should consider testing. Ask your doctor for a FPG or an OGTT. Your doctor will tell you if you have normal blood glucose, prediabetes, or diabetes. If your blood glucose is higher than normal but lower than the diabetes range (called prediabetes), have your blood glucose checked in 1–2 years.

Preventing or Delaying Type 2 Diabetes

A major research study, the Diabetes Prevention Program, confirmed that people who followed a low-fat, low-calorie diet, lost a modest amount of weight, and engaged in regular physical activity (walking briskly for 30 minutes, five times a week, for example) sharply reduced their chances of developing diabetes. These strategies worked well for both men and women and were especially effective for participants aged 60 and older.

Managing Diabetes

If you are diagnosed with diabetes, you can manage it with meal planning, physical activity, and, if needed, medications.

Physical Activity and Diabetes

How can I take care of my diabetes?

Diabetes means that your blood glucose (also called blood sugar) is too high. Your body uses glucose for energy. But having too much glucose in your blood can hurt you. When you take care of your diabetes, you'll feel better. You'll reduce your risk for problems with your kidneys, eyes, nerves, feet and legs, and teeth. You'll also lower your risk for a heart attack or a stroke. You can take care of your diabetes by:

- being physically active;
- following a healthy meal plan; and/or
- taking medicines (if prescribed by your doctor).

What can a physically active lifestyle do for me?

Research has shown that physical activity can:

- lower your blood glucose and your blood pressure;
- lower your bad cholesterol and raise your good cholesterol;
- improve your body's ability to use insulin;
- lower your risk for heart disease and stroke;
- keep your heart and bones strong;
- keep your joints flexible;
- lower your risk of falling;
- help you lose weight;
- reduce your body fat;
- give you more energy; and
- reduce your stress.

Physical activity also plays an important part in preventing type 2 diabetes. A major government study, the Diabetes Prevention Program (DPP), showed that a healthy diet and a moderate exercise program resulting in a 5–7 percent weight loss can delay and possibly prevent type 2 diabetes.

What kinds of physical activity can help me?

Four kinds of activity can help. You can try:

- being extra active every day,
- doing aerobic exercise,
- doing strength training, or
- stretching.

347

Be Extra Active Every Day: Being extra active can increase the number of calories you burn. There are many ways to be extra active.

• Walk around while you talk on the phone.

• Play with the kids.

• Take the dog for a walk.

• Get up to change the television channel instead of using the remote control.

• Work in the garden or rake leaves.

• Clean the house.

• Wash the car.

• Stretch out your chores. For example, make two trips to take the laundry downstairs instead of one.

• Park at the far end of the shopping center lot and walk to the store.

• At the grocery store, walk down every aisle.

• At work, walk over to see a co-worker instead of calling or e-mailing.

• Take the stairs instead of the elevator.

• Stretch or walk around instead of taking a coffee break and eating.

• During your lunch break, walk to the post office or do other errands.

Do Aerobic Exercise: Aerobic exercise is activity that requires the use of large muscles and makes your heart beat faster. You will also breathe harder during aerobic exercise. Doing aerobic exercise for 30 minutes a day, most days of the week, provides many benefits. You can even split up those 30 minutes into several parts. For example, you can take three brisk 10-minute walks, one after each meal.

If you have not exercised lately, see your doctor first to make sure it is okay for you to increase your level of physical activity. Talk with your doctor about how to warm up and stretch before exercise and how to cool down after exercise. Then start slowly with 5–10 minutes a day. Add a little more time each week, aiming for 150 to 200 minutes per week. Try:

• walking briskly

- hiking
- climbing stairs
- swimming or taking a water-aerobics class
- dancing
- riding a bicycle outdoors or a stationary bicycle indoors
- taking an aerobics class
- playing basketball, volleyball, or other sports
- in-line skating, ice skating, or skate boarding
- playing tennis
- cross-country skiing

Do Strength Training: Doing exercises with hand weights, elastic bands, or weight machines two or three times a week builds muscle. When you have more muscle and less fat, you will burn more calories because muscle burns more calories than fat, even between exercise sessions. Strength training can help make daily chores easier, improving your balance and coordination, as well as your bones' health. You can do strength training at home, at a fitness center, or in a class. Your health care team can tell you more about strength training and what kind is best for you.

Stretch: Stretching increases your flexibility, lowers stress, and helps prevent muscle soreness after other types of exercise. Your health care team can tell you what kind of stretching is best for you.

Can I exercise any time I want?

Ask your health care team about the best time of day for you to exercise. Consider your daily schedule, your meal plan, and your diabetes medications in deciding when to exercise.

If you exercise when your blood glucose is above 300, your level can go even higher. It is best not to exercise until your blood glucose is lower. Also, exercise is not recommended if your fasting blood glucose is above 250 and you have ketones in your urine.

Are there any types of physical activity I should not do?

If you have diabetes complications, some exercises can make your problems worse. For example, activities that increase the pressure in the blood vessels of your eyes, such as lifting heavy weights, can make diabetic eye problems worse. If nerve damage from diabetes has made your feet numb, your doctor may suggest that you try swimming instead of walking for aerobic exercise.

Numbness means that you may not feel any pain from sores or blisters on your feet and so may not notice them. Then they can get worse and lead to more serious problems. Make sure you exercise in cotton socks and comfortable, well-fitting shoes that are designed for the activity you are doing. After you exercise, check your feet for cuts, sores, bumps, or redness. Call your doctor if any foot problems develop.

Can physical activity cause low blood glucose?

Physical activity can cause hypoglycemia (low blood glucose) in people who take insulin or certain diabetes pills, including sulfonylureas and meglitinides. Ask your health care team whether your diabetes pills can cause hypoglycemia. Some types of diabetes pills do not.

Hypoglycemia can happen while you exercise, right afterward, or even up to a day later. It can make you feel shaky, weak, confused, irritable, hungry, or tired. You may sweat a lot or get a headache. If your blood glucose drops too low, you could pass out or have a seizure. However, you should still be physically active. These steps can help you be prepared for hypoglycemia:

Before exercise: Be careful about exercising if you have skipped a recent meal. Check your blood glucose. If it is below 100, have a small snack. If you take insulin, ask your health care team whether you should change your dosage before you exercise.

During exercise: Wear your medical identification or other identification. Always carry food or glucose tablets so that you will be ready to treat hypoglycemia. If you will be exercising for more than an hour, check your blood glucose at regular intervals. You may need snacks before you finish.

After exercise: Check to see how exercise affected your blood glucose level.

Treating hypoglycemia. If your blood glucose is 70 or lower, have one of the following right away:

- 2 or 3 glucose tablets
- ½ cup (4 ounces) of any fruit juice
- ½ cup (4 ounces) of a regular (not diet) soft drink
- 1 cup (8 ounces) of milk
- 5 or 6 pieces of hard candy
- 1 or 2 teaspoons of sugar or honey

After 15 minutes, check your blood glucose again. If it is still too low, have another serving. Repeat until your blood glucose is 70 or higher. If it will be an hour or more before your next meal, have a snack as well.

What should I do first?

Check with your doctor. Always talk with your doctor before you start a new physical activity program. Ask about your medications—prescription and over-the-counter—and whether you should change the amount you take before you exercise. If you have heart disease, kidney disease, eye problems, or foot problems, ask which types of physical activity are safe for you.

Decide exactly what you'll do and set some goals. Choose:

- the type of physical activity you want to do;
- the clothes and items you'll need to get ready;
- the days and times you'll add activity;
- the length of each session;
- your warm up and cool down plan for each session;
- alternatives, such as where you'll walk if the weather is bad; and
- your measures of progress.

Find an exercise buddy. Many people find that they are more likely to do something active if a friend joins them. If you and a friend plan to walk together, for example, you may be more likely to do it.

Keep track of your physical activity. Write down when you exercise and for how long in your blood glucose record book. You will be able to track your progress and to see how physical activity affects your blood glucose.

Decide how you will reward yourself. Do something nice for yourself when you reach your activity goals. For example, treat yourself to a movie or buy a new plant for the garden.

What can I do to make sure I stay active?

One of the keys to staying on track is finding some activities you like to do. If you keep finding excuses not to exercise, think about why. Are your goals realistic? Do you need a change in activity? Would another time be more convenient? Keep trying until you find a routine that works for you. Once you make physical activity a habit, you will wonder how you lived without it.

Points to Remember

- Diabetes and prediabetes are diagnosed by checking blood glucose levels.

- Many people with prediabetes develop type 2 diabetes within 10 years.

- If you have prediabetes, you can delay or prevent type 2 diabetes with a low-fat, low-calorie diet, modest weight loss, and regular physical activity.

- If you are 45 or older, you should consider getting tested for diabetes. If you are 45 or older and overweight, it is strongly recommended that you get tested.

- If you are younger than 45, are overweight, and have one or more of the risk factors, you should consider testing.

For More Information

American Diabetes Association
National Service Center
1701 North Beauregard Street
Alexandria, VA 22311
Toll-Free: 800-DIABETES (342-2383)
Fax: 703-549-6995
Website: http://www.diabetes.org
E-mail: askada@diabetes.org

Juvenile Diabetes Research Foundation (JDRF)
120 Wall Street
New York, NY 10005-4001
Toll-Free: 800-533-CURE (2873)
Fax: 212-785-9595
Website: http://www.jdrf.org
E-mail: info@jdrf.org

National Diabetes Education Program (NDEP)
1 Diabetes Way
Bethesda, MD 20814-9692
Toll-Free: 800-438-5383
Phone: 301-496-3583
Website: http://www.ndep.nih.gov
E-mail: ndep@mail.nih.gov

Chapter 48

Hypoglycemia

Hypoglycemia, also called low blood sugar, occurs when your blood glucose (blood sugar) level drops too low to provide enough energy for your body's activities. In adults or children older than ten years, hypoglycemia is uncommon except as a side effect of diabetes treatment, but it can result from other medications or diseases, hormone or enzyme deficiencies, or tumors.

Glucose, a form of sugar, is an important fuel for your body. Carbohydrates are the main dietary sources of glucose. Rice, potatoes, bread, tortillas, cereal, milk, fruit, and sweets are all carbohydrate-rich foods. After a meal, glucose molecules are absorbed into your bloodstream and carried to the cells, where they are used for energy. Insulin, a hormone produced by your pancreas, helps glucose enter cells. If you take in more glucose than your body needs at the time, your body stores the extra glucose in your liver and muscles in a form called glycogen. Your body can use the stored glucose whenever it is needed for energy between meals. Extra glucose can also be converted to fat and stored in fat cells.

When blood glucose begins to fall, glucagon, another hormone produced by the pancreas, signals the liver to break down glycogen and release glucose causing blood glucose levels to rise toward a normal level. If you have diabetes, this glucagon response to hypoglycemia may be impaired, making it harder for your glucose levels to return to the normal range.

National Institute of Diabetes and Digestive and Kidney Diseases (NIDDK), NIH Publication No. 03-3926, March 2003.

Symptoms of Hypoglycemia

- hunger
- nervousness and shakiness
- perspiration
- dizziness or light-headedness
- sleepiness
- confusion
- difficulty speaking
- feeling anxious or weak

Hypoglycemia can also happen while you are sleeping. You might:

- cry out or have nightmares;
- find that your pajamas or sheets are damp from perspiration; or
- feel tired, irritable, or confused when you wake up.

Hypoglycemia: A Side Effect of Diabetes Medications

Hypoglycemia can occur in people with diabetes who take certain medications to keep their blood glucose levels in control. Usually hypoglycemia is mild and can easily be treated by eating or drinking something with carbohydrate. But left untreated, hypoglycemia can lead to loss of consciousness. Although hypoglycemia can happen suddenly, it can usually be treated quickly, bringing your blood glucose level back to normal.

Causes of Hypoglycemia

In people taking certain blood-glucose lowering medications, blood glucose can fall too low for a number of reasons, such as:

- meals or snacks that are too small, delayed, or skipped;
- excessive doses of insulin or some diabetes medications, including sulfonylureas and meglitinides (Alpha-glucosidase inhibitors, biguanides, and thiazolidinediones alone should not cause hypoglycemia but can when used with other diabetes medicines.);
- increased activity or exercise; or
- excessive drinking of alcohol.

Prevention

Your diabetes treatment plan is designed to match your medication dosage and schedule to your usual meals and activities. If you take insulin but then skip a meal, the insulin will still lower your blood glucose, but it will not find the food it is designed to break down. This mismatch might result in hypoglycemia. To help prevent hypoglycemia, you should keep in mind several things.

Your diabetes medications. Some medications can cause hypoglycemia. Ask your health care provider if yours can. Also, always take medications and insulin in the recommended doses and at the recommended times.

Ask your doctor the following questions about your diabetes medications:

- Could my diabetes medication cause hypoglycemia?
- When should I take my diabetes medication?
- How much should I take?
- Should I keep taking my diabetes medication if I am sick?
- Should I adjust my medication before exercise?

Your meal plan. Meet with a registered dietitian and agree on a meal plan that fits your preferences and lifestyle. Do your best to follow this meal plan most of the time. Eat regular meals, have enough food at each meal, and try not to skip meals or snacks.

Your daily activity. Talk to your health care team about whether you should have a snack or adjust your medication before sports or exercise. If you know that you will be more active than usual, or will be doing something that is not part of your normal routine such as shoveling snow, consider having a snack first.

Alcoholic beverages. Drinking, especially on an empty stomach, can cause hypoglycemia, even a day or two later. If you drink an alcoholic beverage, always have a snack or meal at the same time.

Your diabetes management plan. Intensive diabetes management—keeping your blood glucose as close to the normal range as possible to prevent long-term complications—can increase the risk of hypoglycemia. If your goal is tight control, talk to your health care team about ways to prevent hypoglycemia and how best to treat it if it does occur.

Treatment

If you think your blood glucose is too low, use a blood glucose meter to check your level. If it is 70 milligrams per deciliter (mg/dL) or less, have one of these quick fix foods right away to raise your blood glucose:

- 2 or 3 glucose tablets
- ½ cup (4 ounces) of any fruit juice
- ½ cup (4 ounces) of a regular (not diet) soft drink
- 1 cup (8 ounces) of milk
- 5 or 6 pieces of hard candy
- 1 or 2 teaspoons of sugar or honey

After 15 minutes, check your blood glucose again to make sure that it is no longer too low. If it is still too low, have another serving. Repeat these steps until your blood glucose is at least 70. Then, if it will be an hour or more before your next meal, have a snack.

If you take insulin or a medication for diabetes that can cause hypoglycemia, always carry one of the quick-fix foods with you. Wearing a medical identification bracelet or necklace is also a good idea. Exercise can also cause hypoglycemia. Check your blood glucose before you exercise.

Severe hypoglycemia can cause you to lose consciousness. In these extreme cases when you lose consciousness and cannot eat, glucagon

Table 48.1. Normal and Target Blood Glucose Ranges (mg/dL)

Normal blood glucose levels in people who do not have diabetes

Upon waking (fasting)	70 to 110
After meals	70 to 140

Target blood glucose levels in people who have diabetes

Before meals	90 to 130
1 to 2 hours after the start of a meal	less than 180
Hypoglycemia (low blood glucose)	70 or below

can be injected to quickly raise your blood glucose level. Ask your health care provider if having a glucagon kit at home and at work is appropriate for you. This is particularly important if you have type 1 diabetes. Your family, friends, and co-workers will need to be taught how to give you a glucagon injection in an emergency.

Prevention of hypoglycemia while you are driving a vehicle is especially important. Checking blood glucose frequently and snacking as needed to keep your blood glucose above 70 mg/dL will help prevent accidents.

Hypoglycemia and Diabetes: Doing Your Part

Signs and symptoms of hypoglycemia can vary from person to person. Get to know your own signs and describe them to your friends and family so they will be able to help you. If your child has diabetes, tell school staff about hypoglycemia and how to treat it.

If you experience hypoglycemia several times a week, call your health care provider. You may need a change in your treatment plan: less medication or a different medication, a new schedule for your insulin shots or medication, a different meal plan, or a new exercise plan.

Hypoglycemia in People Who Do Not Have Diabetes

Two types of hypoglycemia can occur in people who do not have diabetes: reactive (postprandial, or after meals) and fasting (postabsorptive). Reactive hypoglycemia is not usually related to any underlying disease; fasting hypoglycemia often is.

Symptoms

Symptoms of both types resemble the symptoms that people with diabetes and hypoglycemia experience: hunger, nervousness, perspiration, shakiness, dizziness, light-headedness, sleepiness, confusion, difficulty speaking, and feeling anxious or weak.

If you are diagnosed with hypoglycemia, your doctor will try to find the cause by using laboratory tests to measure blood glucose, insulin, and other chemicals that play a part in the body's use of energy.

Reactive Hypoglycemia

In reactive hypoglycemia, symptoms appear within four hours after you eat a meal.

Diagnosis

To diagnose reactive hypoglycemia, your doctor may:

• ask you about signs and symptoms;

• test your blood glucose while you are having symptoms (The doctor will take a blood sample from your arm and send it to a laboratory for analysis. A personal blood glucose monitor cannot be used to diagnose reactive hypoglycemia.); and/or

• check to see whether your symptoms ease after your blood glucose returns to 70 or above (after eating or drinking).

A blood glucose level of less than 70 mg/dL at the time of symptoms and relief after eating will confirm the diagnosis. The oral glucose tolerance test is no longer used to diagnose hypoglycemia; experts now know that the test can actually trigger hypoglycemic symptoms.

Causes and Treatment

The causes of most cases of reactive hypoglycemia are still open to debate. Some researchers suggest that certain people may be more sensitive to the body's normal release of the hormone epinephrine, which causes many of the symptoms of hypoglycemia. Others believe that deficiencies in glucagon secretion might lead to hypoglycemia.

A few causes of reactive hypoglycemia are certain, but they are uncommon. Gastric (stomach) surgery, for instance, can cause hypoglycemia because of the rapid passage of food into the small intestine. Also, rare enzyme deficiencies diagnosed early in life, such as hereditary fructose intolerance, may cause reactive hypoglycemia.

To relieve reactive hypoglycemia, some health professionals recommend taking the following steps:

• Eat small meals and snacks about every three hours.

• Exercise regularly.

• Eat a variety of foods, including meat, poultry, fish, or vegetarian sources of protein; starchy foods such as whole-grain bread, rice, and potatoes; fruits; vegetables; and dairy products.

• Choose high-fiber foods.

• Avoid or limit foods high in sugar, especially on an empty stomach.

Your doctor can refer you to a registered dietitian for personalized meal planning advice. Although some health professionals recommend a diet high in protein and low in carbohydrates, studies have not proven the effectiveness of this kind of diet for reactive hypoglycemia.

Fasting Hypoglycemia

Diagnosis

Fasting hypoglycemia is diagnosed from a blood sample that shows a blood glucose level of less than 50 mg/dL after an overnight fast, between meals, or after exercise.

Causes and Treatment

Causes include certain medications, alcohol, critical illnesses, hormonal deficiencies, some kinds of tumors, and certain conditions occurring in infancy and childhood.

Medications

Medications, including some used to treat diabetes, are the most common cause of hypoglycemia. Other medications that can cause hypoglycemia include:

- salicylates, including aspirin, when taken in large doses;
- sulfa medicines, which are used to treat infections;
- pentamidine, which treats a very serious kind of pneumonia; and
- quinine, which is used to treat malaria.

If using any of these medications causes your blood glucose to drop, your doctor may advise you to stop using the drug or change the dosage.

Alcohol

Drinking, especially binge drinking, can cause hypoglycemia because your body's breakdown of alcohol interferes with your liver's efforts to raise blood glucose. Hypoglycemia caused by excessive drinking can be very serious and even fatal.

Critical Illnesses

Some illnesses that affect the liver, heart, or kidneys can cause hypoglycemia. Sepsis (overwhelming infection) and starvation are other causes of hypoglycemia. In these cases, treatment targets the underlying cause.

Hormonal Deficiencies

Hormonal deficiencies may cause hypoglycemia in very young children, but usually not in adults. Shortages of cortisol, growth hormone, glucagon, or epinephrine can lead to fasting hypoglycemia. Laboratory tests for hormone levels will determine a diagnosis and treatment. Hormone replacement therapy may be advised.

Tumors

Insulinomas, insulin-producing tumors, can cause hypoglycemia by raising your insulin levels too high in relation to your blood glucose level. These tumors are very rare and do not normally spread to other parts of the body. Laboratory tests can pinpoint the exact cause. Treatment involves both short-term steps to correct the hypoglycemia and medical or surgical measures to remove the tumor.

Conditions Occurring in Infancy and Childhood

Children rarely develop hypoglycemia. If they do, causes may include:

- Brief intolerance to fasting, often in conjunction with an illness that disturbs regular eating patterns. Children usually outgrow this tendency by age 10.

- Hyperinsulinism, which is the excessive production of insulin. This condition can result in transient neonatal hypoglycemia, which is common in infants of mothers with diabetes. Persistent hyperinsulinism in infants or children is a complex disorder that requires prompt evaluation and treatment by a specialist.

- Enzyme deficiencies that affect carbohydrate metabolism. These deficiencies can interfere with the body's ability to process natural sugars, such as fructose and galactose, glycogen, or other metabolites.

- Hormonal deficiencies such as lack of pituitary or adrenal hormones.

Points to Remember

Diabetes-Related Hypoglycemia

- If you think your blood glucose is low, check it and treat the problem right away.

- To treat hypoglycemia, have a serving of a quick-fix food, wait 15 minutes, and check your blood glucose. Repeat the treatment until your blood glucose is above 70.

- Keep quick-fix foods in the car, at work—anywhere you spend time.

- Be careful when you are driving. Check your blood glucose frequently and snack as needed to keep your level above 70 mg/dL.

Hypoglycemia Unrelated to Diabetes

- In reactive hypoglycemia, symptoms occur within four hours of eating. People with this condition are usually advised to follow a healthy eating plan recommended by a registered dietitian.

- Fasting hypoglycemia can be caused by certain medications, critical illnesses, hereditary enzyme or hormonal deficiencies, and some kinds of tumors. Treatment targets the underlying problem.

For More Information

American Diabetes Association
National Service Center
1701 North Beauregard Street
Alexandria, VA 22311
Toll-Free: 800-DIABETES (342-2383)
Fax: 703-549-6995
Website: http://www.diabetes.org
E-mail: askada@diabetes.org

Juvenile Diabetes Research Foundation International
120 Wall Street
New York, NY 10005-4001
Toll-Free: 800-533-2873
Phone: 212-785-9500
Fax: 212-785-9595
E-mail: info@jdrf.org
Website: http://www.jdrf.org

National Diabetes Education Program
1 Diabetes Way
Bethesda, MD 20892-3600
Toll-Free: 800-438-5383
Fax: 703-738-4929
Website: http://www.ndep.nih.gov

Chapter 49

Cancer of the Pancreas

The pancreas is a gland located deep in the abdomen between the stomach and the spine (backbone). The liver, intestine, and other organs surround the pancreas.

The pancreas is about six inches long and is shaped like a flat pear. The widest part of the pancreas is the head, the middle section is the body, and the thinnest part is the tail. The pancreas makes insulin and other hormones. These hormones enter the bloodstream and travel throughout the body. They help the body use or store the energy that comes from food. For example, insulin helps control the amount of sugar in the blood.

The pancreas also makes pancreatic juices. These juices contain enzymes that help digest food. The pancreas releases the juices into a system of ducts leading to the common bile duct. The common bile duct empties into the duodenum, the first section of the small intestine.

Understanding Cancer

Cancer is a group of many related diseases. All cancers begin in cells, the body's basic unit of life. Cells make up tissues, and tissues make up the organs of the body. Normally, cells grow and divide to

"What You Need to Know about Cancer of the Pancreas," National Cancer Institute (NCI), updated September 16, 2002. Revised in January 2007 by Dr. David A. Cooke, M.D., Diplomate, American Board of Internal Medicine.

form new cells as the body needs them. When cells grow old and die, new cells take their place. Sometimes this orderly process breaks down. New cells form when the body does not need them, or old cells do not die when they should. These extra cells can form a mass of tissue called a growth or tumor. Tumors can be benign or malignant.

- **Benign tumors are not cancer.** Usually, doctors can remove them. In most cases, benign tumors do not come back after they are removed. Cells from benign tumors do not spread to tissues around them or to other parts of the body. Most important, benign tumors are rarely a threat to life.

- **Malignant tumors are cancer.** They are generally more serious and may be life-threatening. Cancer cells can invade and damage nearby tissues and organs. Also, cancer cells can break away from a malignant tumor and enter the bloodstream or lymphatic system. That is how cancer cells spread from the original cancer (primary tumor) to form new tumors in other organs. The spread of cancer is called metastasis.

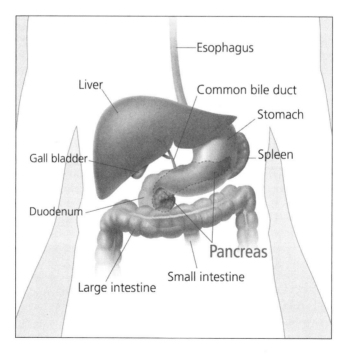

Figure 49.1. *Pancreas and Surrounding Organs*

Most pancreatic cancers begin in the ducts that carry pancreatic juices. Cancer of the pancreas may be called pancreatic cancer or carcinoma of the pancreas. A rare type of pancreatic cancer begins in the cells that make insulin and other hormones. Cancer that begins in these cells is called islet cell cancer.

When cancer of the pancreas spreads (metastasizes) outside the pancreas, cancer cells are often found in nearby lymph nodes. If the cancer has reached these nodes, it means that cancer cells may have spread to other lymph nodes or other tissues, such as the liver or lungs. Sometimes cancer of the pancreas spreads to the peritoneum, the tissue that lines the abdomen.

When cancer spreads from its original place to another part of the body, the new tumor has the same kind of abnormal cells and the same name as the primary tumor. For example, if cancer of the pancreas spreads to the liver, the cancer cells in the liver are pancreatic cancer cells. The disease is metastatic pancreatic cancer, not liver cancer. It is treated as pancreatic cancer, not liver cancer.

Pancreatic Cancer: Who's at Risk?

No one knows the exact causes of pancreatic cancer. Doctors can seldom explain why one person gets pancreatic cancer and another does not. However, it is clear that this disease is not contagious. No one can catch cancer from another person.

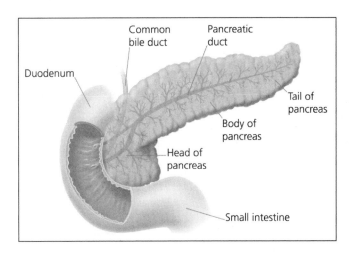

Figure 49.2. Pancreas, Common Bile Duct, and Small Intestine

Research has shown that people with certain risk factors are more likely than others to develop pancreatic cancer. A risk factor is anything that increases a person's chance of developing a disease. Studies have found the following risk factors:

- **Age.** The likelihood of developing pancreatic cancer increases with age. Most pancreatic cancers occur in people over the age of 60.

- **Smoking.** Cigarette smokers are two or three times more likely than nonsmokers to develop pancreatic cancer.

- **Diabetes.** Pancreatic cancer occurs more often in people who have diabetes than in people who do not.

- **Being male.** More men than women are diagnosed with pancreatic cancer.

- **Being African American.** African Americans are more likely than Asians, Hispanics, or Whites to get pancreatic cancer.

- **Family history.** The risk for developing pancreatic cancer triples if a person's mother, father, sister, or brother had the disease. Also, a family history of colon or ovarian cancer increases the risk of pancreatic cancer.

- **Chronic pancreatitis.** Chronic pancreatitis is a painful condition of the pancreas. Some evidence suggests that chronic pancreatitis may increase the risk of pancreatic cancer.

Other studies suggest that exposure to certain chemicals in the workplace or a diet high in fat may increase the chance of getting pancreatic cancer.

Most people with known risk factors do not get pancreatic cancer. On the other hand, many who do get the disease have none of these factors. People who think they may be at risk for pancreatic cancer should discuss this concern with their doctor. The doctor may suggest ways to reduce the risk and can plan an appropriate schedule for checkups.

Symptoms

Pancreatic cancer is sometimes called a silent disease because early pancreatic cancer often does not cause symptoms. But, as the cancer grows, symptoms may include:

- pain in the upper abdomen or upper back;

- yellow skin and eyes, and dark urine from jaundice;
- weakness;
- loss of appetite;
- nausea and vomiting;
- weight loss.

These symptoms are not sure signs of pancreatic cancer. An infection or other problem could also cause these symptoms. Only a doctor can diagnose the cause of a person's symptoms. Anyone with these symptoms should see a doctor so that the doctor can treat any problem as early as possible.

Diagnosis

If a patient has symptoms that suggest pancreatic cancer, the doctor asks about the patient's medical history. The doctor may perform a number of procedures, including one or more of the following:

- **Physical exam.** The doctor examines the skin and eyes for signs of jaundice. The doctor then feels the abdomen to check for changes in the area near the pancreas, liver, and gallbladder. The doctor also checks for ascites, an abnormal buildup of fluid in the abdomen.

- **Lab tests.** The doctor may take blood, urine, and stool samples to check for bilirubin and other substances. Bilirubin is a substance that passes from the liver to the gallbladder to the intestine. If the common bile duct is blocked by a tumor, the bilirubin cannot pass through normally. Blockage may cause the level of bilirubin in the blood, stool, or urine to become very high. High bilirubin levels can result from cancer or from noncancerous conditions.

- **Computed tomography (CT) scan.** An x-ray machine linked to a computer takes a series of detailed pictures. The x-ray machine is shaped like a donut with a large hole. The patient lies on a bed that passes through the hole. As the bed moves slowly through the hole, the machine takes many x-rays. The computer puts the x-rays together to create pictures of the pancreas and other organs and blood vessels in the abdomen.

- **Magnetic resonance imaging (MRI).** A machine that uses powerful magnets to generate radio signals from individual atoms inside the patient's body, linked to a computer, generates very detailed images. The machine has a large tube, which the patient lies inside during the test. It usually takes 20–30 minutes. The machine is quite noisy, and some patients may feel claustrophobic due to the small spaces. The machine can produce highly detailed images of the pancreas and the adjacent organs. The same machine can be used to perform magnetic resonance cholangiopancreatography (MRCP), which generates images of the bile ducts inside the pancreas. This may be performed to help judge whether a patient needs to have an endoscopic retrograde cholangiopancreatography (ERCP) performed.

- **Ultrasonography.** The ultrasound device uses sound waves that cannot be heard by humans. The sound waves produce a pattern of echoes as they bounce off internal organs. The echoes create a picture of the pancreas and other organs inside the abdomen. The echoes from tumors are different from echoes made by healthy tissues. The ultrasound procedure may use an external or internal device, or both types:

  - **Transabdominal ultrasound.** To make images of the pancreas, the doctor places the ultrasound device on the abdomen and slowly moves it around.

  - **Endoscopic ultrasound (EUS).** The doctor passes a thin, lighted tube (endoscope) through the patient's mouth and stomach, down into the first part of the small intestine. At the tip of the endoscope is an ultrasound device. The doctor slowly withdraws the endoscope from the intestine toward the stomach to make images of the pancreas and surrounding organs and tissues.

- **Endoscopic retrograde cholangiopancreatography (ERCP).** The doctor passes an endoscope through the patient's mouth and stomach, down into the first part of the small intestine. The doctor slips a smaller tube (catheter) through the endoscope into the bile ducts and pancreatic ducts. After injecting dye through the catheter into the ducts, the doctor takes x-ray pictures. The x-rays can show whether the ducts are narrowed or blocked by a tumor or other condition.

- **Percutaneous transhepatic cholangiography (PTC).** A dye is injected through a thin needle inserted through the skin into the liver. Unless there is a blockage, the dye should move freely through the bile ducts. The dye makes the bile ducts show up on x-ray pictures. From the pictures, the doctor can tell whether there is a blockage from a tumor or other condition.

- **Biopsy.** In some cases, the doctor may remove tissue. A pathologist then uses a microscope to look for cancer cells in the tissue. The doctor may obtain tissue in several ways. One way is by inserting a needle into the pancreas to remove cells. This is called fine-needle aspiration. The doctor uses x-ray or ultrasound to guide the needle. Sometimes the doctor obtains a sample of tissue during EUS or ERCP. Another way is to open the abdomen during an operation.

A person who needs a biopsy may want to ask the doctor the following questions:

- What kind of biopsy will I have?
- How long will it take? Will I be awake? Will it hurt?
- Are there any risks?
- How soon will I know the results?
- If I do have cancer, who will talk to me about treatment? When?

Staging

When pancreatic cancer is diagnosed, the doctor needs to know the stage, or extent, of the disease to plan the best treatment. Staging is a careful attempt to find out the size of the tumor in the pancreas, whether the cancer has spread, and if so, to what parts of the body.

The doctor may determine the stage of pancreatic cancer at the time of diagnosis, or the patient may need to have more tests. Such tests may include blood tests, a CT scan, ultrasonography, laparoscopy, or angiography. The test results will help the doctor decide which treatment is appropriate.

Treatment

Many people with pancreatic cancer want to take an active part in making decisions about their medical care. They want to learn all they can about their disease and their treatment choices. However, the shock and stress that people may feel after a diagnosis of cancer can make it hard for them to think of everything they want to ask the doctor. Often it helps to make a list of questions before an appointment. To help remember what the doctor says, patients may take notes or ask whether they may use a tape recorder. Some patients also want to have a family member or friend with them when they talk to the doctor— to take part in the discussion, to take notes, or just to listen.

Cancer of the pancreas is very hard to control with current treatments. For that reason, many doctors encourage patients with this disease to consider taking part in a clinical trial. Clinical trials are an important option for people with all stages of pancreatic cancer.

At this time, pancreatic cancer can be cured only when it is found at an early stage, before it has spread. In these patients, surgery, usually followed by chemotherapy, gives the best chance of cure. Unfortunately, most patients are not diagnosed at a stage where this is possible, and the cure rates even amongst those who undergo surgery are disappointing. However, other treatments may be able to control the disease and help patients live longer and feel better. When a cure or control of the disease is not possible, some patients and their doctors choose palliative therapy. Palliative therapy aims to improve quality of life by controlling pain and other problems caused by this disease.

The doctor may refer patients to an oncologist, a doctor who specializes in treating cancer, or patients may ask for a referral. Specialists who treat pancreatic cancer include surgeons, medical oncologists, and radiation oncologists. Treatment generally begins within a few weeks after the diagnosis. There will be time for patients to talk with the doctor about treatment choices, get a second opinion, and learn more about the disease.

Getting a Second Opinion

Before starting treatment, a patient may want a second opinion about the diagnosis and the treatment plan. Some insurance companies require a second opinion; others may cover a second opinion if the patient requests it. Gathering medical records and arranging to see another doctor may take a little time. In most cases, a brief delay to get another opinion will not make therapy less helpful.

There are a number of ways to find a doctor for a second opinion:

- The doctor may refer patients to one or more specialists. At cancer centers, several specialists often work together as a team.

- The Cancer Information Service (800-4-CANCER) can tell callers about treatment facilities, including cancer centers, and other programs supported by the National Cancer Institute, and can send printed information about finding a doctor.

- A local medical society, a nearby hospital, or a medical school can usually provide the name of specialists.

- The American Board of Medical Specialties (ABMS) has a list of doctors who have met certain education and training requirements and have passed specialty examinations. The Official ABMS Directory of Board Certified Medical Specialists lists doctors' names along with their specialty and their educational background. The directory is available in most public libraries. Also, ABMS offers this information on the internet at http://www.abms.org.

Preparing for Treatment

The doctor can describe treatment choices and discuss the results expected with each treatment option. The doctor and patient can work together to develop a treatment plan that fits the patient's needs. Treatment depends on where in the pancreas the tumor started and whether the disease has spread. When planning treatment, the doctor also considers other factors, including the patient's age and general health.

These are some questions a person may want to ask the doctor before treatment begins:

- What is the diagnosis?

- Where in the pancreas did the cancer start?

- Is there any evidence the cancer has spread? What is the stage of the disease?

- Do I need any more tests to check whether the disease has spread?

- What are my treatment choices? Which do you recommend for me? Why?

- What are the expected benefits of each kind of treatment?

- What are the risks and possible side effects of each treatment?

- What is the treatment likely to cost? Is this treatment covered by my insurance plan?

- How will treatment affect my normal activities?

- Would a clinical trial (research study) be appropriate for me?

People do not need to ask all of their questions or understand all of the answers at one time. They will have other chances to ask the doctor to explain things that are not clear and to ask for more information.

Methods of Treatment

People with pancreatic cancer may have several treatment options. Depending on the type and stage, pancreatic cancer may be treated with surgery, radiation therapy, or chemotherapy. Some patients have a combination of therapies.

Surgery may be used alone or in combination with radiation therapy and chemotherapy. The surgeon may remove all or part of the pancreas. The extent of surgery depends on the location and size of the tumor, the stage of the disease, and the patient's general health.

- **Whipple procedure:** If the tumor is in the head (the widest part) of the pancreas, the surgeon removes the head of the pancreas and part of the small intestine, bile duct, and stomach. The surgeon may also remove other nearby tissues.

- **Distal pancreatectomy:** The surgeon removes the body and tail of the pancreas if the tumor is in either of these parts. The surgeon also removes the spleen.

- **Total pancreatectomy:** The surgeon removes the entire pancreas, part of the small intestine, a portion of the stomach, the common bile duct, the gallbladder, the spleen, and nearby lymph nodes.

Sometimes the cancer cannot be completely removed. But if the tumor is blocking the common bile duct or duodenum, the surgeon can create a bypass. A bypass allows fluids to flow through the digestive tract. It can help relieve jaundice and pain resulting from a blockage.

The doctor sometimes can relieve blockage without doing bypass surgery. The doctor uses an endoscope to place a stent in the blocked area. A stent is a tiny plastic or metal mesh tube that helps keep the duct or duodenum open.

After surgery, some patients are fed liquids intravenously (IV) and through feeding tubes placed into the abdomen. Patients slowly return to eating solid foods by mouth. A few weeks after surgery, the feeding tubes are removed.

Questions to Ask the Doctor before Having Surgery

- What kind of operation will I have?

- How will I feel after the operation?
- How will you treat my pain?
- What other treatment will I need?
- How long will I be in the hospital?
- Will I need a feeding tube after surgery? Will I need a special diet?
- What are the long-term effects?
- When can I get back to my normal activities?
- How often will I need checkups?

Radiation therapy (also called radiotherapy) uses high-energy rays to kill cancer cells. A large machine directs radiation at the abdomen. Radiation therapy may be given alone, or with surgery, chemotherapy, or both.

Radiation therapy is local therapy. It affects cancer cells only in the treated area. For radiation therapy, patients go to the hospital or clinic, often five days a week for several weeks. Doctors may use radiation to destroy cancer cells that remain in the area after surgery. They also use radiation to relieve pain and other problems caused by the cancer.

Questions to Ask the Doctor before Having Radiation Therapy

- Why do I need this treatment?
- When will the treatments begin? When will they end?
- How will I feel during therapy? Are there side effects?
- What can I do to take care of myself during therapy? Are there certain foods that I should eat or avoid?
- How will we know if the radiation is working?
- Will I be able to continue my normal activities during treatment?

Chemotherapy is the use of drugs to kill cancer cells. Doctors also give chemotherapy to help reduce pain and other problems caused by pancreatic cancer. It may be given alone, with radiation, or with surgery and radiation. Patients who undergo complete surgical removal of the tumor, plus chemotherapy, appear to have the best odds of being cured.

Chemotherapy is systemic therapy. The doctor usually gives the drugs by injection. Once in the bloodstream, the drugs travel throughout the body. Usually chemotherapy is an outpatient treatment given at the hospital, clinic, doctor's office, or home. However, depending on which drugs are given and the patient's general health, the patient may need to stay in the hospital.

Questions to Ask about Chemotherapy

- Why do I need this treatment?
- What will it do?
- What drugs will I be taking? How will they be given? Will I need to stay in the hospital?
- Will the treatment cause side effects? What can I do about them?
- How long will I be on this treatment?

Side Effects of Treatment

Because cancer treatment may damage healthy cells and tissues, unwanted side effects are common. These side effects depend on many factors, including the type and extent of the treatment. Side effects may not be the same for each person, and they may even change from one treatment session to the next. The health care team will explain possible side effects and how they will help the patient manage the side effects.

Surgery

Surgery for pancreatic cancer is a major operation. Patients need to stay in the hospital for several days afterward. Patients may feel weak or tired. Most need to rest at home for about a month. The length of time it takes to regain strength varies.

The side effects of surgery depend on the extent of the operation, the person's general health, and other factors. Most patients have pain for the first few days after surgery. Pain can be controlled with medicine, and patients should discuss pain relief with the doctor or nurse.

Removal of part, or all, of the pancreas may make it hard for a patient to digest foods. The health care team can suggest a diet plan and medicines to help relieve diarrhea, pain, cramping, or feelings of fullness. During the recovery from surgery, the doctor will carefully monitor the patient's diet and weight. At first, a patient may have only liquids and may receive extra nourishment intravenously or by feeding tube into the intestine. Solid foods are added to the diet gradually.

Patients may not have enough pancreatic enzymes or hormones after surgery. Those who do not have enough insulin may develop diabetes. The doctor can give the patient insulin, other hormones, and enzymes.

Radiation Therapy

Radiation therapy may cause patients to become very tired as treatment continues. Resting is important, but doctors usually advise patients to try to stay as active as they can. In addition, when patients receive radiation therapy, the skin in the treated area may sometimes become red, dry, and tender.

Radiation therapy to the abdomen may cause nausea, vomiting, diarrhea, or other problems with digestion. The health care team can offer medicine or suggest diet changes to control these problems. For most patients, the side effects of radiation therapy go away when treatment is over.

Chemotherapy

The side effects of chemotherapy depend mainly on the drugs and the doses the patient receives as well as how the drugs are given. In addition, as with other types of treatment, side effects vary from patient to patient.

Systemic chemotherapy affects rapidly dividing cells throughout the body, including blood cells. Blood cells fight infection, help the blood to clot, and carry oxygen to all parts of the body. When anticancer drugs damage healthy blood cells, patients are more likely to get infections, may bruise or bleed easily, and may have less energy. Cells in hair roots and cells that line the digestive tract also divide rapidly. As a result, patients may lose their hair and may have other side effects such as poor appetite, nausea and vomiting, diarrhea, or mouth sores. Usually, these side effects go away gradually during the recovery periods between treatments or after treatment is over. The health care team can suggest ways to relieve side effects.

Pain Control

Pain is a common problem for people with pancreatic cancer. The tumor can cause pain by pressing against nerves and other organs.

The patient's doctor or a specialist in pain control can relieve or reduce pain in several ways:

- **Pain medicine.** Medicines often can relieve pain. (These medicines may make people drowsy and constipated, but resting and taking laxatives can help.)

- **Radiation.** High-energy rays can help relieve pain by shrinking the tumor.

- **Nerve block.** The doctor may inject alcohol into the area around certain nerves in the abdomen to block the feeling of pain.

- **Surgery.** The surgeon may cut certain nerves to block pain.

The doctor may suggest other ways to relieve or reduce pain. For example, massage, acupuncture, or acupressure may be used along with other approaches to help relieve pain. Also, the patient may learn relaxation techniques such as listening to slow music, or breathing slowly and comfortably.

Nutrition

People with pancreatic cancer may not feel like eating, especially if they are uncomfortable or tired. Also, the side effects of treatment such as poor appetite, nausea, or vomiting can make eating difficult. Foods may taste different. Nevertheless, patients should try to get enough calories and protein to control weight loss, maintain strength, and promote healing. Also, eating well often helps people with cancer feel better and have more energy.

Careful planning and checkups are important. Cancer of the pancreas and its treatment may make it hard for patients to digest food and maintain the proper blood sugar level. The doctor will check the patient for weight loss, weakness, and lack of energy. Patients may need to take medicines to replace the enzymes and hormones made by the pancreas. The doctor will watch the patient closely and adjust the doses of these medicines. The doctor, dietitian, or other health care provider can advise patients about ways to maintain a healthy diet.

Follow-Up Care

Follow-up care after treatment for pancreatic cancer is an important part of the overall treatment plan. Patients should not hesitate to discuss follow-up with their doctor. Regular checkups ensure that any changes in health are noticed. Any problem that develops can be found and treated. Checkups may include a physical exam, laboratory tests, and imaging procedures.

Support for People with Pancreatic Cancer

Living with a serious disease such as pancreatic cancer is not easy. Some people find they need help coping with the emotional and practical aspects of their disease. Support groups can help. In these groups, patients or their family members get together to share what they have learned about coping with their disease and the effects of treatment. Patients may want to talk with a member of their health care team about finding a support group.

People living with pancreatic cancer may worry about the future. They may worry about caring for themselves or their families, keeping their jobs, or continuing daily activities. Concerns about treatments and managing side effects, hospital stays, and medical bills are also common. Doctors, nurses, and other members of the health care team can answer questions about treatment, diet, working, or other matters. Meeting with a social worker, counselor, or member of the clergy can be helpful to those who want to talk about their feelings or discuss their concerns. Often, a social worker can suggest resources for financial aid, transportation, home care, emotional support, or other services. For patients with a poor prognosis, hospice care can be of enormous benefit to the patient and their family members during the course of their illness.

Additional Information

National Cancer Institute (NCI)
Cancer Information Service
6116 Executive Blvd., Room 3036A
Bethesda, MD 20892-8322
Toll-Free: 800-4-CANCER (422-6237)
Toll-Free TTY: 800-332-8615
Website: http://www.cancer.gov
E-mail: cancergovstaff@mail.nih.gov

Chapter 50

Islet Cell Cancer

Islet cell cancer, a rare cancer, is a disease in which cancer (malignant) cells are found in certain tissues of the pancreas. The pancreas is about six inches long and is shaped like a thin pear, wider at one end and narrower at the other. The pancreas lies behind the stomach, inside a loop formed by part of the small intestine. The broader right end of the pancreas is called the head, the middle section is called the body, and the narrow left end is the tail.

The pancreas has two basic jobs in the body. It produces digestive juices that help break down (digest) food, and hormones (such as insulin) that regulate how the body stores and uses food. The area of the pancreas that produces digestive juices is called the exocrine pancreas. About 95% of pancreatic cancers begin in the exocrine pancreas. The hormone-producing area of the pancreas has special cells called islet cells and is called the endocrine pancreas. Only about 5% of pancreatic cancers start here.

The islet cells in the pancreas make many hormones, including insulin, which help the body store and use sugars. When islet cells in the pancreas become cancerous, they may make too many hormones. Islet cell cancers that make too many hormones are called functioning tumors. Other islet cell cancers may not make extra hormones and are called nonfunctioning tumors. Tumors that do not spread to other

PDQ® Cancer Information Summary. National Cancer Institute; Bethesda, MD. Islet Cell Carcinoma (Endocrine Pancreas) (PDQ®): Treatment–Patient. Updated 07/2005. Available at: http://cancer.gov. Accessed 02/07/2007.

parts of the body can also be found in the islet cells. These are called benign tumors and are not cancer. A doctor will need to determine whether the tumor is cancer or a benign tumor.

A doctor should be seen if there is pain in the abdomen, diarrhea, stomach pain, a tired feeling all the time, fainting, or weight gain without eating too much. If there are symptoms, the doctor will order blood and urine tests to see whether the amounts of hormones in the body are normal. Other tests, including x-rays and special scans, may also be done.

The chance of recovery (prognosis) depends on the type of islet cell cancer the patient has, how far the cancer has spread, and the patient's overall health.

Stage Explanation

Once islet cell cancer is found, more tests will be done to find out if cancer cells have spread to other parts of the body. This is called staging. The staging system for islet cell cancer is still being developed. These tumors are most often divided into one of three groups:

1. Islet cell cancers occurring in one site within the pancreas.

2. Islet cell cancers occurring in several sites within the pancreas.

3. Islet cell cancers that have spread to lymph nodes near the pancreas or to distant sites.

A doctor also needs to know the type of islet cell tumor to plan treatment.

Types of Islet Cell Tumors

Gastrinoma. The tumor makes large amounts of a hormone called gastrin, which causes too much acid to be made in the stomach. Ulcers may develop as a result of too much stomach acid.

Insulinoma. The tumor makes too much of the hormone insulin and causes the body to store sugar instead of burning the sugar for energy. This causes too little sugar in the blood, a condition called hypoglycemia.

Glucagonoma. This tumor makes too much of the hormone glucagon and causes too much sugar in the blood, a condition called hyperglycemia.

Miscellaneous. Other types of islet cell cancer can affect the pancreas and/or small intestine. Each type of tumor may affect different hormones in the body and cause different symptoms.

Recurrent. Recurrent disease means that the cancer has come back (recurred) after it has been treated. It may come back in the pancreas or in another part of the body.

Treatment Option Overview

There are treatments for all patients with islet cell cancer. Three types of treatment are used:

- surgery (taking out the cancer)
- chemotherapy (using drugs to kill cancer cells)
- hormone therapy (using hormones to stop cancer cells from growing)

Surgery is the most common treatment of islet cell cancer. The doctor may take out the cancer and most or part of the pancreas. Sometimes the stomach is taken out (gastrectomy) because of ulcers. Lymph nodes in the area may also be removed and looked at under a microscope to see if they contain cancer.

Chemotherapy uses drugs to kill cancer cells. Chemotherapy may be taken by pill, or it may be put into the body by a needle in the vein or muscle. Chemotherapy is called a systemic treatment because the drug enters the bloodstream, travels through the body, and can kill cancer cells throughout the body.

Hormone therapy uses hormones to stop the cancer cells from growing or to relieve symptoms caused by the tumor.

Hepatic arterial occlusion or embolization uses drugs, or other agents, to reduce, or block, the flow of blood to the liver in order to kill cancer cells growing in the liver.

Treatment by Type

Treatment of islet cell cancer depends on the type of tumor, the stage, and the patient's overall health. Standard treatment may be considered because of its effectiveness in patients in past studies, or participation in a clinical trial may be considered. Not all patients are cured with standard therapy and some standard treatments may have more side effects than are desired. For these reasons, clinical trials are designed to find better ways to treat cancer patients and are based on the most up-to-date information. Clinical trials are ongoing in many parts of the country for patients with islet cell cancer.

Gastrinoma: Treatment may be one of the following:

1. Surgery to remove the cancer.

2. Surgery to remove the stomach (gastrectomy).

3. Surgery to cut the nerve that stimulates the pancreas.

4. Chemotherapy.

5. Hormone therapy.

6. Hepatic arterial occlusion or embolization to kill cancer cells growing in the liver.

Insulinoma: Treatment may be one of the following:

1. Surgery to remove the cancer.

2. Chemotherapy.

3. Hormone therapy.

4. Drugs to relieve symptoms.

5. Hepatic arterial occlusion or embolization to kill cancer cells growing in the liver.

Glucagonoma: Treatment may be one of the following:

1. Surgery to remove the cancer.

2. Chemotherapy.

3. Hormone therapy.

4. Hepatic arterial occlusion or embolization to kill cancer cells growing in the liver.

Miscellaneous Islet Cell Cancer: Treatment may be one of the following:

1. Surgery to remove the cancer.

2. Chemotherapy.

3. Hormone therapy.

4. Hepatic arterial occlusion or embolization to kill cancer cells growing in the liver.

Recurrent Islet Cell Carcinoma: Treatment depends on many factors, including what treatment the patient had before and where the cancer has come back. Treatment may be chemotherapy, or patients may want to consider taking part in a clinical trial.

For More Information

National Cancer Institute (NCI)
Cancer Information Service
6116 Executive Blvd., Room 3036A
Bethesda, MD 20892-8322
Toll-Free: 800-4-CANCER (422-6237)
Toll-Free TTY: 800-332-8615
Website: http://www.cancer.gov
E-mail: cancergovstaff@mail.nih.gov

Chapter 51

Zollinger-Ellison Syndrome

Zollinger-Ellison syndrome (ZES) is a rare disorder that causes tumors in the pancreas and duodenum and ulcers in the stomach and duodenum. The pancreas is a gland located behind the stomach. It produces enzymes that break down fat, protein, and carbohydrates from food, and hormones like insulin that break down sugar. The duodenum is the first part of the small intestine.

The tumors secrete a hormone called gastrin that causes the stomach to produce too much acid, which in turn causes stomach and duodenal ulcers (peptic ulcers). The ulcers caused by ZES are less responsive to treatment than ordinary peptic ulcers. What causes people with ZES to develop tumors is unknown, but approximately 25 percent of ZES cases are associated with a genetic disorder called multiple endocrine neoplasia type 1 (MEN1), which is associated with additional disorders.

The symptoms of ZES include signs of peptic ulcers: gnawing, burning pain in the abdomen; diarrhea; nausea; vomiting; fatigue; weakness; weight loss; and bleeding. Physicians diagnose ZES through blood tests to measure levels of gastrin and gastric acid secretion. They may check for ulcers by doing an endoscopy, which involves looking at the lining of the stomach and duodenum through a lighted tube.

The primary treatment for ZES is medication to reduce the production of stomach acid. Proton pump inhibitors that suppress acid

National Institute of Diabetes and Digestive and Kidney Diseases (NIDDK), NIH Publication No. 04-4692, September 2004.

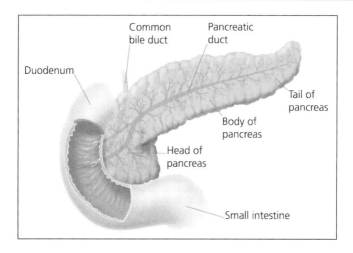

Figure 51.1. Pancreas, Duodenum, and Small Intestine (Source: National Cancer Institute, NIH Publication 01-1560, revised July 2001).

production and promote healing are the first line of treatment and include lansoprazole, omeprazole, pantoprazole, and rabeprazole. H-2 blockers such as cimetidine, famotidine, and ranitidine may also be used, but are less effective in reducing stomach acid. Surgery to treat peptic ulcers or to remove tumors in the pancreas or duodenum are other treatment options. People who have been treated for ZES should be monitored in case the ulcers or tumors recur.

For More Information

National Digestive Diseases Information Clearinghouse
2 Information Way
Bethesda, MD 20892-3570
Toll-Free: 800-891-5389
Fax: 703-738-4929
Website: http://digestive
.niddk.nih.gov
E-mail: nddic@info.niddk.nih.gov

National Organization for Rare Disorders Inc. (NORD)
P.O. Box 1968
Danbury, CT 06813-1968
Toll-Free: 800-999-6673
Phone: 203-744-0100
Fax: 203-798-2291
Website: http://
www.rarediseases.org
E-mail: orphan@rarediseases.org

Part Six

Disorders of the
Ovaries and Testes

Chapter 52

Hypogonadism

Alternative name: Gonadal deficiency

Definition

Hypogonadism is when the sex glands produce little or no hormones. In men, these glands (gonads) are the testes; in women, they are the ovaries.

Causes, Incidence, and Risk Factors

The cause of hypogonadism may be "primary" or "central." In primary hypogonadism, the ovaries or testes themselves do not function properly. Some causes of primary hypogonadism include:

- surgery
- radiation
- genetic and developmental disorders
- liver and kidney disease
- infection
- certain autoimmune disorders

The most common genetic disorders that cause primary hypogonadism are Turner syndrome (in women) and Klinefelter syndrome (in men).

In central hypogonadism, the centers in the brain that control the gonads (hypothalamus and pituitary) do not function properly. Some causes of central hypogonadism include:

- tumors
- surgery
- radiation
- infections
- trauma
- bleeding
- genetic problems
- nutritional deficiencies
- iron excess (hemochromatosis)

A genetic cause of central hypogonadism that also produces an inability to smell is Kallmann syndrome (males). The most common tumors affecting the pituitary area are craniopharyngioma (in children) and prolactinoma (in adults).

Symptoms

In girls, hypogonadism during childhood will result in lack of menstruation and breast development and short height. If hypogonadism occurs after puberty, symptoms include loss of menstruation, low libido, hot flashes, and loss of body hair.

In boys, hypogonadism in childhood results in lack of muscle and beard development and growth problems. In men, the usual complaints are sexual dysfunction, decreased beard and body hair, breast enlargement, and muscle loss.

If a brain tumor is present (central hypogonadism) there may be headaches or visual loss, or symptoms of other hormonal deficiencies (such as hypothyroidism). In the case of the most common pituitary tumor, prolactinoma, there may be a milky breast discharge. People with anorexia nervosa (excessive dieting to the point of starvation) also may have central hypogonadism.

Signs and Tests

Tests may be done that check estrogen level (women) and testosterone level (men) as well as follicle-stimulating hormone (FSH) level and luteinizing hormone (LH) level, the pituitary hormones that stimulate the gonads. Other tests may include a thyroid level; sperm count; prolactin level (milk hormone); blood tests for anemia, chemistries, and iron; and genetic analysis.

Sometimes imaging is necessary, such as a sonogram of the ovaries. If pituitary disease is suspected, a magnetic resonance imaging (MRI) or computed tomography (CT) scan of the brain may be done.

Treatment

Hormone-based medicines are available for men and women. Estrogen comes in the form of a patch or pill. Testosterone can be given by using a patch, a product soaked in by the gums, a gel, or by injection.

For women who have not had their uterus removed, combination treatment with estrogen and progesterone is often recommended to decrease the chances of developing endometrial cancer. In addition, low dose testosterone can be added for women with hypogonadism who have a low sex drive.

In some women, injections or pills can be used to stimulated ovulation. Injections of pituitary hormone may be used to help male patients produce sperm. In others, surgery and radiation therapy may be needed.

Expectations (Prognosis)

Many forms of hypogonadism are potentially treatable and have a good prognosis.

Complications

In women, hypogonadism may cause infertility. Menopause is a form of naturally occurring hypogonadism, which can cause hot flashes, vaginal dryness, and irritability as a woman's estrogen levels fall. The risk of osteoporosis and heart disease increase after menopause.

Some women with hypogonadism opt to take estrogen therapy, particularly those who have early menopause (premature ovarian failure). However, there is a small but significant increase in risk for breast cancer and heart disease with use of hormone replacement for treatment of menopause.

In men, hypogonadism results in loss of sex drive and may cause weakness, impotence, infertility, and osteoporosis. Men normally experience some decline in testosterone as they age, but it is not as dramatic or steep as the decline in sex hormones experienced by women.

Calling Your Health Care Provider

Consult with your doctor if you notice loss of menstruation, breast discharge, problems getting pregnant, hot flashes (women), impotence, loss of body hair, weakness, breast enlargement (men), or problems with your sex drive. Both men and women should call their health care providers if headaches or visual problems occur.

Prevention

Maintain normal body weight and healthy eating habits to prevent anorexia nervosa. Other causes may not be preventable.

Chapter 53

Gynecomastia

What is gynecomastia?

Gynecomastia is defined as breast development or enlargement in males. It may be present on one side or both sides of the body and may cause the breast to be tender. Breast development due to being overweight is referred to as pseudogynecomastia or false gynecomastia. This type of breast development due to weight gain is not the same thing as the condition referred to as gynecomastia.

What causes gynecomastia?

Breast formation in males is most commonly caused by hormonal changes that occur at puberty or as part of the aging process. If the balance between the hormones estrogen and testosterone is changed, breast development can occur. Gynecomastia may also be caused by certain medications (for example, psychiatric medications, ulcer drugs, digoxin) or by an underlying disease (for example, low testosterone state) or a breast cancer tumor.

Who is affected by gynecomastia?

Development of breast tissue in males is most often associated with adolescent boys and aging men. In adolescent boys, breast enlargement is relatively common and typically goes away on its own in 2–3 years. This is often called pubertal gynecomastia.

Why is it important to know about gynecomastia?

Gynecomastia may cause psychological as well as physiologic problems, particularly in adolescent boys. It is therefore important to understand the cause of breast development in males so that proper monitoring and treatment can be done. In addition, breast cancer may develop in males. In these rare cases, as with women, early detection and treatment is important.

What is the role of the endocrinologist?

Diagnosis: Endocrinologists are doctors with specialized training in recognizing and treating hormone-related illnesses and conditions. Sometimes blood tests to measure hormone levels may be necessary to determine the cause of gynecomastia. In most cases, however, a physical examination and medical history of the patient is sufficient.

Treatment: In most cases, treatment is not necessary. At times, medication may be prescribed to reduce breast tenderness. If breast enlargement is due to medication, the medication would be stopped and a different form prescribed. If the breast development is caused by another disease or tumor, treatment of that condition would be necessary. In rare cases, surgery may be used to reduce breast size.

Hormone Foundation

8401 Connecticut Ave., Suite 900
Chevy Chase, MD 20815
Toll-Free: 800-HORMONE (467-6663)
Fax: 301-941-0259
Website: http://www.hormone.org
E-mail: hormone@endo-society.org

To find an endocrinologist near you, visit the "Find-an-Endocrinologist" online physician referral or call 1-800-HORMONE.

Chapter 54

Menstrual Problems

Premenstrual Syndrome (PMS) and Premenstrual Dysphoric Disorder (PMDD)

What is PMS?

Premenstrual syndrome (PMS) is a medical condition that affects some women of childbearing age. More than one in three women suffer from PMS, and one in 20 suffers so severely that their lives are seriously affected. PMS is related to a variety of physical and psychological symptoms that occur just before your menstrual period.

What causes PMS?

The exact cause of PMS is unknown, but it seems to be related to the fluctuating levels of hormones, including estrogen and progesterone, that occur in preparation for menstruation.

What are the symptoms of PMS?

There are many symptoms of PMS, and the number and severity

This information is from: "PMS and PMDD," © 2005 The Cleveland Clinic Foundation, 9500 Euclid Avenue, Cleveland, OH 44195, www.clevelandclinic.org. Additional information is available from the Cleveland Clinic Health Information Center, 216-444-3771, toll-free 800-223-2273 extension 43771, or at http:// www.clevelandclinic.org/health. Additional text under the heading "Amenorrhea," is from the National Institute of Child Health and Human Development (NICHD), September 7, 2006.

of symptoms vary from woman to woman. In addition, the severity of the symptoms can vary from month to month. Common symptoms of PMS include:

- bloating
- breast tenderness
- weight gain
- aggression
- trouble concentrating
- headaches and/or backaches
- skin problems or acne
- fatigue
- tearfulness
- irritability
- anxiety
- mood swings and/or depression

How is PMS diagnosed?

There is no single test to diagnose PMS. However, there are some strategies your doctor may use to help diagnose PMS:

Thyroid test. Because thyroid disorders are common in women of childbearing age, and some of the symptoms of PMS—such as weight gain—are similar to symptoms of thyroid disorders, your doctor may order a test to evaluate thyroid functioning. This can help to rule out a thyroid disorder as a cause of your symptoms.

PMS symptoms diary. Your doctor may ask you to keep a diary of your symptoms, when they occur and for how long. By doing this, you can see if your symptoms correspond to certain times in your monthly cycle. While your symptoms may vary from month to month, a trend likely will appear after tracking your symptoms for a few months.

How is PMS treated?

Treatment for PMS is based on relieving symptoms. Treatment begins with a thorough assessment of your symptoms, as well as their impact on your daily life.

Education. You will be better able to deal with your symptoms if you can relate how you're feeling to your menstrual cycles, knowing that you will feel better once your period starts. Keeping a monthly symptom diary will help you track your symptoms, as well as their severity and how long they last. While symptoms may vary from month to month, this diary can give you a good idea of how your periods affect your physical health and moods. Learning how to cope with the problems in your life may help relieve the stress and irritability you feel before your period. If you experience severe anxiety, irritability, or depression, counseling, and/or medication may be helpful.

Nutrition. A healthy diet is important to overall physical and mental wellness. Making changes in your diet—including reducing the amount of caffeine, salt, and sugar—may help relieve symptoms of PMS. In some cases, nutritional supplements may be recommended. These include Vitamin B_6, calcium, and magnesium.

Exercise. Like a healthy diet, regular exercise can improve your overall health. It also can help relieve and help you cope with the monthly symptoms associated with PMS.

Medications. Over-the-counter pain relievers—such as aspirin and ibuprofen—may help relieve symptoms such as headache, backache, cramps, and breast tenderness. Medications may be prescribed in cases of severe depression or anxiety.

Can PMS be prevented?

PMS itself cannot be prevented, but through education and appropriate treatment of symptoms, most women can find relief. A healthy lifestyle—including exercise and a proper diet—also can help a woman better manage the symptoms of PMS.

What is PMDD?

Premenstrual dysphoric disorder (PMDD) is a severe form of PMS. The symptoms of PMDD are similar to those of PMS, but are severe enough to interfere with work, social activities, and relationships.

How is PMDD diagnosed?

PMDD is diagnosed when at least five of the following symptoms occur seven to ten days before menstruation and go away within a few days of the start of the menstrual period.

- mood swings
- marked anger
- irritability
- tension
- decreased interest in usual activities
- fatigue
- change in appetite
- sleep problems
- physical problems, such as bloating

Before a doctor makes a diagnosis of PMDD, he or she will rule out other emotional disorders, such as major depression or panic disorder, as the cause of the symptoms. In addition, underlying medical or gynecological conditions—such as endometriosis, fibroids, menopause and hormonal problems (such as a thyroid disorder)—that could account for symptoms also must be ruled out.

How common is PMDD?

PMDD occurs in three percent to five percent of menstruating women. Women with a personal or family history of mood disorders—including major depression or postpartum depression—are at greater risk for developing PMDD.

What causes PMDD?

As with PMS, the exact cause of PMDD is not known. Most researchers, however, believe PMDD is brought about by the hormonal changes related to the menstrual cycle. Recent studies have shown a connection between PMDD and low levels of serotonin, a chemical in the brain that helps transmit nerve signals. Certain brain cells that use serotonin as a messenger are involved in controlling mood, attention, sleep and pain. Therefore, chronic changes in serotonin levels can lead to PMDD symptoms.

How is PMDD diagnosed?

Clinical evaluation should include a comprehensive review of the patient's symptoms and medical history, a physical exam, a gynecologic exam, and basic laboratory tests (such as a complete blood count, electrolytes, liver and kidney profile, and thyroid function tests).

Psychiatric evaluation should focus on symptoms of depression, seasonal variation of depression, alcohol and drug use, early victimization and trauma, family history of affective disorder (a group of disorders characterized by a disturbance of mood, accompanied by a manic and depressive syndrome), alcoholism, and current situational stresses.

How is PMDD treated?

Many women gain relief from the symptoms of PMDD with education and lifestyle changes, including exercise, vitamins, and a caffeine-free diet. Medications, including anti-depressants, may be used to treat the emotional symptoms of PMDD. In addition, individual and group counseling, and stress management can be beneficial in helping a woman cope with PMDD.

Amenorrhea

What is amenorrhea?

Amenorrhea is the absence of a menstrual period.

- **Primary amenorrhea** is when a young woman has not yet had a period by age 16.

- **Secondary amenorrhea** describes someone who used to have a regular period, but then it stopped for at least three months (this can include pregnancy).

What are the signs of amenorrhea?

The main sign of amenorrhea is missing a menstrual period. Regular periods are a sign of overall good health. Missing a period may mean that you are pregnant or that something is going wrong. It is important to tell your health care provider if you miss a period so he or she can begin to find out what is happening in your body.

Amenorrhea itself is not a disease, but is usually a symptom of another condition. Depending on that condition, a woman might experience other symptoms, such as headache, vision changes, hair loss, or excess facial hair.

What are the causes of amenorrhea?

Amenorrhea is a symptom of a variety of conditions, ranging from not serious to serious.

Primary Amenorrhea

- Chromosomal or genetic abnormalities can cause the eggs and follicles involved in menstruation to deplete too early in life.

- Hypothalamic or pituitary diseases and physical problems, such as problems with reproductive organs, can prevent periods from starting.

- Moderate or excessive exercise, eating disorders (such as anorexia nervosa), extreme physical or psychological stress, or a combination of these can disrupt the normal menstrual cycle.

Secondary Amenorrhea

- This problem is much more common than primary amenorrhea.

- Common causes include many of those listed for primary amenorrhea, as well as pregnancy, certain contraceptives, breastfeeding, mental stress, and certain medications.

- Hormonal problems involving the hypothalamus, pituitary, thyroid, ovary, or adrenal glands can also cause amenorrhea.

- Women who have very low body weight sometimes stop getting their periods as well.

- Women with premature ovarian failure stop getting their periods before natural menopause.

What is treatment for amenorrhea?

Treatment for amenorrhea depends on the underlying cause. Sometimes lifestyle changes can help if weight, stress, or physical activity is causing the amenorrhea. Other times medications and oral contraceptives can help the problem. For more information, talk to your health care provider.

For More Information

NICHD Information Resource Center
P.O. Box 3006
Rockville, MD 20847
Toll-Free: 800-370-2943
Fax: 301-984-1473
Website: http://www.nichd.nih.gov
E-mail: NICHDIRC@mail.nih.gov

Chapter 55

Polycystic Ovarian Syndrome

Polycystic ovarian syndrome (PCOS) is a health problem that can affect a woman's menstrual cycle, fertility, hormones, insulin production, heart, blood vessels, and appearance. Women with PCOS have these characteristics:

- high levels of male hormones, also called androgens
- an irregular or no menstrual cycle
- may or may not have many small cysts (fluid-filled sacs) in their ovaries

PCOS is the most common hormonal reproductive problem in women of childbearing age.

How many women have PCOS?

An estimated five to 10 percent of women of childbearing age have PCOS.

What causes PCOS?

No one knows the exact cause of PCOS. Women with PCOS frequently have a mother or sister with PCOS. But there is not yet enough evidence to say there is a genetic link to this disorder. Many women with PCOS have a weight problem. So researchers are looking at the

National Women's Health Information Center, December 2004.

relationship between PCOS and the body's ability to make insulin. Insulin is a hormone that regulates the change of sugar, starches, and other food into energy for the body's use or for storage. Since some women with PCOS make too much insulin, it is possible that the ovaries react by making too many male hormones, called androgens. This can lead to acne, excessive hair growth, weight gain, and ovulation problems.

Why do women with PCOS have trouble with their menstrual cycle?

The ovaries are two small organs, one on each side of a woman's uterus. A woman's ovaries have follicles, which are tiny sacs filled with liquid that hold the eggs. These sacs are also called cysts. Each month about 20 eggs start to mature, but usually only one becomes dominant. As the one egg grows, the follicle accumulates fluid in it. When that egg matures, the follicle breaks open to release the egg so it can travel through the fallopian tube for fertilization. When the single egg leaves the follicle, ovulation takes place.

In women with PCOS, the ovary does not make all of the hormones it needs for any of the eggs to fully mature. They may start to grow and accumulate fluid. But no egg becomes large enough. Instead, some may remain as cysts. Since no egg matures or is released, ovulation does not occur, and the hormone progesterone is not made. Without progesterone, a woman's menstrual cycle is irregular or absent. Also, the cysts produce male hormones, which continue to prevent ovulation.

What are the symptoms of PCOS?

These are some of the symptoms of PCOS:

- infrequent menstrual periods, no menstrual periods, and/or irregular bleeding

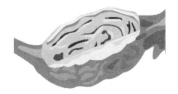 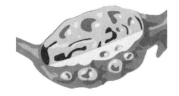

Figure 55.1. Normal Ovary   **Figure 55.2.** Polycystic Ovary

- infertility or inability to get pregnant because of not ovulating
- increased growth of hair on the face, chest, stomach, back, thumbs, or toes
- acne, oily skin, or dandruff
- pelvic pain
- weight gain or obesity, usually carrying extra weight around the waist
- type 2 diabetes
- high cholesterol
- high blood pressure
- male-pattern baldness or thinning hair
- patches of thickened and dark brown or black skin on the neck, arms, breasts, or thighs
- skin tags, or tiny excess flaps of skin in the armpits or neck area
- sleep apnea—excessive snoring and breathing stops at times while asleep

What tests are used to diagnose PCOS?

There is no single test to diagnose PCOS. Your doctor will take a medical history, perform a physical exam—possibly including an ultrasound, check your hormone levels, and measure glucose, or sugar levels, in the blood. If you are producing too many male hormones, the doctor will make sure it is from PCOS. At the physical exam the doctor will want to evaluate the areas of increased hair growth, so try to allow the natural hair growth for a few days before the visit. During a pelvic exam, the ovaries may be enlarged or swollen by the increased number of small cysts. This can be seen more easily by vaginal ultrasound, or screening, to examine the ovaries for cysts and the endometrium. The endometrium is the lining of the uterus. The uterine lining may become thicker if there has not been a regular period.

How is PCOS treated?

Because there is no cure for PCOS, it needs to be managed to prevent problems. Treatments are based on the symptoms each patient is having and whether she wants to conceive or needs contraception. Following are descriptions of treatments used for PCOS.

Birth control pills. For women who do not want to become pregnant, birth control pills can regulate menstrual cycles, reduce male hormone levels, and help to clear acne. However, the birth control pill does not cure PCOS. The menstrual cycle will become abnormal again if the pill is stopped. Women may also think about taking a pill that only has progesterone, like Provera, to regulate the menstrual cycle and prevent endometrial problems. But progesterone alone does not help reduce acne and hair growth.

Diabetes medications. The medicine, Metformin, also called Glucophage, which is used to treat type 2 diabetes, also helps with PCOS symptoms. Metformin affects the way insulin regulates glucose and decreases the testosterone production. Abnormal hair growth will slow down and ovulation may return after a few months of use. These medications will not cause a person to become diabetic.

Fertility medications. The main fertility problem for women with PCOS is the lack of ovulation. Even so, her husband's sperm count should be checked and her tubes checked to make sure they are open before fertility medications are used. Clomiphene (pills) and gonadotropins (shots) can be used to stimulate the ovary to ovulate. PCOS patients are at increased risk for multiple births when using these medications. In vitro fertilization (IVF) is sometimes recommended to control the chance of having triplets or more. Metformin can be taken with fertility medications and helps to make PCOS women ovulate on lower doses of medication.

Medicine for increased hair growth or extra male hormones. If a woman is not trying to get pregnant, there are some other medicines that may reduce hair growth. Spironolactone is a blood pressure medicine that has been shown to decrease the male hormone's effect on hair. Propecia, a medicine taken by men for hair loss, is another medication that blocks this effect. Both of these medicines can affect the development of a male fetus and should not be taken if pregnancy is possible. Other non-medical treatments such as electrolysis or laser hair removal are effective at getting rid of hair. A woman with PCOS can also take hormonal treatment to keep new hair from growing.

Surgery. Although it is not recommended as the first course of treatment, surgery called ovarian drilling is available to induce ovulation. The doctor makes a very small incision above or below the navel, and inserts a small instrument that acts like a telescope into the abdomen. This is called laparoscopy. The doctor then punctures the ovary with a small needle carrying an electric current to destroy a small portion of the ovary. This procedure carries a risk of developing scar tissue on the ovary. This surgery can lower male hormone levels and help with ovulation. But these effects may only last a few months. This treatment does not help with increased hair growth and loss of scalp hair.

A healthy weight. Maintaining a healthy weight is another way women can help manage PCOS. Since obesity is common with PCOS, a healthy diet and physical activity help maintain a healthy weight, which will help the body lower glucose levels, use insulin more efficiently, and may help restore a normal period. Even loss of 10% of her body weight can help make a woman's cycle more regular.

How does PCOS affect a woman while pregnant?

There appears to be a higher rate of miscarriage, gestational diabetes, pregnancy-induced high blood pressure, and premature delivery in women with PCOS. Researchers are studying how the medicine metformin prevents or reduces the chances of having these problems while pregnant, in addition to looking at how the drug lowers male hormone levels and limits weight gain in women who are obese when they get pregnant. No one yet knows if metformin is safe for pregnant women. Because the drug crosses the placenta, doctors are concerned that the baby could be affected by the drug. Research is ongoing.

Does PCOS put women at risk for other conditions?

Women with PCOS can be at an increased risk for developing several other conditions. Irregular menstrual periods and the absence of ovulation cause women to produce the hormone estrogen, but not the hormone progesterone. Without progesterone, which causes the endometrium to shed each month as a menstrual period, the endometrium becomes thick, which can cause heavy bleeding or irregular bleeding. Eventually, this can lead to endometrial hyperplasia or cancer. Women with PCOS are also at higher risk for diabetes, high cholesterol, high blood pressure, and heart disease. Getting the symptoms under control at an earlier age may help to reduce this risk.

Does PCOS change at menopause?

Researchers are looking at how male hormone levels change as women with PCOS grow older. They think that as women reach menopause, ovarian function changes and the menstrual cycle may become more normal. But even with falling male hormone levels, excessive hair growth continues, and male pattern baldness or thinning hair gets worse after menopause.

For More Information

American Association of Clinical Endocrinologists (AACE)
1000 Riverside Ave., Suite 205
Jacksonville, FL 32204
Phone: 904-353-7878
Fax: 904-353-8185
Website: http://www.aace.com
E-mail: info@aace.com

American Society for Reproductive Medicine (ASRM)
1209 Montgomery Highway
Birmingham, AL 35216-2809
Phone: 205-978-5000
Fax: 205-978-5005
Website: http://www.asrm.org
E-mail: asrm@asrm.org

Hormone Foundation
8401 Connecticut Ave., Suite 900
Chevy Chase, MD 20815
Toll-Free: 800-HORMONE (467-6663)
Fax: 301-941-0259
Website: http://www.hormone.org
E-mail: hormone@endo-society.org

InterNational Council on Infertility Information Dissemination, Inc. (INCIID)
P.O. Box 6836
Arlington, VA 22206
Phone: 703-379-9178
Fax: 703-379-1593

Website: http://www.inciid.org
E-mail: alert@inciid.org

National Women's Health Information Center (NWHIC)
8270 Willow Oaks Corporate Dr.
Fairfax, VA 22031
Toll-Free: 800-994-WOMAN (9662)
Toll-Free TDD: 888-220-5446
Website: http://www.4woman.gov

Chapter 56

Premature Ovarian Failure

What is premature ovarian failure (POF)?

Health care providers use the term POF to describe a stop in normal functioning of the ovaries in a woman under the age of 40. Many women naturally experience a decline in fertility at age 40; this age may also mark the beginning of irregularities in their menstrual cycles that signal the onset of menopause. For women with POF, the fertility decline and menstrual irregularities occur before age 40, sometimes even in the teens. Some health care providers also use the term primary ovarian insufficiency to describe this condition.

In the past, health care providers called this condition premature menopause, but this term is not an accurate description of what happens in a woman with POF. A woman who has gone through natural menopause will rarely ever have another period; a woman with POF is much more likely to have periods, even though they might not come regularly. There is virtually no chance for a woman who has gone through menopause naturally to get pregnant; in some cases, a woman with POF can still get pregnant.

What causes POF?

Although researchers have a general idea of what causes POF, in most cases the exact cause remains unclear. To understand what

"Do I Have Premature Ovarian Failure (POF)?" National Institute of Child Health and Human Development (NICHD), August 29, 2006.

happens in POF, you need to understand what happens in a woman's body when it's functioning normally.

In general, a woman's reproductive health involves her:

- **Hypothalamus** (pronounced high-poe-THAL-amus)—part of the brain that functions as the main control for the body's reproductive system. The hypothalamus works like a thermostat in a furnace, in that it controls the levels of different hormones and other chemicals in the body. If the hypothalamus detects that there is too little of a hormone in the body, it orders the body to make more.

- **Pituitary** (pronounced pitt-OO-ih-terry) gland—the body's master gland. The pituitary sends out hormones, or chemical signals to control the other glands in the body. The pituitary gets orders from the hypothalamus about what the body needs.

- **Ovaries**—the source of eggs in a woman's body. The ovaries have follicles, which are tiny, fluid-filled sacs that hold the eggs. The ovaries also make hormones that help to maintain a woman's health, such as estrogen, progesterone, and testosterone. The ovaries receive the chemical signals from the pituitary and respond by making certain hormones. In POF, the ovaries stop working correctly in both their egg production role, and in their hormone production role.

- **Uterus**—where a woman carries a baby, also called the womb. The uterus has different layers; its innermost layer or lining is called the endometrium—*endo* means inside and *metrium* (pronounced MEE-tree-um) means womb. The endometrium functions as a bed for an embryo when a woman is pregnant. If no pregnancy occurs during the cycle, then the endometrium is shed as a menstrual flow, or a period, and the cycle starts all over again.

These parts interact with one another to coordinate a woman's monthly menstrual cycle.

- The hypothalamus keeps track of the level of estradiol (pronounced ess-trah-DYE-awl) in the body. Estradiol is the natural estrogen that a woman's body makes, so it will be called estrogen from now on.

- When the level gets low, the hypothalamus sends an order to the pituitary gland telling it that the body needs more estrogen.

- The pituitary gets the order and responds by sending out follicle stimulating hormone (FSH), a hormone that causes the follicles on the ovary to grow and mature. Mature follicles make estrogen and other substances, such as inhibin. The pituitary continues to make FSH until the mature ovarian follicles make enough estrogen. If the follicles do not make enough estrogen, the level of FSH goes even higher.

- When the level of estrogen gets high enough, the hypothalamus and pituitary know that there is a mature egg in one of the follicles. To get this egg to the uterus so that it can be fertilized, the pituitary sends out a large burst of luteinizing hormone (LH). LH breaks open the mature follicle to release the egg, which allows it to move toward the uterus. The level of LH is only high during the time an egg is being released. This LH burst is the basis for home ovulation detection kits. Because LH may be high throughout much of the menstrual cycle in women who have POF, home ovulation detection kits are unreliable in these women.

- The empty follicle is then transformed into a yellowish, corpus luteum (pronounced CORE-puss loo-tee-um). *Corpus* means body and *luteum* means yellow. The corpus luteum makes progesterone, the hormone that prepares the uterus for pregnancy.

- Increased levels of progesterone cause the endometrium to change in preparation for pregnancy, should it occur. Once the endometrium is properly prepared, it can support an embryo and allow the embryo to grow.

- If the egg is fertilized, it sends out a hormone called human chorionic gonadotropin (HCG) to let the body know that it is there. HCG causes the corpus luteum to continue to make progesterone, the hormone needed for pregnancy. Pregnancy tests measure the level of HCG. If HCG is present, then it is likely that a woman is pregnant.

- If there is no signal, that is, no HCG is present because the egg was not fertilized, the corpus luteum stops making progesterone. Without progesterone, the endometrium starts to break down, and the woman's body sheds it as her period.

What happens differently in POF?

Currently, researchers are unable to pinpoint exactly what happens in POF to stop normal function of the ovaries in most cases.

Remember that the FSH levels are high when the ovaries fail to produce enough estrogen. LH levels also stay high in many cases, even during the occasional times that follicles successfully grow. Mature follicles in the ovaries make estrogen, as well as other substances, including the protein inhibin. Because women with POF have low levels of estrogen, scientists are focusing their attention on the follicles in the ovary in their study of POF.

Follicles in the ovaries start out as microscopic seeds, called primordial (pronounced prime-OR-dee-ul) follicles. These seeds are not yet follicles, but can grow into them. In general, a woman is born with about two million primordial follicles, which should be enough to last her until she goes through menopause. But this may not be the case for a woman with POF. Women with POF may fall into one of two groups.

Follicle Depletion: A woman with follicle depletion has no responsive follicles left in her ovaries. There is no way for the body to make more primordial follicles. And, currently, there is no way for scientists to make primordial follicles. Although scientists have not identified all the causes of follicle depletion, some known causes include:

- Chemotherapy or radiation therapy—strong treatments for cancer.

- An abnormal or missing X chromosome—the X chromosome stores genetic material that helps build a person. It also helps to determine whether a person is a male or a female. Females need two normal X chromosomes to make enough primordial follicles, and to use them properly. If a critical part of either X chromosome is missing, or if an entire X chromosome is missing, the body may not make enough primordial follicles to begin with, or it may use them up too quickly. This problem is the cause of POF in two percent to three percent of women with the condition.

- Even when it appears that all a woman's follicles are depleted, it is possible that a very small number of surviving follicles can, without warning, begin to function on their own. This spontaneous function can cause ovulation or a menstrual period; if insemination occurs, this function could lead to pregnancy, although such a situation is uncommon. Currently, health care providers cannot predict which women with POF will experience this recovery of ovarian function.

Follicle Dysfunction: A woman with follicle dysfunction still has follicles in her ovaries, but for unknown reasons they are not working properly. Currently, scientists do not have a safe and effective way to make follicles start working normally again. Although they have yet to identify all the causes of follicle dysfunction, some known causes include:

- An autoimmune attack: The immune system normally protects the body from invading bacteria and viruses. In some women, though, for reasons researchers do not understand, the immune system attacks developing follicles, which prevents the follicles from working the way they should. Current research suggests that this type of problem occurs in five percent of women with POF.

- A low number of follicles: Even though only one mature follicle releases an egg each month, that follicle usually has less mature follicles developing along with it. Scientists do not understand exactly how, but these supporting follicles seem to play a role in helping the mature follicle function normally. If these extra follicles are missing, the dominant follicle becomes luteinized and will not mature and release an egg properly. Current research estimates that this problem may occur in up to 60 percent of women with POF, but this is not a definite number.

Research also shows that ten percent to 20 percent of women with POF have a family history of the condition, which could mean that some cases of POF have a genetic component. But, inheritance patterns show that POF is not a purely genetic disorder. Research into the causes of POF is ongoing, in hopes that knowing why it occurs will also help in developing treatments for the disorder.

How many women have POF?

POF affects approximately:

- one in 10,000 women by age 20
- one in 1,000 women by age 30
- one in 250 women by age 35
- one in 100 women by age 40

What are the symptoms of POF?

The most common first symptom of POF is having irregular periods. Health care providers sometimes dismiss irregular or skipped periods (sometimes called amenorrhea—pronounced AY-men-or-ee-uh) as being related to stress; but a woman's monthly cycle is actually an important sign of her health, in the same way that blood pressure or temperature are signs of health. If you have irregular periods or skip periods, you should tell your health care provider, so that he or she can begin to determine the cause of these problems.

Some women with POF also experience other symptoms with POF. These symptoms are similar to those experienced by women who are going through natural menopause and include (but are not limited to):

- hot flashes
- night sweats
- irritability
- poor concentration
- decreased interest in sex
- pain during sex
- drying of the vagina
- infertility

How do I know if I have POF?

One of the most common signs of POF is having irregular periods. Women should pay close attention to their menstrual cycles, so that they can alert their health care provider when changes occur in their periods.

If you are under age 40 and your periods are irregular, or if you miss your period altogether for three months or more, your health care provider may measure the level of FSH in your blood, to determine if you have primary ovarian insufficiency in its early stages, or possibly even fully developed POF. Remember that FSH signals the ovaries to make estrogen. If the ovaries are not working properly, as is the case in POF, the level of FSH in the blood increases. A higher level of FSH in the blood is a strong sign of POF. But, irregular periods alone are not a sure sign that you have POF—research shows that fewer than ten percent of women who have irregular or skipped periods have high FSH levels and POF.

To do an FSH test, your health care provider will collect some of your blood and send it to a laboratory. At the lab, a technician will check the level of FSH. If the level of FSH is in the menopausal range, it is likely that you have POF.

Chapter 57

Precocious Puberty

Puberty, usually occurring during adolescence, is when kids develop physically and emotionally into young men and women. Usually, this starts to happen no earlier than about 7 to 8 years of age for girls and 9 years of age for boys (the average age is about 10 for girls and 12 for boys). But what if a younger child—for example, a 5-year-old girl—begins showing the signs of puberty? How would it affect her?

Precocious puberty—the onset of signs of puberty before age 7 or 8 in girls and age 9 in boys—can be physically and emotionally difficult for children and can sometimes be the sign of an underlying health problem.

What are the signs of precocious puberty?

In girls, the telltale signs of precocious puberty include any of the following before 7 or 8 years of age:

- breast development

- pubic or underarm hair

- development rapid height growth—a growth "spurt"

- onset of menstruation
- acne
- "mature" body odor

In boys, the signs of precocious puberty before 9 years of age include:

- enlargement of the testicles or penis
- pubic, underarm, or facial hair development
- rapid height growth—a growth "spurt"
- voice deepening
- acne
- "mature" body odor

Many children who show some of the early signs of puberty have what's known as "partial" precocious puberty. Some girls, usually beginning between the ages of 6 months and 3 years, may show breast development that later disappears or may persist without other physical changes of puberty.

Similarly, some girls and boys may experience early growth of pubic and/or underarm hair that isn't associated with other changes in sexual development. Children with "partial" precocious puberty may require evaluation to rule out "true" precocious puberty or other health problems, but they generally need no treatment and usually will show the other expected signs of puberty at the usual age.

How does precocious puberty affect a child?

When puberty ends, growth in height stops. Because their skeletons mature and bone growth stops at an earlier age than normal, kids with precocious puberty usually don't achieve their full adult height potential. Their early growth spurt may make them initially tall when compared with their peers, but they may stop growing too soon and end up at a shorter height than they would have otherwise.

Going through puberty early can also be difficult for a child emotionally and socially. For example, girls with precocious puberty may be confused or embarrassed about physical changes such as getting their periods or having enlarged breasts well before any of their peers. But the hardest part may be the teasing that children with the condition—especially girls—may experience.

Even emotions and behavior may change in children with precocious puberty. Girls can become moody and irritable. Boys can become more aggressive and also develop a sex drive inappropriate for their age.

What causes precocious puberty?

The onset of puberty is normally triggered by the hypothalamus (the area of the brain that helps control pituitary gland function). It signals the pituitary gland (a pea-sized gland near the base of the brain) to release hormones that stimulate the ovaries (in girls) or testicles (in boys) to make sex hormones.

Sometimes, precocious puberty stems from a structural problem in the brain (such as a tumor), brain injury due to head trauma, an infection (such as meningitis), or a problem in the ovaries or thyroid gland that triggers the onset of puberty ahead of schedule—but this usually isn't the case.

For the majority of girls, there's no underlying medical problem—they simply start puberty too early for no known reason. In boys, the condition is less common, and more likely to be associated with an underlying medical problem than it is in girls.

In about 5% of boys, precocious puberty is inherited. Starting puberty early can be passed to the son from the father or to the son from the maternal grandfather through the mother (who will not be affected by the disorder). But less than 1% of girls affected by precocious puberty have inherited the condition.

How is precocious puberty diagnosed?

Talk to your child's doctor if your child shows any signs of early sexual maturation before age 7 or 8 in girls or age 9 in boys, including breast development, rapid height growth, menstruation, acne, enlarged testicles or penis, or pubic or underarm hair.

The physical changes boys and girls go through during puberty are usually evident to a doctor during an exam. To confirm a diagnosis of precocious puberty, your child's doctor may order blood and urine tests to detect elevated levels of sex hormones. And x-rays of your child's wrist and hand can show whether the bones are maturing too rapidly.

Imaging and scanning tests such as computed tomography (CT) scans, magnetic resonance imaging (MRI), and ultrasound studies can help rule out specific causes of precocious puberty, such as a tumor in the brain, ovary, or testicle.

How is precocious puberty treated?

If your child's doctor suspects that your little one has precocious puberty, he or she may refer you to a pediatric endocrinologist (a doctor who specializes in growth and hormonal disorders in children) for further evaluation and treatment.

Once it's diagnosed, the goal of treating precocious puberty is to halt or even reverse sexual development and stop the rapid growth and bone maturation that can eventually result in adult short stature. Depending upon the cause, there are two possible approaches to treatment:

1. Treating the underlying cause or disease, such as a tumor.

2. Lowering the high levels of sex hormones with medication to stop sexual development from progressing.

In some cases, treatment of an underlying health problem can stop the precocious puberty from progressing. But in most cases, because there's no other disease triggering the condition, treatment usually consists of hormone therapy that stops sexual development.

The currently approved hormone treatment is with drugs called luteinizing hormone-releasing hormone (LHRH) analogs—synthetic hormones that block the body's production of the sex hormones that are causing the early puberty. Dramatic results are usually seen within a year of starting treatment with an LHRH analog, which is generally safe and usually causes no side effects in children. In girls, breast size may decrease—or at least there will be no further development. In boys, the penis and testicles may shrink back to the size expected for their age. Growth in height will also slow down to a rate expected for children before puberty. A child's behavior usually becomes more age appropriate as well.

Caring for Your Child

Give your child a simple, truthful explanation about what's happening. Explain that these changes are normal for older kids and teens, but that his or her body has started developing a little too early. Keep your child informed about his or her treatment and what can be expected along the way.

Also be sure to watch for signs that teasing or other difficulties associated with precocious puberty may be affecting your child's emotional development. Common warning signs to discuss with your child's doctor include:

- poor grades
- problems at school
- loss of interest in daily activities
- depression

How you cope with the issue can also determine how successfully your child will cope. The goal is to prevent your child from dwelling on sexual development or developing a poor self-image or low self-esteem. To create a supportive environment, try not to focus your comments on your child's appearance; instead, offer praise for achievements in school or sports and support your child's participation in other activities.

The important thing to remember is that children with precocious puberty can be treated. Doctors can help your child preserve his or her adult height potential as well as limit the emotional and social difficulties your child may face from maturing early.

Part Seven

Other Disorders of Endocrine and Metabolic Functioning

Chapter 58

Inborn Errors of Metabolism

Section 58.1

Understanding Inborn Errors of Metabolism

The topic of inborn errors of metabolism is challenging for most physicians. The number of known metabolic disorders is probably as large as the number of presenting symptoms that may indicate metabolic disturbances. Furthermore, physicians know they may not encounter certain rare inborn errors of metabolism during a lifetime of practice. Nonetheless, with a collective incidence of 1 in 1,500 persons, at least one of these disorders will be encountered by almost all practicing physicians.[1-3]

Improvements in medical technology and greater knowledge of the human genome are resulting in significant changes in the diagnosis, classification, and treatment of inherited metabolic disorders. Many known inborn errors of metabolism will be recognized earlier or treated differently because of these changes. It is important for primary care physicians to recognize the clinical signs of inborn errors of metabolism and to know when to pursue advanced laboratory testing or referral to a children's subspecialty center.

Early Diagnosis and Screening in Asymptomatic Infants

The principles of population screening to identify persons with biologic markers of disease and to apply interventions to prevent disease progression are well established. Screening tests must be timely and effective with a high predictive value. Current approaches to detecting inborn errors of metabolism revolve around laboratory screening for certain disorders in asymptomatic newborns, follow-up and verification of abnormal laboratory results, prompt physician recognition in symptomatic persons of disorders not screened for in newborn screening, and rapid implementation of appropriate therapies.

The increasing application of new technologies such as electrospray ionization-tandem mass spectrometry to newborn screening[4] in asymptomatic persons allows earlier identification of clearly defined inborn errors of metabolism. It also detects some conditions of uncertain clinical significance.[5] The inborn errors of metabolism detected by tandem mass spectrometry generally include aminoacidemias, urea cycle disorders, organic acidurias, and fatty acid oxidation disorders. Earlier recognition of these inborn errors of metabolism has the potential to reduce morbidity and mortality rates in affected infants.[6]

Tandem mass spectrometry has been introduced or mandated in many states, with some states testing for up to seven conditions and others screening for up to 40 conditions. Therefore, physicians must be aware of variability in newborn screening among individual hospitals and states. Current state-by-state information on newborn screening programs can be obtained through the internet resource GeNeS-R-US (Genetic and Newborn Screening Resource Center of the United States; http://genes-r-us.uthscsa.edu/).[7] Primary care physicians are most likely to be the first to inform parents of an abnormal result from a newborn screening program. In many instances, primary care physicians may need to clarify preliminary laboratory results or explain the possibility of a false-positive result.[6]

Editor's note: Chapter 9 of this Sourcebook contains state-by-state information on newborn screening programs.

Early Diagnosis in Symptomatic Infants

Within a few days or weeks after birth, a previously healthy neonate may begin to show signs of an underlying metabolic disorder. Although the clinical picture may vary, infants with metabolic disorders typically present with lethargy, decreased feeding, vomiting, tachypnea (from acidosis), decreased perfusion, and seizures. As the metabolic illness progresses, there may be increasing stupor or coma associated with progressive abnormalities of tone (hypotonia, hypertonia), posture (fisting, opisthotonos), and movements (tongue-thrusting, lip-smacking, myoclonic jerks), and with sleep apnea.[8] Metabolic screening tests should be initiated. Elevated plasma ammonia levels, hypoglycemia, and metabolic acidosis, if present, are suggestive of inborn errors of metabolism. In addition, the parent or physician may notice an unusual odor in an infant with certain inborn errors of metabolism (for example, maple syrup urine disease, phenylketonuria [PKU], hepatorenal tyrosinemia type 1, isovaleric acidemia). A disorder similar to Reye syndrome (for example,

Table 58.1. Inborn Errors of Metabolism and Associated Symptoms*
(Continued on next page)

Symptoms	Disorder	Incidence
Diarrhea		
	Lactase deficiency	common
	Mitochondrial disorders (for example, Pearson syndrome [rare])	1:30,000
	Abetalipoproteinemia	rare
	Enteropeptidase deficiency	rare
	Lysinuric protein intolerance	rare
	Sucrase-isomaltase deficiency	rare
Exercise intolerance		
	Fatty acid oxidation disorders	1:10,000
	Glycogenolysis disorders	1:20,000
	Mitochondrial disorder (for example, lipoamide dehydrogenase deficiency [rare])	1:30,000
	Myoadenylate deaminase deficiency	1:100,000
Familial myocardial infarct/stroke		
	5,10-methylenetetrahydrofolate reductase deficiency	common
	Familial hypercholesterolemia	1:500
	Fabry disease	1:80,000 to 1:117,000
	Homocystinuria	1:200,000
Muscle cramps/ spasticity		
	Multiple carboxylase deficiency (for example, holocarboxylase synthetase [rare]) and biotinidase deficiencies	1:60,000
	Metachromatic leukodystrophy	1:100,000
	HHH[a] syndrome	rare
Peripheral neuropathy		
	Mitochondrial disorders	1:30,000
	Peroxisomal disorders (for example, Zellweger syndrome, neonatal adrenoleukodystrophy, Refsum disease)	1:50,000
	Metachromatic leukodystrophy	1:100,000
	Congenital disorders of glycosylation	rare

Table 58.1. Inborn Errors of Metabolism and Associated Symptoms*
(continued)

Symptoms	Disorder	Incidence
Recurrent emesis		
	Galactosemia	1:40,000
	3-oxothiolase deficiency	1:100,000
	D-2-hydroxyglutaricaciduria	rare
Symptoms of pancreatitis	Mitochondrial disorder (for example, cytochrome-c oxidase deficiency; MELAS[a] syndrome; Pearson syndrome [all rare])	1:30,000
	Glycogenosis, type I	1:70,000
	Hyperlipoproteinemia, types I and IV	rare
	Lipoprotein lipase deficiency	rare
	Lysinuric protein intolerance	rare
Upward gaze paralysis	Mitochondrial disorders (for example, Leigh disease, Kearns-Sayre syndrome [rare])	1:30,000
	Niemann-Pick disease, type C	rare

Note: Disorders are listed as possible diagnostic considerations in order of descending incidence. Incidence in the general U.S. population is comparable to international estimates; however, disorders may occur more often in select ethnic populations. Rare is defined as an estimated incidence of fewer than 1:250,000 persons.

[a]HHH = hyperornithinemia-hyperammonemia-homocitrullinuria; MELAS = mitochondrial encephalopathy, lactic acidosis, and stroke-like episodes.

*Inborn errors of metabolism can induce disease manifestations in any organ at various stages of life, from newborn to adulthood. Whereas advanced newborn screening programs using tandem mass spectrometry will detect some inherited metabolic disorders before clinical signs appear, most of these disorders will be detected by the primary care physician before the diagnosis is made. Reliable determination of certain metabolic disorders varies between laboratories. Changes in screening reflect a growing field.

Information from references 1 through 3.

nonspecific hepatic encephalopathy, possibly with hypoglycemia) may be present secondary to abnormalities of gluconeogenesis, fatty acid oxidation, the electron transport chain, or organic acids.

Most metabolic disorders associated with organ system manifestations are not detected by tandem mass spectrometry screening. These highly diverse presentations of inborn errors of metabolism may be associated with dysfunction of the central nervous system (CNS), liver, kidney, eye, bone, blood, muscle, gastrointestinal tract, and integument. Infants with symptoms of acute or chronic encephalopathy usually require a focused but systematic evaluation by a children's neurologist and appropriate testing (for example, magnetic resonance imaging, additional genetic or metabolic analysis). Subspecialty referral is likewise necessary for infants or children presenting with hepatic, renal, or cardiac syndromes; dysmorphic syndromes; ocular findings; or significant orthopedic abnormalities.

A "pattern recognition" approach helps guide the physician toward a differential diagnosis and targeted biochemical and molecular testing.[9] However, this approach is not to be confused with the identification of congenital malformations, particularly those related to chromosomal disorders. Patients generally have a normal appearance in the early stages of most inborn metabolic disorders. Because most inborn errors of metabolism are single-gene disorders, chromosomal testing usually is not indicated.

Considerations in Older Infants and Children

Older infants with inborn errors of metabolism may demonstrate paroxysmal stupor, lethargy, emesis, failure to thrive, or organomegaly. Neurologic findings of neurometabolic disorders are acquired macrocephaly or microcephaly (CNS storage, dysmyelination, atrophy), hypotonia, hypertonia and/or spasticity, seizures, or other movement disorders. General non-neurologic manifestations of neurometabolic disorders include skeletal abnormalities and coarse facial features (for example, with mucopolysaccharidoses), macular or retinal changes (with leukodystrophies, poliodystrophies, mitochondrial disorders), corneal clouding (with Hurler syndrome, galactosemia), skin changes (for example, angiokeratomas in Fabry disease), or hepatosplenomegaly (with various storage diseases).

Consistent features of metabolic disorders in toddlers and preschool-age children include stagnation or loss of cognitive milestones; loss of expressive language skills; progressive deficits in attention, focus, and concentration; and other behavioral changes. The physician should attempt to make fundamental distinctions between primary-genetic and secondary-acquired causes of conditions that present as developmental delay or failure to thrive. Clues can be extracted through careful family, social, environmental, and nutritional history-taking. Syndromes with metabolic disturbances may lead to the identification of clinically recognizable genetic disorders. Referral to a geneticist often is indicated to further evaluate physical findings of primary genetic determinants.

Initial laboratory investigations for older children are the same as for infants. Infants and children presenting with acute metabolic decompensation precipitated by periods of prolonged fasting should be evaluated further for those organic acid, fatty acid oxidation, or peroxisomal disorders that are not detected by tandem mass spectrometry or certain regional neonatal screening programs.

Cerebrospinal fluid (CSF) may be helpful in the evaluation of certain metabolic disorders after neuroimaging studies and basic blood and urine analyses have been completed. Common CSF studies include cells (to rule out inflammatory disorders), glucose (plus plasma glucose to evaluate for blood-brain barrier or glucose transporter disorders), lactate (as a marker of energy metabolism or mitochondrial disorders), total protein, and quantitative amino acids. Nuclear magnetic resonance spectroscopy can provide a noninvasive, in vivo evaluation of proton-containing metabolites and can lead to the diagnosis of certain rare, but potentially treatable, neurometabolic disorders.[10] Electron microscopic evaluation of a skin biopsy is a highly sensitive screening tool that provides valuable clues to stored membrane material or ultrastructural organelle changes.[11]

Table 58.2 lists some of the more common inborn errors of metabolism, classified by type of metabolic disorder. Such prototypical inborn errors of metabolism include PKU, ornithine transcarbamylase deficiency, methylmalonicaciduria, medium-chain acyl-CoA dehydrogenase (MCAD) deficiency, galactosemia, and Gaucher disease.

Phenylketonuria (PKU)

PKU is an autosomal-recessive disorder most commonly caused by a mutation in the gene coding for phenylalanine hydroxylase, an enzyme responsible for the conversion of phenylalanine to tyrosine. Sustained phenylalanine concentrations higher than 20 milligrams (mg) per deciliter (dL) (1,211 millimole [mmol] per liter [L]) usually correlate with classic symptoms of PKU, such as impaired head circumference growth, poor cognitive function, irritability, and lighter skin

Table 58.2. Examples of Inborn Errors of Metabolism by Disorder (*continued on next 2 pages*)

Amino acid metabolism

Phenylketonuria: ~Incidence: 1:15,000
Inheritance: Autosomal recessive
Metabolic error: Phenylalanine hydroxylase (greater than 98 percent);
    Biopterin metabolic defects (less than 2 percent)
Key manifestation: Mental retardation, acquired microcephaly
Key laboratory test: Plasma phenylalanine concentration
Therapy approach: Diet low in phenylalanine hydroxylase

Maple syrup urine disease: ~Incidence 1:150,000 (1:1,000 in Mennonites)
Inheritance: Autosomal recessive
Metabolic error: Branched-chain a-keto acid dehydrogenase
Key manifestation: Acute encephalopathy, metabolic acidosis, mental retardation
Key laboratory test: Plasma amino acids and urine organic acids;
    Dinitrophenylhydrazine for ketones
Therapy approach: Restriction of dietary branched-chain amino acids

Carbohydrate metabolism

Galactosemia: ~Incidence 1:40,000
Inheritance: Autosomal recessive
Metabolic error: Galactose 1-phosphate uridyltransferase (most common);
    galactokinase; epimerase
Key manifestation: Hepatocellular dysfunction, cataracts
Key laboratory test: Enzyme assays, galactose and galactose 1-phosphate assay,
    molecular assay
Therapy approach: Lactose-free diet

Glycogen storage disease, type I[a] (von Gierke disease): ~Incidence: 1:100,000
Inheritance: Autosomal recessive
Metabolic error: Glucose-6-phosphatase
Key manifestation: Hypoglycemia, lactic acidosis, ketosis
Key laboratory test: Liver biopsy enzyme assay
Therapy approach: Corn starch and continuous overnight feeds

Fatty acid oxidation

Medium-chain acyl-CoA dehydrogenase deficiency: ~Incidence: 1:15,000
Inheritance: Autosomal recessive
Metabolic error: Medium-chain acyl-CoA dehydrogenase
Key manifestation: Nonketotic hypoglycemia, acute encephalopathy, coma, sudden infant death
Key laboratory test: Urine organic acids, acylcarnitine, gene test
Therapy approach: Avoid hypoglycemia, avoid fasting

Table 58.2. (continued) Examples of Inborn Errors of Metabolism by Disorder (*continued on next page*)

Lactic acidemia

Pyruvate dehydrogenase deficiency: ~Incidence: 1:200,000
Inheritance: X-linked
Metabolic error: E_1 subunit defect most common
Key manifestation: Hypotonia, psychomotor retardation, failure to thrive, seizures, lactic acidosis
Key laboratory test: Plasma lactate; Skin fibroblast culture for enzyme assay
Therapy approach: Correct acidosis; high-fat, low-carbohydrate diet

Lysosomal storage

Gaucher disease: ~Incidence: 1:60,000; type 1; 1:900 in Ashkenazi Jews
Inheritance: Autosomal recessive
Metabolic error: b-glucocerebrosidase
Key manifestation: Coarse facial features, hepatosplenomegaly
Key laboratory test: Leukocyte b-glucocerebrosidase assay
Therapy approach: Enzyme therapy, bone marrow transplant

Fabry disease: ~Incidence: 1:80,000 to 1:117,000
Inheritance: X-linked
Metabolic error: a-galactosidase A
Key manifestation: Acroparesthesias, angiokeratomas hypohidrosis, corneal opacities, renal insufficiency
Key laboratory test: Leukocyte a-galactosidase A assay
Therapy approach: Enzyme replacement therapy

Hurler syndrome: ~Incidence: 1:100,000
Inheritance: Autosomal recessive
Metabolic error: a-l-iduronidase
Key manifestation: Coarse facial features, hepatosplenomegaly
Key laboratory test: Urine mucopolysaccharides; Leukocyte a-l-iduronidase assay
Therapy approach: Bone marrow transplant

Organic aciduria

Methylmalonicaciduria: ~Incidence: 1:20,000
Inheritance: Autosomal recessive
Metabolic error: Methylmalonyl-CoA mutase, cobalamin metabolism
Key manifestation: Acute encephalopathy, metabolic acidosis, hyperammonemia
Key laboratory test: Urine organic acids; Skin fibroblasts for enzyme assay
Therapy approach: Sodium bicarbonate, carnitine, vitamin B_{12}, low-protein diet, liver transplant

Table 58.2. (continued) Examples of Inborn Errors of Metabolism by Disorder

Organic aciduria (continued)

Propionic aciduria: ~Incidence: 1:50,000
Inheritance: Autosomal recessive
Metabolic error: Propionyl-CoA carboxylase
Key manifestation: Metabolic acidosis, hyperammonemia
Key laboratory test: Urine organic acids
Therapy approach: Dialysis, bicarbonate, sodium benzoate, carnitine, low-protein diet, liver transplant

Peroxisomes

Zellweger syndrome: ~Incidence: 1:50,000
Inheritance: Autosomal recessive
Metabolic error: Peroxisome membrane protein
Key manifestation: Hypotonia, seizures, liver dysfunction
Key laboratory test: Plasma very-long-chain fatty acids
Therapy approach: No specific treatment available

Urea cycle

Ornithine transcarbamylase deficiency: ~Incidence: 1:70,000
Inheritance: X-linked
Metabolic error: Ornithine transcarbamylase
Key manifestation: Acute encephalopathy
Key laboratory test: Plasma ammonia, plasma amino acids; Urine orotic acid; Liver (biopsy) enzyme concentration
Therapy approach: Sodium benzoate, arginine, low-protein diet, essential amino acids; dialysis in acute stage

pigmentation. Infants diagnosed with PKU are treated with a special low-phenylalanine formula. Tyrosine is given at approximately 25 mg per kilogram (kg) of weight per day; amino acids are given at about three grams (g) per kg per day in infancy and two g per kg per day in childhood. Infants and children must be monitored regularly during the developmental period, and it is recommended that strict dietary therapy be continued for life. Special considerations for pregnant women with PKU include constant monitoring of phenylalanine concentrations to prevent intrauterine fetal malformation.[12]

Ornithine Transcarbamylase Deficiency

Ornithine transcarbamylase deficiency is the most common urea cycle disorder. Signs of ornithine transcarbamylase deficiency in infant boys include severe emesis, hyperammonemia, and progressive encephalopathy. Heterozygous girls, who demonstrate partial expression of the X-linked ornithine transcarbamylase deficiency disorder, may present with symptoms such as mild hyperammonemia and notable avoidance of dietary protein. Acute treatment options include sodium benzoate, sodium phenylacetate, and arginine. Certain persons may benefit from liver transplantation.

Methylmalonicaciduria Disorders

The most common genetic causes of methylmalonicaciduria are deficiencies in methylmalonyl-CoA mutase activity and in enzymatic synthesis of cobalamin. Pernicious anemia and dietary cobalamin deficiency also can result in abnormal methylmalonic acid metabolism. Metabolic ketoacidosis is the clinical hallmark of methylmalonic aciduria in infants. Therapy consists of protein restriction, restriction of methylmalonate precursors, and pharmacologic doses of vitamin B_{12}.

Medium-Chain Acyl-CoA Dehydrogenase (MCAD) Deficiency

The most common fatty acid oxidation disorder is MCAD deficiency. The majority of infants diagnosed with MCAD deficiency are homozygous for the A985G missense mutation and have northwestern European ancestry. Infants with MCAD deficiency appear to develop normally but present with rapidly progressive hypoglycemia, lethargy, and seizures, typically secondary to acute vomiting or fasting. Treatment of MCAD deficiency includes frequent cornstarch feeds and avoidance of fasting. Parents must have a basic understanding of the metabolic deficit in their child and should carry a letter from their treating physicians to alert emergency caregivers about the need for urgent attention in a crisis situation.

Galactosemia

There are three known enzymatic errors in galactose metabolism. The most common defect is confirmed by measuring decreased activity of erythrocyte galactose 1-phosphate uridyltransferase (GALT). Clinical manifestations of galactosemia include lethargy, hypotonia, jaundice, hypoglycemia, elevated liver enzymes, and coagulopathy. It is important to distinguish the galactosemia disease genotype (G/G) from asymptomatic variant genotypes (for example, G/D, G/N, D/D), which can be picked up as "positive" in newborn screening.

The main treatment for infants with the G/G mutation or very low GALT activity is lactose-free formula followed by dietary restriction of all lactose-containing foods later in life. Untreated infants who survive the neonatal period may have severe growth failure, mental retardation, cataracts, ovarian failure, and liver cirrhosis. Despite early and adequate intervention, some children still may develop milder signs of these clinical manifestations.

Gaucher Disease

Type 1 Gaucher disease, the most common lysosomal storage disorder, typically presents with hepatosplenomegaly, pancytopenia, and destructive bone disease. Types 2 and 3 Gaucher disease present with strabismus, bulbar signs, progressive cognitive deterioration, and myoclonic seizures. Treatment options for type 1 Gaucher disease include regular infusions with recombinant human acid b-glucosidase.

Importance of Early Treatment

Often, empiric therapeutic measures are needed before a definitive diagnosis is available. In a critically ill infant, aggressive treatment before the definitive confirmation of diagnosis is lifesaving and may reduce neurologic sequelae. Infants with a treatable organic acidemia (for example, methylmalonic acidemia) may respond to one mg of intramuscular vitamin B_{12}. Metabolic acidosis should be treated aggressively with sodium bicarbonate. Seizures in infancy should be treated initially with traditional antiepileptic drugs, but patients with rare inborn errors of metabolism may respond to other treatments (for example, oral pyridoxine in a dosage of five mg per kg per day) if rare disorders such as pyridoxine-dependent epilepsy are clinically suspected by the consulting neurologist.

Long-Term Treatment

Traditional therapies for metabolic diseases include dietary therapy such as protein restriction, avoidance of fasting, or cofactor supplements (Table 58.2). Evolving therapies include organ transplantation and enzyme replacement. Efforts to provide treatment through somatic gene therapy are in early stages, but there is hope that this approach will provide additional therapeutic possibilities. Even when no effective therapy exists or when an infant dies from a metabolic disorder, the family still needs an accurate diagnosis for clarification, reassurance, genetic counseling, and potential prenatal screening. Additional resources, including information about regional biochemical genetic consultation services, are available online.[13-15]

References

1. Beaudet AL, Scriver CR, Sly WS, Valle D. Molecular bases of variant human phenotypes. In: Scriver CR, ed. *The Metabolic and Molecular Bases of Inherited Disease. 8th ed.* New York: McGraw-Hill, 2001:3-51.

2. Applegarth DA, Toone JR, Lowry RB. Incidence of inborn errors of metabolism in British Columbia, 1969-1996. *Pediatrics* 2000;105:e10.

3. Meikle PJ, Hopwood JJ, Clague AE, Carey WF. Prevalence of lysosomal storage disorders. *JAMA* 1999;281:249-54.

4. Wilcken B, Wiley V, Hammond J, Carpenter K. Screening newborns for inborn errors of metabolism by tandem mass spectrometry. *N Engl J Med* 2003;348:2304-12.

5. Holtzman NA. Expanding newborn screening: how good is the evidence? *JAMA* 2003;290:2606-8.

6. Waisbren SE, Albers S, Amato S, Ampola M, Brewster TG, Demmer L, et al. Effect of expanded newborn screening for biochemical genetic disorders on child outcomes and parental stress. *JAMA* 2003;290: 2564-72.

7. University of Texas Health Science Center at San Antonio. National Newborn Screening and Genetics Resource Center. Accessed online January 10, 2006, at: http://genes-r-us.uthscsa .edu.

8. Clarke JT. *A Clinical Guide to Inherited Metabolic Diseases. 2nd ed.* New York: Cambridge University Press, 2002.

9. Blau N, Duran M, Blaskovics ME, Gibson KM. *Physician's Guide to the Laboratory Diagnosis of Metabolic Diseases. 2nd ed.* New York: Springer, 2003.

10. Novotny E, Ashwal S, Shevell M. Proton magnetic resonance spectroscopy: an emerging technology in pediatric neurology research. *Pediatr Res* 1998;44:1-10.

11. Prasad A, Kaye EM, Alroy J. Electron microscopic examination of skin biopsy as a cost-effective tool in the diagnosis of lysosomal storage diseases. *J Child Neurol* 1996;11:301-8.

12. Levy HL, Ghavami M. Maternal phenylketonuria: a metabolic teratogen. *Teratology* 1996;53:176-84.

13. GeneTests. National Institutes of Health. Accessed online January 10, 2006, at: http://www.genetests.org.

14. National Human Genome Research Institute. National Institutes of Health. Accessed online January 10, 2006, at: http://www.genome.gov/.

15. American Society of Human Genetics. Accessed online January 10, 2006, at: http://www.ashg.org.

Section 58.2

Galactosemia

What is galactosemia?

Galactosemia is an inherited disorder that prevents a person from processing the sugar galactose, which is found in many foods. Galactose also exists as part of another sugar, lactose, found in all dairy products.

Normally when a person consumes a product that contains lactose, the body breaks the lactose down into galactose and glucose. Galactosemia means too much galactose builds up in the blood. This accumulation of galactose can cause serious complications such as an enlarged liver, kidney failure, cataracts in the eyes, or brain damage. If untreated, as many as 75 percent of infants with galactosemia will die.

Duarte galactosemia is a variant of classic galactosemia. Fortunately, the complications associated with classic galactosemia have not been associated with Duarte galactosemia. There is some disagreement over the need for dietary restriction in the treatment of children with Duarte galactosemia. Consult your healthcare professional for his or her advice on this topic.[1]

What are the symptoms of galactosemia?

Galactosemia usually causes no symptoms at birth, but jaundice, diarrhea, and vomiting soon develop, and the baby fails to gain weight. Although galactosemic children are started on dietary restrictions at birth, there continues to be a high incidence of long-term complications involving speech and language, fine and gross motor skill delays, and specific learning disabilities. Ovarian failure may occur in girls.[2]

What causes galactosemia?

Classic galactosemia is a rare genetic metabolic disorder. A child born with classic galactosemia inherits a gene for galactosemia from both parents, who are carriers. A child with Duarte galactosemia inherits a gene for classic galactosemia (G) from one parent and a Duarte variant gene (D) from the other parent.

How is galactosemia diagnosed?

Diagnosis for both classic and Duarte galactosemia is made usually within the first week of life by a blood test from a heel prick as part of a standard newborn screening.

How is galactosemia treated?

Treatment requires the strict exclusion of lactose and galactose from the diet. A person with galactosemia will never be able to properly digest foods containing galactose. There is no chemical or drug substitute for the missing enzyme at this time. An infant diagnosed with galactosemia will simply be changed to a formula that does not contain galactose. With care and continuing medical advances, most children with galactosemia can now live normal lives.

If my child has been diagnosed with galactosemia, what should I ask our doctor?

Speak to your doctor about your child's dietary restrictions.

Who is at risk for galactosemia?

The gene defect for galactosemia is a recessive genetic trait. This faulty gene only emerges when two carriers have children together and pass it to their offspring. For each pregnancy of two such carriers, there is a 25 percent chance that the child will be born with the disease and a 50 percent chance that the child will be a carrier for the gene defect.[3]

References

1. Galactosemia.org. "What is Duarte Galactosemia." <http://www.galactosemia.org/galactosemia.asp>. Viewed 11/20/2006.

2. Galactosemia.org "What is Classic Galactosemia." <http://www.galactosemia.org/galactosemia.asp>. Viewed 11/20/2006.

3. SaveBabies.org. "Galactosemia (GALT)." <http://www.savebabies.org/diseasedescriptions/galactosemia.php>. Viewed 11/20/2006.

Section 58.3

Maple Syrup Urine Disease

"Maple Syrup Urine Disease," © 2006 Washington State Department of Health Newborn Screening Program. Reprinted with permission.

Primary Defect

Maple syrup urine disease (MSUD) is a deficiency or absence of an enzyme needed to break down the branched chain amino acids, leucine, isoleucine, and valine. This results in increased serum levels of these amino acids and ketoacid intermediates.

Screening Test

Historically screening has been based on measurement of leucine in the dried blood spot using a bacterial inhibition assay similar to the original Guthrie assay for phenylketonuria (PKU). Screening is now possible using tandem mass spectrometry to measure the amino acids. Predictive values are not documented but should be high.

Etiology and Prevalence

MSUD is a genetic, autosomal recessive disease. A number of specific genetic defects have been identified. With some, residual enzyme activity may occur, resulting in moderation of symptoms.

About one in every 200,000 babies in the United States is born with MSUD.

If Untreated

MSUD is lethal for the classical form (absent enzyme activity), usually in the first month of life. If residual enzyme activity is present, children develop mental and physical retardation.

Therapy

Treatment for MSUD involves dietary restriction of branched chain amino acids. This requires specialized medical and nutritional intervention.

Treatment

With treatment, the outcome is variable being related to age and neurological symptoms at the time therapy is initiated. Treated infants may have retardation related to onset of symptoms before screening test results are communicated. A highly coordinated screening system is essential since irreversible damage or death can occur within the first two weeks of life.

Section 58.4

Phenylketonuria (PKU)

National Institute of Child Health and Human Development
(NICHD), August 25, 2006.

What is phenylketonuria (PKU)?

Phenylketonuria (pronounced fee-nill-key-toe-NURR-ee-uh), or PKU, is an inherited disorder of metabolism that can cause mental retardation if not treated. In PKU, the body cannot process a portion of the protein called phenylalanine (Phe), which is in almost all foods. If the Phe level gets too high, the brain can become damaged. All babies born in U.S. hospitals are now routinely tested for PKU soon after birth, making it easier to diagnose and treat them early.

What are the symptoms of PKU?

Children with untreated PKU may appear normal at birth. By age three to six months, they begin to lose interest in their surroundings. By age one year, they are developmentally delayed and their skin has less pigmentation than someone without the condition. If Phe is not restricted in the diet, those with PKU develop severe mental retardation.

What are the treatments for PKU?

The most effective treatment for PKU is a special diet of foods that help control the amount of Phe consumed (some Phe is needed for normal growth and development). People with PKU who are on this diet from birth, or shortly thereafter, develop normally and often have no symptoms of PKU. The PKU diet includes fruits, vegetables, and some low-protein breads, pastas, and cereals. There is also a special formula, made without Phe, that people with PKU drink to help them get the vitamins and minerals they cannot get from their food. Generally, people with PKU cannot eat high-protein foods such as meat, milk, eggs, and nuts. An NIH Consensus Panel recommends that people with PKU stay on the diet for life to promote overall health and to prevent decline in mental function.

Are there other concerns for those with PKU?

Pregnant women who know they have PKU need to keep good control of the level of Phe in their diets beginning before and continuing throughout pregnancy. High levels of Phe in the blood can cause developmental problems and birth defects (such as small brain size and heart defects) in the fetus.

Additional Information about PKU

Children's PKU Network (CPN)
3790 Via De la Valle, Suite 120
Del Mar, CA 92014
Phone: 858-509-0767
Fax: 858-509-0768
Website: http://www.pkunetwork.org
E-mail: pkunetwork@aol.com

MUMS: National Parent to Parent Network
150 Custer Court
Green Bay, WI 54301-1243
Toll-Free: 877-336-5333 (Parents only please)
Phone: 920-336-5333
Fax: 920-339-0995
Website: http://www.netnet.net/mums
E-mail: mums@netnet.net

National Institute of Child Health and Human Development (NICHD)
31 Center Drive
Bethesda, MD 20892-2425
Toll Free: 800-370-2943
Toll-Free TTY: 888-320-6942
Fax: 301-984-1473
Website: http://www.nichd.nih.gov

Section 58.5

Urea Cycle Disorders

This section includes: "What Is a Urea Cycle Disorder?" "What Are the Symptoms?" "What Kinds of Disorders Are There?" and "What Are the Treatment Options?" Reprinted by permission of the National Urea Cycle Disorders Foundation, http://www.nucdf.org. © 2006 National Urea Cycle Disorders Foundation. All rights reserved. This section concludes with "Homocystinuria Facts" from "Homocystinuria," © 2006 Washington State Department of Health Newborn Screening Program. Reprinted with permission.

What is a urea cycle disorder?

A urea cycle disorder (UCD) is a genetic disorder caused by a deficiency of one of the enzymes in the urea cycle which is responsible for removing ammonia from the blood stream. The urea cycle involves a series of biochemical steps in which nitrogen, a waste product of protein metabolism, is removed from the blood and converted to urea. Normally, the urea is transferred into the urine and removed from the body. In urea cycle disorders, the nitrogen accumulates in the form of ammonia, a highly toxic substance, and is not removed from the body resulting in hyperammonemia. Ammonia then reaches the brain through the blood, where it causes irreversible brain damage, coma, and/or death.

Urea cycle disorders are included in the category of inborn errors of metabolism. There is no cure. Inborn errors of metabolism represent a substantial cause of brain damage and death among newborns and infants. Because many cases of urea cycle disorders remain undiagnosed and infants born with the disorders die without a definitive diagnosis, the exact incidence of these cases is unknown and underestimated. It is believed that up to 20% of sudden infant death syndrome (SIDS) cases may be attributed to an undiagnosed inborn error of metabolism such a urea cycle disorder. In April 2000, research experts at the Urea Cycle Consensus Conference estimated the incidence of the disorders at one in 10,000 births. This represents a significant increase in case diagnosis in the last few years. Research studies have now been initiated to more accurately determine the incidence and prevalence of UCD.

What are the symptoms?

The neonatal period: Children with severe urea cycle disorders typically show symptoms after the first 24 hours of life. The baby may be irritable at first, or refuse feedings, followed by vomiting and increasing lethargy. Soon after, seizures, hypotonia (poor muscle tone, floppiness), respiratory distress (respiratory alkalosis), and coma may occur. These symptoms are caused by rising ammonia levels in the blood. Sepsis and Reye syndrome are common misdiagnoses. If untreated, these severely affected infants will die. Severe neonatal symptoms are more commonly seen in both boys and girls with ornithine transcarbamylase (OTC) and carbamoyl phosphate synthetase (CPS) deficiency, but can also occur with citrullinemia or argininosuccinate lyase deficiency (ASA).

Childhood: Children with mild or moderate urea cycle enzyme deficiencies may not show recognizable symptoms until early childhood. Earliest symptoms may include failure to thrive, inconsolable crying, agitation or hyperactive behavior, sometimes accompanied by screaming, self-injurious behavior, and refusal to eat meat or other high-protein foods. Later symptoms may include frequent episodes of vomiting, especially following high-protein meals, lethargy and delirium, and finally, if the condition is undiagnosed and untreated, hyperammonemic coma or death may occur. Undiagnosed children may be referred to child psychologists because of their behavior and eating problems. Childhood episodes of hyperammonemia (high ammonia levels in the blood) may be brought on by viral illnesses including chickenpox, colds or flu, teething, growth spurts, high-protein meals, or even exhaustion. Common misdiagnoses include Reye syndrome. Childhood onset can be seen in both boys and girls affected by any of the urea cycle disorders.

Early clinical manifestations of arginase (AG) deficiency (similar to those of the other disorders), may be seen as early as one year of age, but some children with AG remain asymptomatic at four years of age. AG symptoms are usually progressive and include growth failure, spastic tetraplegia (lower limbs more severely affected than upper limbs), seizures, psychomotor retardation, and hyperactivity.

Major characteristics of N-acetylglutamate synthetase (NAGS) deficiency, considered the rarest urea cycle disorder, include severe hyperammonemia, deep encephalopathy despite only mild hyperammonemia, recurrent diarrhea and acidosis, movement disorder, hypoglycemia, and hyperornithinemia.[1]

Adulthood: Recently, the number of adults being diagnosed with urea cycle disorders has increased at an alarming rate. These individuals have survived undiagnosed to adulthood, probably due to less severe enzyme deficiencies. These individuals exhibit stroke-like symptoms, episodes of lethargy, and delirium. These adults are likely to be referred to neurologists or psychiatrists because of their psychiatric symptoms. However, without proper diagnosis and treatment, these individuals are at risk for permanent brain damage, coma, and death. Adult-onset symptoms have been observed following viral illnesses, childbirth, dieting, use of valproic acid (an anti-epileptic drug which causes excess ammonia), and chemotherapy.

OTC carriers: Approximately 85% of adult female carriers (heterozygotes) for OTC deficiency are asymptomatic (exhibit no symptoms). The remainder (15% of adult female carriers) show symptoms including protein intolerance, headache, episodes of confusion or inability to concentrate, behavioral or neurological abnormalities, cyclical vomiting, and episodes of hyperammonemia. Studies have shown carriers to be of normal to above-normal intelligence, but some have been shown to demonstrate subtle deficits in fine motor, visual-spatial, and non-verbal functions.[2] Concerns are beginning to emerge with carriers with regard to common health issues (diabetes, hypercholesterolemia, cancer) and effects that treatments or drugs used to treat these common conditions may have on urea cycle function.

What kinds of disorders are there?

There are six enzyme disorders of the urea cycle, collectively known as inborn errors of urea synthesis, or urea cycle enzyme defects. Each is referred to by the initials of the missing enzyme:

- CPS—carbamyl phosphate synthetase
- NAGS—N-acetylglutamate synthetase
- OTC—ornithine transcarbamylase
- AS—argininosuccinic acid synthetase (citrullinemia)
- AL/ASA—argininosuccinate lyase (argininosuccinic aciduria)
- AG—arginase

Additionally, there are three transporter defects:

- mitochondrial ornithine carrier (hyperornithinemia-hyperammonemia-hypercitrullinuria, or HHH syndrome)

- mitochondrial aspartate/glutamate carrier (citrullinemia type II)

- dibasic amino acid carrier (hyperdibasic amino aciduria, or lysinuric protein intolerance)

Neonatal onset disorders represent severe enzyme deficiencies or complete absence of enzyme function. Individuals with childhood or adult onset disease have partial enzyme deficiency. The percentage, or amount of enzyme function, varies widely between individuals with partial enzyme deficiencies. All of these disorders are transmitted genetically as autosomal recessive genes—each parent contributes a defective gene to the child—except for ornithine transcarbamylase deficiency (OTC). OTC deficiency is acquired in one of three ways: as an X-linked trait from the mother, who may be an undiagnosed carrier; in some cases of female children, the disorder can also be inherited from the defect on the father's X-chromosome; and finally, OTC deficiency may be acquired as a new, spontaneous mutation occurring in the fetus. Recent research has shown that some female carriers of the disease may become symptomatic with the disorder later in life, suffering high ammonia levels and experiencing classic symptoms. Several undiagnosed women have died during childbirth as a result of high ammonia levels, and on autopsy were determined to have been unknown symptomatic carriers of the disorder.

What are the treatment options?

The treatment of urea cycle disorders consists of dietary management to limit ammonia production in conjunction with medications and/or supplements which provide alternative pathways for the removal of ammonia from the bloodstream. A careful balance of dietary protein, carbohydrates, and fats is necessary to insure that the body receives adequate calories for energy needs, as well as adequate essential amino acids (for cell growth and development). Dietary protein must be carefully monitored and some restriction is necessary; too much dietary protein causes excessive ammonia production. However, if protein intake is too restrictive or insufficient calories are provided, the body will break down lean muscle mass (called catabolism) to obtain the amino acids or energy it requires; this catabolism creates excessive ammonia. Therefore, the correct nutritional balance for each individual in each stage of growth is critical in avoiding hyperammonemic crises. Frequent blood tests (serum ammonia, plasma quantitative amino acids) are required to monitor the disorders and are an important tool for optimizing treatment.

Treatment may include supplementation with special amino acid formulas (Cyclinex, UCD I and II), developed specifically for urea cycle disorders, which can be prescribed to provide approximately 50% of the daily dietary protein allowance. Some patients may require individual branched chain amino acid supplementation. Metabolic nutritionists routinely prescribe calorie modules such as Pro-Phree, Polycose, and Moducal to be used in combination with the amino acid formulas. Pharmaceutical grade (not over-the-counter) L-citrulline (for OTC and CPS deficiency) or L-arginine free base (ASA and citrullinemia) is also required. These are not to be used in arginase (AG) deficiency. Multiple vitamins and calcium supplements are also recommended.

Sodium phenylbutyrate (trade name Buphenyl) is the primary medication being used to treat urea cycle disorders. The Urea Cycle Disorders Foundation played a key role in initiating and supporting the research at Johns Hopkins University to develop the medication. Sodium benzoate is also used in some patients, solely or in conjunction with Buphenyl; both are ammonia scavengers—providing alternative pathways for removal of ammonia from the bloodstream and helping to prevent hyperammonemia. One or both of these medications is administered three to four times per day in order to insure continual removal of toxic ammonia from the bloodstream.

Children with urea cycle disorders often lack appetite (due to excess serotonin in the brain suppressing appetite), and some may benefit from receiving medications and some feedings either via gastrostomy tube (G-tube), a tube surgically implanted in the stomach, or nasogastric tube (NG-tube), a tube manually inserted through the nose into the stomach. The access these tubes provide often makes a critical difference in metabolic stability and in averting hyperammonemic crises; medications and formulas can still be administered when children have flu or colds, or other illness. Some centers have reported as much as 70% reduction in hospital admissions after placement of G-tubes or parents were trained to use NG-tubes.

Optimal treatment of urea cycle disorders requires a medical team consisting minimally of a geneticist and/or metabolic specialist and nutritionist specifically experienced in successful management of the disorders. These teams are usually found at university hospitals. Specialty consultation and second opinions from experts in the field of UCD can be obtained by families who live in areas where optimal medical care is not available.

When optimal treatment fails, or for neonatal onset CPS and OTC deficiency, liver transplant becomes an option. Liver transplants have been done successfully as a cure for the disorder (although L-arginine supplementation is still necessary in argininosuccinate lyase deficiency posttransplant). The transplant alternative must be carefully considered and evaluated with medical professionals to determine the potential of success compared to the serious risks and potential for new medical concerns, including the possibility of fatal viruses (Epstein-Barr, Cytomegalovirus [CMV]), risk of developmental delay, or lymphoproliferative disease as a side effect of immunosuppression and immunosuppressants.

Homocystinuria Facts

Primary Defect

Homocystinuria is the deficiency or absence of an enzyme necessary for the breakdown of the amino acid methionine results in build up of methionine in the blood and elevated excretion of homocystine in the urine.

Screening Test

Historically screening has been based on measurement of methionine in the dried blood spot using a bacterial inhibition assay similar to the original Guthrie assay for phenylketonuria (PKU). Screening is now possible using tandem mass spectrometry (MS/MS). Predictive value should be high. Because of delayed accumulation of methionine if residual enzyme activity is present, screening may be more effective at two to four weeks of age for these infants.

Etiology and Prevalence

Homocystinuria is a genetic, autosomal recessive disease. A number of specific genetic defects have been identified. With some, residual enzyme activity may occur, resulting in moderation of symptoms and delay in accumulation of elevated levels of methionine.

About one in every 200,000 babies in the United States is born with homocystinuria.

If Untreated

There is wide variation in the clinical course for affected infants. Clinical features include: circulatory blood clotting (thromboembolism) and physical and mental developmental disabilities. Approximately half of the affected individuals die by age 25 due to thromboembolism. Developmental delay and physical defects affect most. The most common defect (cystathionine b-synthase deficiency) can be classified as either responsive or non-responsive to treatment with vitamin B_6. This may be related to residual enzyme activity needed for response. Those who are not responsive have a more severe clinical course.

Therapy

Treatment includes vitamin B_6 supplementation for those who are responsive; dietary restriction of methionine with supplementation of cystine for those who are not. Other treatment is focused on clinical features such as aspirin to combat thromboembolism.

Treatment

With treatment, mortality and mental retardation are prevented or reduced. Clinical variability of other features remains.

References

1. S. Brusilow, A. Horwich, "Urea Cycle Enzyme," *The Metabolic and Molecular Bases of Inherited Disease*, Vol II p. 1810–1962: McGraw Hill.

2. A. Gropman, M. Batshaw: *Cognitive outcome in urea cycle disorders. Molecular Genetics and Metabolism* Vol 81, Sup 1, Apr 2004, p. 58–62.

Additional Information

National Urea Cycle Disorders Foundation
4841 Hill Street
La Canada, CA 91011
Toll-Free: 800-38-NUCDF (68233)
Fax: 818-248-9770
Website: http://www.nucdf.org
E-mail: info@nucdf.org

Washington State Department of Health
Newborn Screening Program
P.O. Box 557291610
Shoreline, WA 98155-0729
Toll-Free: 866-660-9050
Phone: 206-418-5410
Fax: 206-418-5415
Website: http://www.doh.wa.gov/EHSPHL/PHL/Newborn/pubs/
2006_en_brochure.pdf
E-mail: NBSProg@doh.wa.gov

Chapter 59

Glycogen-Storage Diseases

Glucose-6-Phosphate Dehydrogenase Deficiency

What other names do people use for glucose-6-phosphate dehydrogenase deficiency?

- deficiency of glucose-6-phosphate dehydrogenase
- G6PDD
- G6PD deficiency
- von Gierke disease

What is glucose-6-phosphate dehydrogenase deficiency?

Glucose-6-phosphate dehydrogenase deficiency is a genetic disorder that occurs most often in males. This condition mainly affects red blood cells, which carry oxygen from the lungs to tissues throughout the body. In affected individuals, a defect in an enzyme called glucose-6-phosphate dehydrogenase causes red blood cells to break down prematurely. This destruction of red blood cells is called hemolysis.

This chapter includes text from: "Glucose-6-phosphate dehydrogenase deficiency," Genetics Home Reference, National Library of Medicine, May 2006; "Pompe Disease Information Page," National Institute of Neurological Disease and Stroke (NINDS), September 2006; and "McArdle Syndrome," © 2007 A.D.A.M., Inc. Reprinted with permission. Additional information from the National Organization on Rare Disorders (NORD) is cited separately within the chapter.

The most common medical problem associated with glucose-6-phosphate dehydrogenase deficiency is hemolytic anemia, which occurs when red blood cells are destroyed faster than the body can replace them. This type of anemia leads to paleness, yellowing of the skin and whites of the eyes (jaundice), dark urine, fatigue, shortness of breath, and a rapid heart rate. In people with glucose-6-dehydrogenase deficiency, hemolytic anemia is most often triggered by bacterial or viral infections or by certain drugs (such as some antibiotics and medications used to treat malaria). Hemolytic anemia can also occur after eating fava beans or inhaling pollen from fava plants (a reaction called favism).

Glucose-6-dehydrogenase deficiency is also a significant cause of mild to severe jaundice in newborns. Many people with this disorder, however, never experience any signs or symptoms.

How common is glucose-6-phosphate dehydrogenase deficiency?

An estimated 400 million people worldwide have glucose-6-phosphate dehydrogenase deficiency. This condition occurs most frequently in certain parts of Africa, Asia, and the Mediterranean. It affects about one in ten African-American males in the United States.

What genes are related to glucose-6-phosphate dehydrogenase deficiency?

Mutations in the G6PD gene cause glucose-6-phosphate dehydrogenase deficiency. The G6PD gene provides instructions for making an enzyme called glucose-6-phosphate dehydrogenase. This enzyme is involved in the normal processing of carbohydrates. It also protects red blood cells from the effects of potentially harmful molecules called reactive oxygen species. Reactive oxygen species are byproducts of normal cellular functions. Chemical reactions involving glucose-6-phosphate dehydrogenase produce compounds that prevent reactive oxygen species from building up to toxic levels within red blood cells.

If mutations in the G6PD gene reduce the amount of glucose-6-phosphate dehydrogenase or alter its structure, this enzyme can no longer play its protective role. As a result, reactive oxygen species can accumulate and damage red blood cells. Factors such as infections, certain drugs, or ingesting fava beans can increase the levels of reactive oxygen species, causing red blood cells to be destroyed faster than the body can replace them. A reduction in the amount of red blood cells causes the signs and symptoms of hemolytic anemia.

Researchers believe that carriers of a G6PD mutation may be partially protected against malaria, an infectious disease carried by a certain type of mosquito. A reduction in the amount of functional glucose-6-dehydrogenase appears to make it more difficult for this parasite to invade red blood cells. Glucose-6-phosphate dehydrogenase deficiency occurs most frequently in areas of the world where malaria is common.

How do people inherit glucose-6-phosphate dehydrogenase deficiency?

This condition is inherited in an X-linked recessive pattern. A condition is considered X-linked if the mutated gene that causes the disorder is located on the X chromosome, one of the two sex chromosomes. In males (who have only one X chromosome), one altered copy of the gene in each cell is sufficient to cause the condition. In females (who have two X chromosomes), a mutation must be present in both copies of the gene to cause the disorder. Males are affected by X-linked recessive disorders much more frequently than females. A striking characteristic of X-linked inheritance is that fathers cannot pass X-linked traits to their sons.

Pompe Disease

Pompe disease is a rare (estimated at one in every 40,000 births), inherited, and often fatal disorder that disables the heart and muscles. It is caused by mutations in a gene that makes an enzyme called alpha-glucosidase (GAA). Normally, the body uses GAA to break down glycogen, a stored form of sugar used for energy. But in Pompe disease, mutations in the GAA gene reduce or completely eliminate this essential enzyme. Excessive amounts of glycogen accumulate everywhere in the body, but the cells of the heart and skeletal muscles are the most seriously affected. Researchers have identified up to 70 different mutations in the GAA gene that cause the symptoms of Pompe disease, which can vary widely in terms of age of onset and severity. The severity of the disease and the age of onset are related to the degree of enzyme deficiency.

Early-onset (or infantile Pompe disease) is the result of complete or near complete deficiency of GAA. Symptoms begin in the first months of life, with feeding problems, poor weight gain, muscle weakness, floppiness, and head lag. Respiratory difficulties are often complicated by lung infections. The heart is grossly enlarged. More than half of all infants with Pompe disease also have enlarged tongues. Most babies with Pompe disease die from cardiac or respiratory complications before their first birthday.

Late-onset (juvenile or adult) Pompe disease is the result of a partial deficiency of GAA. The onset can be as early as the first decade of childhood or as late as the sixth decade of adulthood. The primary symptom is muscle weakness progressing to respiratory weakness and death from respiratory failure after a course lasting several years. The heart may be involved, but it will not be grossly enlarged. A diagnosis of Pompe disease can be confirmed by screening for the common genetic mutations or measuring the level of GAA enzyme activity in a blood sample—a test that has 100 percent accuracy. Once Pompe disease is diagnosed, testing of all family members and consultation with a professional geneticist is recommended. Carriers are most reliably identified via genetic mutation analysis.

Is there any treatment?

Individuals with Pompe disease are best treated by a team of specialists (such as cardiologist, neurologist, and respiratory therapist) knowledgeable about the disease, who can offer supportive and symptomatic care. The discovery of the GAA gene has led to rapid progress in understanding the biological mechanisms and properties of the GAA enzyme. As a result, an enzyme replacement therapy has been developed that has shown, in clinical trials with infantile-onset patients, to decrease heart size, maintain normal heart function, improve muscle function, tone, and strength, and reduce glycogen accumulation. A drug called alglucosidase alfa (Myozyme®), has received FDA approval for the treatment of Pompe disease.

What is the prognosis?

Without enzyme replacement therapy, the hearts of babies with infantile-onset Pompe disease progressively thicken and enlarge. These babies die before the age of one year from either cardiorespiratory failure or respiratory infection. For individuals with late-onset Pompe disease, the prognosis is dependent upon the age of onset. In general, the later the age of onset, the slower the progression of the disease. Ultimately, the prognosis is dependent upon the extent of respiratory muscle involvement.

What research is being done?

The National Institute of Neurological Disorders and Stroke (NINDS), and other Institutes of the National Institutes of Health (NIH), conduct research related to Pompe disease in laboratories at the NIH, and also support additional research through grants to major medical institutions across the country. Much of this research focuses on finding better ways to prevent, treat, and ultimately cure disorders such as Pompe disease.

Forbes Disease

Information under this heading is excerpted with permission from several Rare Disease Reports produced by the National Organization for Rare Disorders® (NORD), P.O. Box 1968, Danbury, CT 06913-1968, (800)-999-NORD (6673). © 2007 NORD. All rights reserved. Full-text reports for these and many other disorders, which include information on symptoms, causes, treatments, and clinical trials, can be purchased individually or by subscription on the NORD website at http://www.rarediseases.org.

Synonyms of Forbes disease include:

- amylo-1,6-glucosidase deficiency
- Cori disease
- debrancher deficiency
- glycogen-storage disease III
- glycogenosis type III
- limit dextrinosis

Forbes disease (GSD-III) is one of several glycogen-storage disorders (GSD) that are inherited as autosomal recessive traits. Symptoms are caused by a lack of the enzyme amylo-1,6 glucosidase (debrancher enzyme). This enzyme deficiency causes excess amounts of an abnormal glycogen (the stored form of energy that comes from carbohydrates) to be deposited in the liver, muscles and, in some cases, the heart.

There are two forms of this disorder. GSD-IIIA affects about 85% of patients with Forbes disease and involves both the liver and the muscles. GSD-IIIB affects only the liver.

Andersen Disease (GSD IV)

Synonyms of Andersen disease include:

- amylopectinosis

- Andersen glycogenosis

- brancher deficiency

- branching enzyme deficiency

- glycogen-storage disease IV

- glycogenosis type IV

Andersen disease belongs to a group of rare genetic disorders of glycogen metabolism, known as glycogen-storage diseases. Glycogen is a complex carbohydrate that is converted into the simple sugar glucose for the body's use as energy. Glycogen-storage diseases are characterized by deficiencies of certain enzymes involved in the metabolism of glycogen, leading to an accumulation of abnormal forms or amounts of glycogen in various parts of the body, particularly the liver and muscle.

Andersen disease is also known as glycogen-storage disease (GSD) type IV. It is caused by deficient activity of the glycogen-branching enzyme, resulting in accumulation of abnormal glycogen in the liver, muscle, and/or other tissues. In most affected individuals, symptoms and findings become evident in the first months of life. Such features typically include failure to grow and gain weight at the expected rate (failure to thrive) and abnormal enlargement of the liver and spleen (hepatosplenomegaly). In such cases, the disease course is typically characterized by progressive liver (hepatic) scarring (cirrhosis) and liver failure, leading to potentially life-threatening complications. In rare cases, however, progressive liver disease may not develop. In addition, several neuromuscular variants of Andersen disease have been described that may be evident at birth, in childhood, or adulthood. The disease is inherited as an autosomal recessive trait.

McArdle Syndrome

Alternative names: Glycogen-storage disease type V; myophosphorylase deficiency; muscle glycogen phosphorylase deficiency; PGYM deficiency.

Definition

McArdle syndrome is the inability to break down glycogen. Glycogen an important source of energy that is stored in muscle tissue.

Causes, Incidence, and Risk Factors

McArdle syndrome results from a defect in a gene that makes a protein called glycogen phosphorylase. As a result, the body cannot break down glycogen in the muscles. This may lead to weakness, cramps, and muscle pain.

The disease is an autosomal recessive genetic disorder. This means that you get a copy of the defective gene from both parents. A person who gets a defective gene from only one parent usually does not develop this syndrome. A family history of McArdle syndrome increases the risk.

Symptoms

The symptoms usually begin as a young adult. They may include:

- muscle pain
- muscle cramps
- muscle stiffness
- muscle weakness
- intolerance for exercise
- exercise can produce a burgundy-colored urine (myoglobinuria)

The symptoms can be reduced by avoiding strenuous exercise.

Signs and Tests

The following tests may be performed:

- lactic acid in blood
- myoglobin in urine

- serum creatine kinase
- muscle biopsy
- electromyography (EMG)
- magnetic resonance imaging (MRI)
- genetic testing (enzyme and DNA)

Treatment

There is no specific treatment, but the symptoms can be managed by controlling exercise and physical activity. For example, avoid excessive or intense exercise.

Expectations (Prognosis)

People with McArdle syndrome can live a normal life by managing their physical activity.

Complications

Exercise may produce muscle pain, or even breakdown of skeletal muscle, a condition called rhabdomyolysis. This is associated with burgundy-colored urine and a risk for kidney failure, if severe.

Calling Your Health Care Provider

Contact your health care provider if you have repeated episodes of sore or cramped muscle after exercise, especially if accompanied by burgundy or pink urine.

Consider genetic counseling if you have a family history of McArdle disease.

Hers Disease

Information under this heading is excerpted with permission from several Rare Disease Reports produced by the National Organization for Rare Disorders® (NORD), P.O. Box 1968, Danbury, CT 06913-1968, (800)-999-NORD (6673). © 2007 NORD. All rights reserved. Full-text reports for these and many other disorders, which include information on symptoms, causes, treatments, and clinical trials, can be purchased individually or by subscription on the NORD website at http://www.rarediseases.org.

Synonyms of Hers disease include:

- glycogen-storage disease VI

- glycogenosis type VI

- hepatophosphorylase deficiency glycogenosis

- liver phosphorylase deficiency

- phosphorylase deficiency glycogen-storage disease

Hers disease is a genetic metabolic disorder caused by a deficiency of the enzyme, liver phosphorylase. This enzyme is necessary to break down (metabolize) glycogen, a carbohydrate that is stored in the liver and muscle and used for energy. Deficiency of this enzyme results in the abnormal accumulation of glycogen in the body. Hers disease is one of a group of disorders known as the glycogen-storage disorders. It is characterized by enlargement of the liver (hepatomegaly), moderately low blood sugar (hypoglycemia), elevated levels of acetone and other ketone bodies in the blood (ketosis), and moderate growth retardation. Symptoms are not always evident during childhood, and children are usually able to lead normal lives.

Glycogen-Storage Disease Type VII

Information under this heading is excerpted with permission from several Rare Disease Reports produced by the National Organization for Rare Disorders® (NORD), P.O. Box 1968, Danbury, CT 06913-1968, (800)-999-NORD (6673). © 2007 NORD. All rights reserved. Full-text reports for these and many other disorders, which include information on symptoms, causes, treatments, and clinical trials, can be purchased individually or by subscription on the NORD website at http://www.rarediseases.org.

Synonyms of glycogen-storage disease type VII include:

- GSD VII

- muscle phosphofructokinase deficiency

- PFKM deficiency

- Tarui disease

Glycogen-storage diseases are a group of disorders in which stored glycogen cannot be metabolized into glucose to supply energy for the body. Glycogen-storage disease type VII (GSD VII) is characterized by weakness, pain, and stiffness during exercise. GSD VII is caused by abnormalities in the muscle phosphofructokinase gene that results in a deficiency of the phosphofructokinase enzyme. This enzyme deficiency leads to a reduced amount of energy available to muscles during exercise. GSD VII is inherited as an autosomal recessive genetic disorder.

Additional Information

Association for Glycogen-Storage Disease
P.O. Box 896
Durant, IA 52747
Phone: 563-785-6038
Website: http://www.agsdus.org

CLIMB (Children Living with Inherited Metabolic Diseases)
Climb Building
176 Nantwich Road
Crewe CW2 6BG
United Kingdom
Phone: +44-87-0-7700-325
Fax: +44-87-0-7700-327
Website: http://www.CLIMB.org.uk
E-mail: infosvcs@climb.org.uk

Muscular Dystrophy Association
3300 E. Sunrise Dr.
Tucson, AZ 85718
Toll-Free: 800-344-4863
Phone: 520-529-2000
Website: http://www.mdausa.org
E-mail: mda@mdausa.org

Endocrine and Metabolic Diseases Information Service
6 Information Way
Bethesda, MD 20892-3569
Toll-Free: 888-828-0904
Fax: 703-738-4929
Website: http://www.endocrine.niddk.nih.gov
E-mail: endoandmeta@info.niddk.nih.gov

National Digestive Diseases Information Clearinghouse
2 Information Way
Bethesda, MD 20892-3570
Toll-Free: 800-891-5389
Fax: 703-738-4929
Website: http://digestive.niddk.nih.gov
E-mail: nddic@info.niddk.nih.gov

Chapter 60

Inherited Metabolic Storage Disorders

Chapter Contents

Section 60.1

Lipid Storage Diseases

"Lipid Storage Diseases Fact Sheet," National Institute of Neurological Disorders and Stroke (NINDS), NIH Publication No. 05-2628, July 18, 2006.

What are lipid storage diseases?

Lipid storage diseases, or the lipidoses, are a group of inherited metabolic disorders in which harmful amounts of fatty materials called lipids accumulate in some of the body's cells and tissues. People with these disorders either do not produce enough of one of the enzymes needed to metabolize lipids, or they produce enzymes that do not work properly. Over time, this excessive storage of fats can cause permanent cellular and tissue damage, particularly in the brain, peripheral nervous system, liver, spleen, and bone marrow.

What are lipids?

Lipids are fat-like substances that are important parts of the membranes found within and between each cell and in the myelin sheath that coats and protects the nerves. Lipids include oils, fatty acids, waxes, steroids (such as cholesterol and estrogen), and other related compounds.

These fatty materials are stored naturally in the body's cells, organs, and tissues. Minute bodies within the cells called lysosomes regularly convert, or metabolize, the lipids and proteins into smaller components to provide energy for the body. Disorders that store this intracellular material are called lysosomal storage diseases. In addition to lipid storage diseases, other lysosomal storage diseases include the mucolipidoses in which excessive amounts of lipids and sugar molecules are stored in the cells and tissues, and the mucopolysaccharidoses in which excessive amounts of sugar molecules are stored.

How are lipid storage diseases inherited?

Lipid storage diseases are inherited from one or both parents who carry a defective gene that regulates a particular protein in a class of the body's cells. They can be inherited two ways:

- *Autosomal recessive inheritance* occurs when both parents carry and pass on a copy of the faulty gene, but neither parent is affected by the disorder. Each child born to these parents has a 25 percent chance of inheriting both copies of the defective gene, a 50 percent chance of being a carrier, and a 25 percent chance of not inheriting either copy of the defective gene. Children of either gender can be affected by an autosomal recessive this pattern of inheritance.

- *X-linked (or sex-linked) recessive inheritance* occurs when the mother carries the affected gene on the X chromosome that determines the child's gender and passes it to her son. Sons of carriers have a 50 percent chance of inheriting the disorder. Daughters have a 50 percent chance of inheriting the X-linked chromosome but usually are not severely affected by the disorder. Affected men do not pass the disorder to their sons, but their daughters will be carriers for the disorder.

How are these disorders diagnosed?

Diagnosis is made through clinical examination, biopsy, genetic testing, molecular analysis of cells or tissue to identify inherited metabolic disorders, and enzyme assays (testing a variety of cells or body fluids in culture for enzyme deficiency). In some forms of the disorder, a urine analysis can identify the presence of stored material. Some tests can also determine if a person carries the defective gene that can be passed to her or his children. This process is known as genotyping.

Biopsy for lipid storage disease involves removing a small sample of the liver or other tissue and studying it under a microscope. In this procedure, a physician will administer a local anesthetic and then remove a small piece of tissue either surgically or by needle biopsy (a small piece of tissue is removed by inserting a thin, hollow needle through the skin). The biopsy is usually performed at an outpatient testing facility.

Genetic testing can help individuals who have a family history of lipid storage disease determine if they are carrying a mutated gene that causes the disorder. Other genetic tests can determine if a fetus has the disorder or is a carrier of the defective gene. Prenatal testing is usually done by chorionic villus sampling, in which a very small sample of the placenta is removed and tested during early pregnancy. The sample, which contains the same deoxyribonucleic acid (DNA) as the fetus, is removed by catheter or fine needle inserted through the cervix or by a fine needle inserted through the abdomen. Results are usually available within two weeks.

What are the types of lipid storage diseases?

Gaucher Disease: Gaucher disease is the most common of the lipid storage diseases. It is caused by a deficiency of the enzyme glucocerebrosidase. Fatty material can collect in the spleen, liver, kidneys, lungs, brain, and bone marrow. Symptoms may include enlarged spleen and liver, liver malfunction, skeletal disorders and bone lesions that may cause pain, severe neurologic complications, swelling of lymph nodes and (occasionally) adjacent joints, distended abdomen, a brownish tint to the skin, anemia, low blood platelets, and yellow spots in the eyes. Persons affected most seriously may also be more susceptible to infection. The disease affects males and females equally.

Gaucher disease has three common clinical subtypes. Type 1 (or non-neuronopathic type) is the most common form of the disease. Depending on disease onset and severity, type 1 patients may live well into adulthood. Many patients have a mild form of the disease or may not show any symptoms. Type 2 (or acute infantile neuronopathic Gaucher disease) typically begins within three months of birth. Type 3 (the chronic neuronopathic form) can begin at any time in childhood or even in adulthood. It is characterized by slowly progressive but milder neurologic symptoms compared to the acute or type 2 version. Patients often live to their early teen years and often into adulthood.

Niemann-Pick Disease: Niemann-Pick (NP) disease is actually a group of autosomal recessive disorders caused by an accumulation of fat and cholesterol in cells of the liver, spleen, bone marrow, lungs, and, in some patients, brain. Neurological complications may include ataxia, eye paralysis, brain degeneration, learning problems, spasticity, feeding and swallowing difficulties, slurred speech, loss of muscle tone, hypersensitivity to touch, and some corneal clouding. A characteristic cherry-red halo develops around the center of the retina in 50 percent of patients.

Niemann-Pick disease is currently subdivided into four categories. Onset of type A, the most severe form, is in early infancy. Infants appear normal at birth but develop an enlarged liver and spleen, swollen lymph nodes, nodes under the skin (xanthoma), and profound brain damage by six months of age. The spleen may enlarge to as much as ten times its normal size and can rupture. These children become progressively weaker, lose motor function, may become anemic, and are susceptible to recurring infection. They rarely live beyond 18 months. This form of the disease occurs most often in Jewish families. In the second group, called type B (or juvenile onset), enlargement of the liver and spleen characteristically occurs in the pre-teen years. Most patients also develop ataxia, peripheral neuropathy, and pulmonary difficulties that progress with age, but the brain is generally not affected. Type B patients may live a comparatively long time but many require supplemental oxygen because of lung involvement. Niemann-Pick types A and B result from accumulation of the fatty substance called sphingomyelin, due to deficiency of acid sphingomyelinase.

Niemann-Pick disease also includes two other variant forms called types C and D. These may appear early in life or develop in the teen or even adult years. Niemann-Pick disease types C and D are not caused by a deficiency of sphingomyelinase but by a lack of the NPC1 or NPC2 proteins. As a result, various lipids and cholesterol accumulate inside nerve cells and cause them to malfunction. Patients with types C and D have only moderate enlargement of their spleens and livers. Brain involvement may be extensive, leading to inability to look up and down, difficulty in walking and swallowing, and progressive loss of vision and hearing. Type D patients typically develop neurologic symptoms later than those with type C and have a progressively slower rate of loss of nerve function. Most type D patients share a common ancestral background in Nova Scotia. The life expectancies of patients with types C and D vary considerably. Some patients die in childhood while others, who appear to be less severely affected, live into adulthood.

There is currently no cure for Niemann-Pick disease. Treatment is supportive. Children usually die from infection or progressive neurological loss. Bone marrow transplantation has been attempted in a few patients with type B. Patients with types C and D are frequently placed on a low-cholesterol diet and/or cholesterol lowering drugs, although research has not shown these interventions to change cholesterol metabolism or halt disease progression.

Fabry Disease: Fabry disease, also known as alpha-galactosidase-A deficiency, causes a buildup of fatty material in the autonomic nervous system, eyes, kidneys, and cardiovascular system. Fabry disease is the only X-linked lipid storage disease. Males are primarily affected although a milder form is common in females, some of whom may have severe manifestations similar to those seen in affected males. Onset of symptoms is usually during childhood or adolescence. Neurological symptoms include burning pain in the arms and legs, which worsens in hot weather or following exercise, and the buildup of excess material in the clear layers of the cornea (resulting in clouding but no change in vision). Fatty storage in blood vessel walls may impair circulation, putting the patient at risk for stroke or heart attack. Other symptoms include heart enlargement, progressive kidney impairment leading to renal failure, gastrointestinal difficulties, decreased sweating, and fever. Angiokeratomas (small, non-cancerous, reddish-purple elevated spots on the skin) may develop on the lower part of the trunk of the body and become more numerous with age.

Patients with Fabry disease often die prematurely of complications from heart disease, renal failure, or stroke. Drugs such as phenytoin and carbamazepine are often prescribed to treat pain that accompanies Fabry disease. Metoclopramide or Lipisorb (a nutritional supplement) can ease gastrointestinal distress that often occurs in Fabry patients, and some individuals may require kidney transplant or dialysis. Recent experiments indicate that enzyme replacement can reduce storage, ease pain, and improve organ function in patients with Fabry disease.

Farber Disease: Farber disease, also known as Farber lipogranulomatosis or ceramidase deficiency, describes a group of rare autosomal recessive disorders that cause an accumulation of fatty material in the joints, tissues, and central nervous system. The disorder affects both males and females. Disease onset is typically in early infancy but may occur later in life. Children who have the classic form of Farber disease develop neurological symptoms within the first few weeks of life. These symptoms may include moderately impaired mental ability and problems with swallowing. The liver, heart, and kidneys may also be affected. Other symptoms may include vomiting, arthritis, swollen lymph nodes, swollen joints, joint contractures (chronic shortening of muscles or tendons around joints), hoarseness, and xanthoma which thicken around joints as the disease progresses. Patients with breathing difficulty may require insertion of a breathing tube. Most children with the disease die by age two, usually from lung disease. In one of the most severe forms of the disease, an enlarged liver and spleen (hepatosplenomegaly) can be diagnosed soon after birth. Children born with this form of the disease usually die within six months.

There is no specific treatment for Farber disease. Corticosteroids may be prescribed to relieve pain. Bone marrow transplants may improve granulomas (small masses of inflamed tissue) on patients with little or no lung or nervous system complications. Older patients may have granulomas surgically reduced or removed.

Gangliosidoses: The gangliosidoses are two distinct genetic groups of diseases. Both are autosomal recessive and affect males and females equally.

The G_{M1} gangliosidoses are caused by a deficiency of beta-galactosidase, with resulting abnormal storage of acidic lipid materials in cells of the central and peripheral nervous systems, but particularly in the nerve cells. G_{M1} has three forms: early infantile, late infantile, and adult. Symptoms of early infantile G_{M1} (the most severe subtype, with onset shortly after birth) may include neurodegeneration, seizures, liver and spleen enlargement, coarsening of facial features, skeletal irregularities, joint stiffness, distended abdomen, muscle weakness, exaggerated startle response to sound, and problems with gait. About half of affected patients develop cherry-red spots in the eye. Children may be deaf and blind by age one and often die by age three from cardiac complications or pneumonia. Onset of late infantile G_{M1} is typically between ages one and three years. Neurological symptoms include ataxia, seizures, dementia, and difficulties with speech. Onset of adult G_{M1} is between ages three and thirty. Symptoms include muscle atrophy, neurological complications that are less severe and progress at a slower rate than in other forms of the disorder, corneal clouding in some patients, and dystonia (sustained muscle contractions that cause twisting and repetitive movements or abnormal postures). Angiokeratomas may develop on the lower part of the trunk of the body. Most patients have a normal size liver and spleen.

The G_{M2} gangliosidoses also cause the body to store excess acidic fatty materials in tissues and cells, most notably in nerve cells. These disorders result from a deficiency of the enzyme beta-hexosaminidase. The G_{M2} disorders include:

- *Tay-Sachs disease* (also known as G_{M2} variant B). Tay-Sachs and its variant forms are caused by a deficiency in the enzyme beta-hexosaminidase A. The incidence is particularly high among Eastern European and Ashkenazi Jewish populations, as well as certain French Canadians and Louisianan Cajuns. Affected children appear to develop normally for the first few months of life. Symptoms begin by six months of age and include progressive loss of mental ability, dementia, decreased eye contact, increased startle reflex to noise, progressive loss of hearing leading to deafness, difficulty in swallowing, blindness, cherry-red spots in the retinas, and some paralysis. Seizures may begin in the child's second year. Children may eventually need a feeding tube and they often die by age four from recurring infection. No specific treatment is available. Anticonvulsant medications may initially control seizures. Other supportive treatment includes proper nutrition and hydration and techniques to keep the airway open. A much rarer form of the disorder, which occurs in patients in their twenties and early thirties, is characterized by unsteadiness of gait and progressive neurological deterioration.

- *Sandhoff disease* (variant AB). This is a severe form of Tay-Sachs disease. Onset usually occurs at the age of six months and is not limited to any ethnic group. Neurological symptoms may include progressive deterioration of the central nervous system, motor weakness, early blindness, marked startle response to sound, spasticity, myoclonus (shock-like contractions of a muscle), seizures, macrocephaly (an abnormally enlarged head), and cherry-red spots in the eye. Other symptoms may include frequent respiratory infections, murmurs of the heart, doll-like facial features, and an enlarged liver and spleen. There is no specific treatment for Sandhoff disease. As with Tay-Sachs disease, supportive treatment includes keeping the airway open and proper nutrition and hydration. Anticonvulsant medications may initially control seizures. Children generally die by age three from respiratory infections.

Krabbe Disease: Krabbe disease (also known as globoid cell leukodystrophy and galactosylceramide lipidosis) is an autosomal recessive disorder caused by deficiency of the enzyme galactosylceramidase. The disease most often affects infants, with onset before age six months, but can occur in adolescence or adulthood. The buildup of undigested fats affects the growth of the nerve's protective myelin sheath and causes severe degeneration of mental and motor skills. Other symptoms include muscle weakness, hypertonia (reduced ability of a muscle to stretch), myoclonic seizures (sudden, shock-like contractions of the limbs), spasticity, irritability, unexplained fever, deafness, optic atrophy and blindness, paralysis, and difficulty when swallowing. Prolonged weight loss may also occur. The disease may be diagnosed by its characteristic grouping of certain cells, nerve demyelination and degeneration, and destruction of brain cells. In infants, the disease is generally fatal before age two. Patients with a later onset form of the disease have a milder course of the disease and live significantly longer. No specific treatment for Krabbe disease has been developed, although early bone marrow transplantation may help some patients.

Metachromatic Leukodystrophy: Metachromatic leukodystrophy, or MLD, is a group of disorders marked by storage buildup in the white matter of the central nervous system and in the peripheral nerves and to some extent in the kidneys. Similar to Krabbe disease, MLD affects the myelin that covers and protects the nerves. This autosomal recessive disorder is caused by a deficiency of the enzyme arylsulfatase A. Both males and females are affected by this disorder.

MLD has three characteristic phenotypes: late infantile, juvenile, and adult. The most common form of the disease is late infantile, with onset typically between 12 and 20 months following birth. Infants may appear normal at first but develop difficulty in walking and a tendency to fall, followed by intermittent pain in the arms and legs, progressive loss of vision leading to blindness, developmental delays, impaired swallowing, convulsions, and dementia before age two. Children also develop gradual muscle wasting and weakness and eventually lose the ability to walk. Most children with this form of the disorder die by age five. Symptoms of the juvenile form typically begin between ages three and ten. Symptoms include impaired school performance, mental deterioration, ataxia, seizures, and dementia. Symptoms are progressive with death occurring 10 to 20 years following onset. In the adult form, symptoms begin after age 16 and may include impaired concentration, depression, psychiatric disturbances, ataxia, seizures, tremor, and dementia. Death generally occurs within six to fourteen years after onset of symptoms.

There is no cure for MLD. Treatment is symptomatic and supportive. Bone marrow transplantation may delay progression of the disease in some cases.

Wolman Disease: Wolman disease, also known as acid lipase deficiency, is a severe lipid storage disease that is usually fatal by age one. This autosomal recessive disorder is marked by accumulation of cholesteryl esters (normally a transport form of cholesterol) and triglycerides (a chemical form in which fats exist in the body) that can build up significantly and cause damage in the cells and tissues. Both males and females are affected by this severe disorder. Infants are normal and active at birth but quickly develop progressive mental deterioration, enlarged liver and grossly enlarged spleen, distended abdomen, gastrointestinal problems including steatorrhea (excessive amounts of fats in the stools), jaundice, anemia, vomiting, and calcium deposits in the adrenal glands, causing them to harden.

Cholesteryl Ester Storage Disease: Another type of acid lipase deficiency is cholesteryl ester storage disease. This extremely rare disorder results from storage of cholesteryl esters and triglycerides in cells in the blood and lymph and lymphoid tissue. Children develop an enlarged liver leading to cirrhosis and chronic liver failure before adulthood. Children may also have calcium deposits in the adrenal glands and may develop jaundice late in the disorder. There is no specific treatment for Wolman disease or cholesteryl ester storage disease.

How are these disorders treated?

Currently there is no specific treatment available for most of the lipid storage disorders but highly effective enzyme replacement therapy is available for patients with type 1 Gaucher disease and some patients with type 3 Gaucher disease. Patients with anemia may require blood transfusions. In some patients, the enlarged spleen must be removed to improve cardiopulmonary function. The drugs phenytoin and carbamazepine may be prescribed to help treat pain (including bone pain) for patients with Fabry disease. Restricting one's diet does not prevent lipid buildup in cells and tissues.

What research is being done?

Investigators at the National Institute of Neurological Disorders and Stroke (NINDS) identified the gene that is altered in the majority of patients with type C and D Niemann-Pick disease. In the year 2000, scientists discovered a second gene that is mutated in a minority of patients with type C Niemann-Pick disease. NINDS researchers have developed highly effective enzyme replacement therapy for Gaucher and Fabry diseases. These researchers are now developing improved research techniques, including a mouse model of Fabry disease. Gene therapy in this model appears to be especially encouraging.

Among other potential therapies for lipid storage diseases under way, NINDS scientists are studying the effectiveness and safety of the medicine called OGT-918, which has been shown to slow the production of the lipid that builds up in Gaucher disease. Scientists hope the drug, which passes through the blood-brain barrier into the brain, will reduce lipid storage and therefore the neurological symptoms of the disease. Other NINDS investigators are evaluating the safety and effectiveness of continued replacement of the enzyme alpha-galactosidase-A in patients with Fabry disease. In a preliminary 24-week clinical trial, this therapy was found to reduce pain, improve renal function, and reverse heart problems among Fabry patients.

NINDS scientists are also studying the mechanisms by which the lipids accumulating in these storage diseases cause harm to the body. The goal of this research is to develop novel approaches to the treatment of these disorders.

Among several current projects being funded by the NINDS, scientists are studying ways to deliver genes and proteins into the brain in animal models of Krabbe disease. Other NINDS-sponsored scientists are examining the possible role of the protein psychosine in the neuro-inflammatory response seen in this disease and hope to identify potential therapeutic drugs for use in human trials. Researchers are investigating the mechanisms of intracellular cholesterol delivery and metabolism in Niemann-Pick type C disease and hope to develop a diagnostic tool for the disorder. Other researchers are studying dysfunctional cholesterol processing (seen in Niemann-Pick disease) as a key feature in the development of several neurodegenerative disorders.

For More Information

March of Dimes Birth Defects Foundation
1275 Mamaroneck Avenue
White Plains, NY 10605
Toll-Free: 888-MODIMES (663-4637)
Phone: 914-428-7100
Fax: 914-428-8203
Website: http://www.marchofdimes.com
E-mail: askus@marchofdimes.com

National Organization for Rare Disorders (NORD)
P.O. Box 1968
Danbury, CT 06813-1968
Toll-Free: 800-999-NORD (6673)
Phone: 203-744-0100
Fax: 203-798-2291
Website: http://www.rarediseases.org
E-mail: orphan@rarediseases.org

Section 60.2

Gaucher Disease

The text in this section is from Genetics Home Reference of the
National Library of Medicine, August 2005.

What is Gaucher disease?

Gaucher disease is an inherited disorder that affects many of the
body's organs and tissues. In people with this condition, the body is
unable to break down a certain type of fat (lipid) called glucocerebroside.

Genetic changes are related to the following types of Gaucher disease:

- Gaucher disease, type 1

- Gaucher disease, type 2

- Gaucher disease, type 3

- Gaucher-like disease

The signs and symptoms of Gaucher disease vary widely among
affected individuals. The major features of this disorder include enlargement of the liver and spleen (hepatosplenomegaly), a low number of red blood cells (anemia), easy bruising caused by a decrease in
blood platelets (thrombocytopenia), and bone disease. Gaucher disease
can also affect the heart and lungs.

The subtypes of Gaucher disease are grouped by their signs and
symptoms. Type 1 is called non-neuronopathic Gaucher disease because the nervous system is usually not affected. The features of this
disorder range from mild to severe and may appear early in life or in
adulthood.

Types 2 and 3 Gaucher disease are known as neuronopathic forms
of the disorder because they are characterized by problems that affect the nervous system. In addition to the signs and symptoms described, these conditions can cause seizures and brain damage. Type
2 Gaucher disease usually causes severe medical problems beginning

in infancy. Type 3 Gaucher disease also affects the nervous system, but tends to progress more slowly than type 2. Gaucher-like disease chiefly affects the heart, but may also cause bone disease and mild enlargement of the spleen.

How common is Gaucher disease?

This disease is seen in 1 in 50,000 to 100,000 people in the general population. Type 1 Gaucher disease is the most common form of the disorder, and occurs more frequently in people of Ashkenazi (eastern and central European) Jewish heritage than in those with other backgrounds. The disorder affects 1 in 500 to 1,000 people of Ashkenazi Jewish heritage. Types 2 and 3 Gaucher disease and Gaucher-like disease are uncommon, and do not occur more frequently in people of Ashkenazi Jewish descent.

What genes are related to Gaucher disease?

Mutations in the GBA gene cause Gaucher disease. Mutations in the GBA gene lead to extremely low levels of an enzyme called beta-glucocerebrosidase. This enzyme usually breaks down a lipid called glucocerebroside into a sugar (glucose) and a simpler fat molecule. Without functional beta-glucocerebrosidase, glucocerebroside can build up in the body's cells. The abnormal accumulation of this substance damages tissues and organs, causing the characteristic features of Gaucher disease.

How do people inherit Gaucher disease?

This condition is inherited in an autosomal recessive pattern, which means two copies of the gene in each cell are altered. Most often, the parents of an individual with an autosomal recessive disorder are carriers of one copy of the altered gene but do not show signs and symptoms of the disorder.

What other names do people use for Gaucher disease?

- cerebroside lipidosis syndrome
- Gaucher splenomegaly
- Gaucher syndrome
- GD

- glucocerebrosidase deficiency
- glucocerebrosidosis
- glucosylceramidase deficiency
- glucosylceramide beta-glucosidase deficiency
- glucosylceramide lipidosis
- glucosyl cerebroside lipidosis
- kerasin histiocytosis
- kerasin lipoidosis
- kerasin thesaurismosis
- lipoid histiocytosis (kerasin type)

Gaucher Disease, Type 1

Gaucher disease is an inherited disorder that affects many of the body's organs and tissues. In people with this condition, the body is unable to break down a certain type of fat (lipid) called glucocerebroside. The features of type 1 Gaucher disease range from mild to severe and may appear early in life or in adulthood. Gaucher disease, type 1 is a subtype of Gaucher disease.

The signs and symptoms of type 1 Gaucher disease include an enlarged liver and spleen (hepatosplenomegaly), low red blood cell counts (anemia), easy bruising caused by a decrease in blood platelets (thrombocytopenia), bone pain, and skeletal abnormalities. Brown spots at the edges of the cornea (the front surface of the eye) are also a feature of this disorder.

Type 1 Gaucher disease is known as a non-neuronopathic form of the disorder because it does not typically affect the nervous system; however, bone disease may lead to neurologic problems such as compression of the spinal cord.

How common is Gaucher disease, type 1?

Gaucher disease is seen in 1 in 50,000 to 100,000 people in the general population. Type 1 Gaucher disease is the most common form of this disorder. Type 1 occurs more frequently in people of Ashkenazi (eastern and central European) Jewish heritage than in those with other backgrounds. This disease is seen in 1 in 500 to 1,000 people in the Ashkenazi Jewish population.

What genes are related to Gaucher disease, type 1?

Mutations in the GBA gene cause Gaucher disease, type 1. Mutations in the GBA gene lead to extremely low levels of an enzyme called beta-glucocerebrosidase. This enzyme usually breaks down a lipid called glucocerebroside into a sugar (glucose) and a simpler fat molecule. Without functional beta-glucocerebrosidase, glucocerebroside can build up in the body's cells. The abnormal accumulation of this substance damages tissues and organs, causing the characteristic features of Gaucher disease.

How do people inherit Gaucher disease, type 1?

This condition is inherited in an autosomal recessive pattern, which means two copies of the gene in each cell are altered. Most often, the parents of an individual with an autosomal recessive disorder are carriers of one copy of the altered gene but do not show signs and symptoms of the disorder. Approximately 1 in 18 people of Ashkenazi Jewish descent carry one altered copy of the GBA gene.

Gaucher Disease, Type 2

Gaucher disease is an inherited disorder that affects many of the body's organs and tissues. In people with this condition, the body is unable to break down a certain type of fat (lipid) called glucocerebroside. Type 2 Gaucher disease is characterized by onset in infancy and severe involvement of the central nervous system (the brain and spinal cord). Gaucher disease, type 2 is a subtype of Gaucher disease.

As in other types of Gaucher disease, signs and symptoms of type 2 include enlargement of the liver and spleen (hepatosplenomegaly). Type 2 is known as the acute neuronopathic form of the disease because the central nervous system is also affected, causing progressive brain damage, seizures, paralysis of the eye muscles, abnormal muscle tone, and choking spells. These signs and symptoms first appear in infancy. People with type 2 Gaucher disease usually live only into early childhood.

How common is Gaucher disease, type 2?

This rare condition is seen in fewer than 1 in 500,000 births. Unlike type 1, type 2 Gaucher disease is not more frequent in the Ashkenazi (central and eastern European) Jewish population.

What genes are related to Gaucher disease, type 2?

Mutations in the GBA gene cause Gaucher disease, type 2. Mutations in the GBA gene lead to extremely low levels of an enzyme called beta-glucocerebrosidase. This enzyme usually breaks down a lipid called glucocerebroside into a sugar (glucose) and a simpler fat molecule. Without functional beta-glucocerebrosidase, glucocerebroside can build up in the body's cells. The abnormal accumulation of this substance damages tissues and organs causing the characteristic features of Gaucher disease.

How do people inherit Gaucher disease, type 2?

This condition is inherited in an autosomal recessive pattern, which means two copies of the gene in each cell are altered. Most often, the parents of an individual with an autosomal recessive disorder are carriers of one copy of the altered gene but do not show signs and symptoms of the disorder.

Gaucher Disease, Type 3

Gaucher disease is an inherited disorder that affects many of the body's organs and tissues. In people with this condition, the body is unable to break down a certain type of fat (lipid) called glucocerebroside. Type 3 Gaucher disease is characterized by involvement of the central nervous system (the brain and spinal cord) and a slower, more favorable course than type 2. Gaucher disease, type 3 is a subtype of Gaucher disease.

The signs and symptoms of type 3 Gaucher disease usually appear in childhood or adolescence and vary widely among affected individuals. Characteristic features include an enlarged liver and spleen (hepatosplenomegaly), low red blood cell counts (anemia), bruising due to a low number of blood platelets (thrombocytopenia), and bone pain. Type 3 is known as the chronic neuronopathic form of the disease because the central nervous system is also affected, causing loss of muscle coordination (ataxia), seizures, paralysis of the eye muscles, and dementia. People with type 3 Gaucher disease can live into adulthood, but may have a shortened life span.

How common is Gaucher disease, type 3?

This rare condition affects fewer than 1 in 100,000 births. Type 3 is also known as the Norrbottnian type of Gaucher disease because many cases have been reported in the province of Norrbotten in northern Sweden.

What genes are related to Gaucher disease, type 3?

Mutations in the GBA gene cause Gaucher disease, type 3. Mutations in the GBA gene lead to extremely low levels of an enzyme called beta-glucocerebrosidase. This enzyme usually breaks down a lipid called glucocerebroside into a sugar (glucose) and a simpler fat molecule. Without functional beta-glucocerebrosidase, glucocerebroside can build up in the body's cells. The abnormal accumulation of this substance damages tissues and organs, causing the characteristic features of Gaucher disease.

How do people inherit Gaucher disease, type 3?

This condition is inherited in an autosomal recessive pattern, which means two copies of the gene in each cell are altered. Most often, the parents of an individual with an autosomal recessive disorder are carriers of one copy of the altered gene but do not show signs and symptoms of the disorder.

Gaucher-Like Disease

Gaucher disease is an inherited disorder that affects many of the body's organs and tissues. In people with this condition, the body is unable to break down a certain type of fat (lipid) called glucocerebroside. Gaucher-like disease has different signs and symptoms than the three other recognized types of Gaucher disease, although they are caused by mutations in the same gene. Gaucher-like disease is a subtype of Gaucher disease.

This disorder is known as the cardiovascular form of Gaucher disease because it chiefly affects the heart, causing the heart valves to harden (calcify). Other signs and symptoms include cloudiness of the front part of the eye (the cornea), difficulty with eye movements, bone disease, and mild spleen enlargement (splenomegaly).

How common is Gaucher-like disease?

This disease is very rare; it has been reported in only a few patients worldwide.

What genes are related to Gaucher-like disease?

Mutations in the GBA gene cause Gaucher-like disease. Gaucher-like disease occurs when a person has a specific, rare mutation in two copies of the GBA gene that leads to extremely low levels of an enzyme called beta-glucocerebrosidase. This enzyme usually breaks down a lipid called glucocerebroside into a sugar (glucose) and a simpler fat molecule. Without functional beta-glucocerebrosidase, glucocerebroside can build up in the body's cells. The abnormal accumulation of this substance damages tissues and organs, causing the characteristic features of Gaucher-like disease.

How do people inherit Gaucher-like disease?

This condition is inherited in an autosomal recessive pattern, which means two copies of the gene in each cell are altered. Most often, the parents of an individual with an autosomal recessive disorder are carriers of one copy of the altered gene but do not show signs and symptoms of the disorder.

For More Information about Gaucher Disease

Children's Gaucher Research Fund
P.O. Box 2123
Granite Bay, CA 95746-2123
Phone: 916-797-3700
Fax: 916-797-3707
Website: http://www.childrensgaucher.org
E-mail: research@childrensgaucher.org

National Gaucher Foundation
2227 Idlewood Rd., Suite 12
Tucker, GA 30084
Toll-Free: 800-504-3189
Fax: 770-934-2911
Website: http://www.gaucherdisease.org
E-mail: rhonda@gaucherdisease.org

Section 60.3

Hurler Syndrome

Definition of Hurler Syndrome

Hurler syndrome is an inherited metabolic storage disorder that can cause severe damage to the brain, heart, bones, and other organs and tissues.

Hurler syndrome is one of a group of inherited metabolic storage disorders in which the lack of an enzyme affects various organs and tissues, including the brain. Enzymes are proteins that play many roles, including metabolizing (breaking down) substances in the body. In metabolic storage disorders, the body lacks an enzyme needed to metabolize a substance, such as a sugar. Instead, the substance builds up in the body and causes damage.

Mucopolysaccharidosis (MPS)

An MPS disorder, Hurler syndrome is also called mucopolysaccharidosis I (MPS-I). It is one of a subgroup of metabolic disorders known as MPS disorders. MPS disorders are caused by a mutation (mistake) in a certain gene. A gene carries an inherited code of instructions that tell the body how to make every cell and substance in the body. The mutated gene in MPS disorders affects an enzyme called alpha-L-iduronidase (IDUA). This enzyme breaks down complex sugars called glycosaminoglycan (GAG). The body needs GAG to build bones and tissues, so a healthy body is always making and breaking down GAG. In people with MPS disorders, the body keeps making GAG but does not have the enzyme to break them down. The GAG is stored in cells throughout the body. As they build up, they damage organs and tissues.

Inheriting Hurler Syndrome

Hurler syndrome occurs in about one of every 100,000 babies born. A child inherits the syndrome when he or she gets two abnormal genes that affect the IDUA enzyme, one from each parent. If only one parent passes on the gene mutation, the child will not have the disease. Instead, the child will be a carrier and may pass the gene mutation to his or her own children.

Signs and Symptoms of Hurler Syndrome

As GAG builds up in the body, signs and symptoms of the damage GAG causes begin to appear. These may include:

- problems with mental function (mental retardation);
- heart problems, including changes in the valves;
- hearing problems and frequent ear infections;
- large head size, broad forehead, and heavy eyebrows;
- deformed bones and stiff joints, especially the spine, hips, knees, wrists, and fingers;
- short size;
- breathing problems.

Signs and symptoms usually appear within the first year of life and grow worse over time. If the disease is not stopped, children with Hurler syndrome usually die by five to ten years of age.

Diagnosis

Tests doctors may use to diagnose Hurler syndrome include:

- urine tests for extra GAG;
- tests of blood and/or skin samples to see if the body is making the IDUA enzyme;
- genetic tests for mutations to the gene for the IDUA enzyme;
- x-rays to check for damage to the spine;
- electrocardiogram (EKG) or echocardiogram to check heart function and valve problems.

Families affected by Hurler syndrome may want to talk with a genetic counselor about family planning and the chances of having children with the disorder. Early diagnosis can enable early treatment of a child after birth, which can make a difference in outcomes.

Hurler Syndrome Treatments

The goal of treatment for Hurler syndrome is to give the body the missing enzyme so it can break down GAG. The two main treatments for children with Hurler syndrome are enzyme replacement therapy and a bone marrow or cord blood transplant.

Enzyme Replacement Therapy

For enzyme replacement therapy, a patient is given a drug that has the IDUA enzyme his or her body is missing. The drug is called laronidase, or Aldurazyme. Treatment with laronidase can improve problems with breathing, growth, the bones, joints, and heart. However, there is no evidence that it has any effect on mental development problems caused by Hurler syndrome.

- Enzyme replacement therapy may be a good option for children who have a form of MPS I disorder that does not cause mental retardation (Scheie syndrome or Hurler/Scheie syndrome).

- Some children with Hurler syndrome may be treated with both enzyme therapy and a transplant. This approach is being studied in a clinical trial.

Bone Marrow or Cord Blood Transplant

A bone marrow or cord blood transplant (also called a BMT) is the only known treatment that can stop the progression of mental damage caused by Hurler syndrome.

Transplant for Hurler Syndrome

A transplant replaces the abnormal cells in the bone marrow (the cells with the mutated gene) with healthy cells from a family member or unrelated donor or cord blood unit. The healthy cells provide a source of the enzyme needed to break down GAG and stop further damage to the body.

In general, a transplant has the best chance of success when it is done soon after diagnosis. Getting a transplant early is important to stop damage caused by the disorder before it becomes severe. Children who receive a transplant early enough can have normal or near-normal mental development. Damage to the organs is stopped and hearing may improve.

However, transplants for children who have already developed severe damage have had disappointing results. If the disorder has caused organ damage, a child has a higher risk of developing life-threatening complications from transplant. In addition, a transplant may not undo damage the disease has already done, especially to the nervous system. However, in some children, there have been improvements in some organs, such as the liver, airway, and heart. The child must live with and be treated for the damage that already exists. For example, most children will need multiple surgeries to treat problems with bones, joints, and other tissues.

Transplant Risks

A transplant is an intense treatment, and some possible side effects can be life-threatening. For children with Hurler syndrome, three of the most serious risks of transplant are:

- Graft-versus-host disease (GVHD): A common transplant complication that can range from mild to severe. For patients who receive a transplant to treat leukemia, GVHD may be linked with a beneficial graft-versus-leukemia effect. However, there is no benefit to GVHD for patients with Hurler syndrome.

- Graft failure: Graft failure is when the donated cells (the graft) do not grow and make new blood cells for the body (engraft). Graft failure can be life-threatening. If the child's own cells return, he or she may survive, but the progress of the disease will not be stopped. Graft failure is a bigger risk for children being treated for Hurler syndrome than for many other diseases.

- Bleeding in the lungs (pulmonary hemorrhage): Children with Hurler syndrome have an increased risk for this serious complication. Bleeding in the lungs can affect how well the child can breathe. In some cases, a child may need a breathing tube and a breathing machine (ventilator).

Learning about Hurler Syndrome and Transplant

In the 1980s and 1990s, doctors conducted research studies to learn whether transplant could help children with Hurler syndrome. Their studies showed that transplant could be life-saving for some children. The studies also showed that some children had normal or near-normal mental development after transplant. Children had a better chance of normal mental development after transplant if they:

- were younger when they received the transplant; and

- had good mental development at the time of transplant—their mental functions had not yet been severely damaged.

It is a good idea to ask your doctor for help interpreting these data and any other survival outcomes data you find. Your doctor can provide context for these data and discuss your specific situation with you.

Transplants Using Family Donors

One study included 54 children with Hurler syndrome who received a transplant from a family member between 1983 and 1995.[1] In this study, at five years:

- Of the 28 children who were to receive a transplant from a matched brother or sister, 21 survived (75%). Two patients died during the transplant preparative treatment and did not receive the transplant. The transplant engrafted in all 21 of the children who survived.

- Of the 26 children who received a transplant from a partly matched (haploidentical) parent, 14 survived (53%). However, the donor's cells did not engraft in five of these fourteen children. Instead, the children's own (defective) cells returned and the disease was not stopped.

- Transplant stopped damage to mental function for some, but not all, children. Stable mental function was more likely in children who received a transplant before 24 months of age and in children who had better mental function before transplant.

Transplants Using Unrelated Donors

Another study included 40 children who received unrelated donor transplants between 1989 and 1994.[2]

- At two years, 20 children were alive (49%).

- The donor's cells engrafted in 13 of these children. Five children had their own (defective) cells return, and two had a mixture of donor's cells and their own.

- Transplant stopped damage to mental function for some, but not all, children. Stable mental function was more likely in children who received a transplant before 29 months of age and in children who had better mental function before transplant.

Between 1987 and 2003, the National Marrow Donor Program (NMDP) facilitated 101 unrelated donor transplants for children with Hurler syndrome. The estimated rate of survival at five years was 53%. The median age of the children at the time of transplant was 18 months. (The median is the middle point, with half of the children younger and half older.)

Cord Blood Transplants

Recent studies have also shown good results for transplants using cord blood. Cord blood transplants may be an important option for children with Hurler syndrome, because many do not have a suitable donor in their family and they need to have a transplant quickly. A suitable cord blood unit may be more quickly available than an unrelated adult donor.

One study reported on 20 children treated for Hurler syndrome with cord blood from unrelated donors between 1995 and 2002.[3]

- At the time of the report (333 days to more than seven years after transplant), 17 patients were alive (85%).

- The transplant engrafted in all 17 children who survived.

- All children had stable or improved mental development after transplant.

- The median age of the children at the time of transplant was 16 months, younger than in other studies. The younger age of the children in this study may have contributed to these improved results.

Making Treatment Decisions

If your child has Hurler syndrome, it is important to see a doctor who is an expert in this disorder. If your doctor has not treated other patients with Hurler syndrome, ask him or her to refer you to an expert for consultation. Since Hurler syndrome gets worse quickly, it is important to see an expert as soon as possible. If transplant is a treatment option for your child, talk with your doctor about the risks, limits, and possible benefits of transplant.

References

1. Peters C, Shapiro EG, Anderson J, et al. Hurler syndrome: II. Outcome of HLA-genotypically identical sibling and HLA-haploidentical related donor bone marrow transplantation in fifty-four children. The Storage Disease Collaborative Study Group. *Blood*. 1998; 91(7):2601–2608.

2. Peters C, Balthazor M, Shapiro EG, et al. Outcome of unrelated donor bone marrow transplantation in 40 children with Hurler syndrome. *Blood*. 1996; 87(11):4894–4902.

3. Staba SL, Escolar ML, Poe M, et al. Cord-blood transplants from unrelated donors in patients with Hurler syndrome. *N Engl J Med*. 2004; 350:1960–1969.

Section 60.4

Globoid-Cell Leukodystrophy (Krabbe Disease)

Definition of Globoid-Cell Leukodystrophy

Globoid-cell leukodystrophy (GLD) is also called Krabbe disease (pronounced crab-A). GLD is an inherited metabolic storage disorder that affects the muscles, vision and mental abilities. It is life-threatening.

Globoid-cell leukodystrophy is one of a group of inherited metabolic storage disorders in which the lack of an enzyme affects various organs and tissues, including the brain. Enzymes are proteins that play many roles, including metabolizing (breaking down) substances in the body. In metabolic storage disorders, the body lacks an enzyme needed to metabolize a substance, such as a sugar. Instead, the substance builds up in the body and causes damage.

A Type of Leukodystrophy

GLD is one of a subgroup of metabolic disorders called the leukodystrophies. The leukodystrophies are caused by a variety of gene mutations (mistakes). Genes carry an inherited code of instructions that tells the body how to make every cell and substance in the body. In the leukodystrophies, the gene mutations lead to damage of the myelin.

Myelin is the fatty substance that forms a sheath around the axons that carry signals to and from nerves in the central nervous system (brain and spinal cord). The myelin sheath is similar to the insulation on a wire. It enables the axons to carry signals very quickly. When the myelin sheath is damaged, the signals slow down or may stop completely.

If the signals from the brain and spinal cord have trouble getting to the rest of the body, a person can have problems controlling the body's movements. If the signals between nerves in the brain are slowed or stopped, a person can have problems with memory, learning, speaking and understanding speech, and other mental functions.

Globoid-Cell Leukodystrophy

In people with GLD, the gene mutation affects an enzyme called galactocerebrosidase (GALC). Lack of GALC causes the buildup of a substance that damages cells that make myelin. This results in damage to the central nervous system. A person gets the disorder when he or she inherits a gene with the mutation from both parents. The disorder can appear soon after birth (early-onset GLD or Krabbe disease) or in older children or adults (late-onset GLD). The disorder is rare. About 40 cases of GLD are diagnosed in the United States each year.

Signs and Symptoms of GLD

Early-Onset GLD: Symptoms of early-onset GLD usually appear in babies between two and twelve months of age. Symptoms include:

- unexplained crying
- fevers
- stiffness

- seizures
- slow development

These symptoms get worse quickly, and children usually die before the age of two years. The early-onset form of the disorder occurs much more often than the late-onset form.

Late-Onset GLD: Late-onset GLD can appear in people of any age. The symptoms include:

- weakness
- stiffness
- problems seeing
- problems walking
- loss of mental ability

Without treatment, the symptoms of late-onset GLD get worse and become life-threatening. Symptoms grow worse more slowly in late-onset GLD, but the time for symptoms to become severe varies greatly.

Diagnosis

GLD can be diagnosed by testing a sample of blood or skin cells to measure activity levels of the enzyme GALC. Patients with GLD show very low GALC activity levels. A doctor may also do a lumbar puncture (spinal tap) to get a sample of the fluid around the spinal cord. In patients with GLD, this fluid has very high levels of protein. Families affected by GLD may want to talk with a genetic counselor about family planning and the chances of having children with the disorder.

Transplant for GLD

The only known treatment that has some effect on the progression of the disease is a bone marrow or cord blood transplant (also called a BMT). The healthy cells received in a transplant can make the GALC enzyme the body was missing. Though it has serious risks and is not an option for all patients, a transplant can be life-saving and prevent severe disability for some people with GLD.

Transplants for late-onset GLD have had a better chance of good results than transplants for early-onset GLD. This is because late-onset GLD gets worse more slowly than early-onset GLD. It takes months for the transplanted cells to make enough healthy cells to correct a patient's metabolism, and the disorder can continue to cause damage during that time. The best results in people with late-onset GLD have occurred when they receive a transplant early in the course of the disease, before severe symptoms develop.

Babies with early-onset GLD may be helped by a transplant if they receive it within the first one or two months of life. This is before symptoms appear in most cases. Most babies diagnosed early are tested for GLD because an older sibling is affected with the disorder. Early diagnosis can be important to the success of transplants for early-onset GLD. Transplants for babies who are three months of age or older, and already show symptoms, have had poor results.

Transplant Outcomes

It is a good idea to ask your doctor for help interpreting these data and any other survival outcomes data you find. Your doctor can provide context for these data and discuss your specific situation with you. Doctors are conducting research to learn about when and how transplant can help people with GLD. The disorder is rare and studies of transplant outcomes for people with GLD have included small numbers of patients. In one study of five children with GLD, four received bone marrow transplants from matched related donors, and one received an unrelated umbilical cord blood transplant.[1]

- Four children had late-onset GLD—After transplant, damage to the central nervous system was stopped and many of their symptoms improved.

- One child had early-onset GLD—This child had a transplant at two months of age. At 16 months of age, he had no signs of central nervous system damage, though he had some stiffness, and his skills development was behind the norm for his age.

Cord Blood Transplants for Early-Onset GLD

Cord blood transplants may be an important option for children with GLD because many do not have a suitable donor in their family, and they need a transplant quickly. A suitably matched cord blood unit may be easier to find and more quickly available than an unrelated adult donor.

A study of babies with early-onset GLD treated with umbilical cord blood transplants showed that cord blood transplant can be an effective treatment, but early transplant remains very important.[2] This study reported results for 25 babies who received cord blood transplants between 1998 and 2004. At the time of the report in 2005:

- Eleven babies had no symptoms and received transplants within the first two months of life. All eleven survived and had normal vision, hearing, and thinking skills for their age, but some had mild to severe problems with motor skills such as walking or picking up objects.

- Fourteen babies already had symptoms of disease and received transplants between four and eleven months of age. Six children (43%) survived, but their symptoms remained severe and in some cases continued to get worse.

Making Treatment Decisions

If you or your child has GLD, it is important to see a doctor who is an expert in this disorder. If your doctor has not treated other patients with GLD, ask him or her to refer you to an expert for consultation. Since GLD can get worse quickly, it is important to see an expert as soon as possible. If transplant is a treatment option, talk with your doctor about the risks, limits, and possible benefits of transplant.

References

1. Krivit W, Shapiro EG, Peters C, et al. Hematopoietic stem-cell transplantation in globoid-cell leukodystrophy. *N Engl J Med*. 1998; 338(16):1119–1126.

2. Escolar ML, Poe MD, Provenzale JM, et al. Transplantation of umbilical-cord blood in babies with infantile Krabbe's disease. *N Engl J Med*. 2005; 352(20):2069–2081.

For Additional Information on GLD

National Institute of Neurological Disorders and Stroke (NINDS)
P.O. Box 5801
Bethesda, MD 20824
Toll-Free: 800-352-9424
Phone: 301-496-5751
Fax: 301-468-5981
Website: http://www.ninds.nih.gov
E-mail: braininfo@ninds.nih.gov

United Leukodystrophy Foundation
2304 Highland Drive
Sycamore, IL 60178
Toll-Free: 800-728-5483
Phone: 815-895-3211
Fax: 815-895-2432
Website: http://www.ulf.org
E-mail: office@ulf.org

Section 60.5

Metachromatic Leukodystrophy (MLD)

"Metachromatic Leukodystrophy (MLD) and Transplant," © 2006 National Marrow Donor Program. Reprinted with permission. For additional information from the National Marrow Donor Program, visit http://www.marrow.org.

Definition of Metachromatic Leukodystrophy A Metabolic Storage Disorder

Metachromatic leukodystrophy (MLD) is an inherited metabolic storage disorder that affects motor skills, balance, vision, and mental skills.

Metachromatic leukodystrophy is one of a group of inherited metabolic storage disorders in which the lack of an enzyme affects various organs and tissues, including the brain. Enzymes are proteins that play many roles, including metabolizing (breaking down) substances in the body. In metabolic storage disorders, the body lacks an enzyme needed to metabolize a substance, such as a sugar. Instead, the substance builds up in the body and causes damage.

A Type of Leukodystrophy

MLD is one of a subgroup of metabolic disorders called the leukodystrophies. The leukodystrophies are caused by a variety of gene mutations (mistakes). Genes carry an inherited code of instructions that tells the body how to make every cell and substance in the body.

In the leukodystrophies, the gene mutations lead to damage of the myelin.

Myelin is the fatty substance that forms a sheath around the axons that carry signals to and from nerves in the central nervous system (brain and spinal cord). The myelin sheath is similar to the insulation on a wire. It enables the axons to carry signals very quickly. When the myelin sheath is damaged, the signals slow down or may stop completely.

If the signals from the brain and spinal cord have trouble getting to the rest of the body, a person can have problems controlling the body's movements. If the signals between nerves in the brain are slowed or stopped, a person can have problems with memory, learning, speaking and understanding speech, and other mental functions.

Metachromatic Leukodystrophy

In people with MLD, the gene mutation affects an enzyme called arylsulfatase A. This enzyme breaks down substances called sulfatides. Sulfatides are one of the ten substances that make up myelin. Without the arylsulfatase-A enzyme, sulfatides build up and damage the myelin sheath, causing problems with the central nervous system and peripheral nervous system. The peripheral nervous system is the nerves throughout the body that carry signals to and from the central nervous system.

A person gets MLD when he or she inherits a gene with the mutation from both parents. MLD appears most often in babies and young toddlers, but it also occurs in older children and adults. MLD is rare. About 1 in 100,000 people has this disorder.

Signs and Symptoms of MLD

Late-Infantile MLD: The most common and severe form of MLD is the late-infantile form. The symptoms of the late-infantile form of MLD appear when children are six to twenty-four months old. The first symptoms include problems with walking or other motor skills. Symptoms get worse quickly. Painful muscle cramps and problems with speech, movement, and the ability to learn get worse until the child becomes paralyzed and blind. Children with this form of MLD usually die before ten years of age.

Juvenile MLD: The juvenile form of MLD appears in children between the ages of four and twelve, sometimes earlier. Early symptoms include problems with learning or with walking. As the disease progresses, symptoms include behavior problems, trouble following directions, and worsening problems with walking and speech. Eventually the child becomes paralyzed and blind. Some children with juvenile MLD survive into adulthood, though others die sooner.

Adult MLD: The adult form of MLD can appear in teenagers or adults of any age. The first symptoms are often changes in personality and poor school or job performance. Adult MLD is often mistaken for other disorders such as schizophrenia or depression. As the disorder progresses, problems with memory and other mental skills, speech, controlling movement, and eating get worse slowly. People with adult MLD may sometimes live ten to thirty years or more after symptoms appear.

Diagnosis

Tests a doctor may use to help diagnose MLD include:

- blood or skin tests to check for low levels of arylsulfatase-A enzyme activity;
- brain scans using magnetic resonance imaging (MRI) to check for abnormalities;
- lumbar puncture (spinal tap) to check the fluid around the spinal cord for high levels of protein;
- urine tests to check for high levels of sulfatides and other signs of possible MLD;
- tests to check the function of the nerves (nerve velocity conduction studies).

Families affected by MLD may want to talk with a genetic counselor about family planning and the chances of having children with the disorder. Early diagnosis may enable early treatment before symptoms occur, which can be important to outcomes.

Transplant for MLD

The only known treatment that can affect the progression of MLD is a bone marrow or cord blood transplant (also called a BMT). The healthy cells received in a transplant can make the arylsulfatase A the body was missing.

Though it has serious risks and is not an option for all patients, a transplant can be life-saving. It can stop damage to the central nervous system, preventing severe mental disability for some people with MLD. A transplant is most likely to benefit a person early in the course of MLD who shows few or no symptoms. Some of the limits of transplant for MLD include:

- Problems that have already appeared will remain after transplant. Damage the disease has already done is not reversed.

- Patients who already have severe symptoms are unlikely to benefit from transplant. Their symptoms are likely to continue to get worse.

- A transplant cannot stop damage to the peripheral nervous system. Problems with controlling movement are likely to continue to get worse after transplant.

- It takes time (sometimes as long as a year) for the transplanted cells to make enough healthy cells to correct a patient's metabolism. During this time, the disorder can continue to cause damage.

The results described here are from reports of individual patients; no larger clinical studies are available. It is a good idea to ask your doctor for help interpreting these data and any other survival outcomes data you find. Your doctor can provide context for these data and discuss your specific situation with you.

Transplant Outcomes for Late-Infantile MLD

Most transplants that have been done to treat young children with the late-infantile form of MLD have not been successful in preventing severe damage. This is because the late-infantile form gets worse quickly once problems have developed. However, some children with late-infantile MLD have benefited from a transplant.[1] Good results are more likely when a transplant is done early, before symptoms appear. Most children who are diagnosed early are tested for MLD because they have an older sibling affected with the disorder.

Transplants for Juvenile and Adult MLD

The juvenile and adult forms of MLD get worse at a slower rate. Transplants for these forms have helped some people. The best results have appeared in people who received a transplant before symptoms of disease appeared or at an early stage of the disease. In published reports of transplants for older children and young adults with MLD, transplant has succeeded in stopping central nervous system damage for some patients. Those patients' mental abilities stayed the same or in some cases improved somewhat. In other patients, transplant did not stop the disease and damage continued after transplant.[2, 3, 4, 5]

Outcomes for Unrelated Donor Transplants

Between 1987 and 2003, the National Marrow Donor Program (NMDP) facilitated transplants using unrelated donors for 37 patients with MLD. At five years the likelihood of survival for these patients was 54%. Information about whether the patients had the early, juvenile, or adult forms is not available. The age of patients at the time of transplant ranged from three months to thirty-three years, with a median age of five years. (The median is the middle point, with half of the patients younger and half older.)

Making Treatment Decisions

If you or your family member has MLD, it is important to see a doctor who is an expert in MLD. If your doctor has not treated other patients with MLD, ask him or her to refer you to an expert for consultation. If transplant is a treatment option, talk with your doctor about the risks, limits and possible benefits of transplant.

Even after a successful transplant, a patient will face physical problems from MLD. However, a transplant may offer a person with MLD a chance to live a longer life as well as to keep his or her ability to think and learn.

References

1. Krivit W, Shapiro E, Kennedy W, et al. Treatment of late infantile metachromatic leukodystrophy by bone marrow transplantation. *N Engl J Med*. 1990; 322(1):28–32.

2. Kapaun P, Dittmann RW, Granitzny B, et al. Slow progression of juvenile metachromatic leukodystrophy 6 years after bone marrow transplantation. *Journal Child Neurol*. 1999; 14(4):222–228.

3. Malm G, Ringden O, Winiarski J, et al. Clinical outcome in four children with metachromatic leukodystrophy treated by

bone marrow transplantation. *Bone Marrow Transplant*. 1996; 17(6):1003–1008.

4. Navarro C, Fernandez JM, Dominguez C, Fachal C, Alvarez M. Late juvenile metachromatic leukodystrophy treated with bone marrow transplantation; a 4-year follow-up study. *Neurology*. 1996; 46(1):254–256.

5. Solders G, Celsing G, Hagenfeldt L, Ljungman P, Isberg B, Ringden O. Improved peripheral nerve conduction, EEG and verbal IQ after bone marrow transplantation for adult meta-chromatic leukodystrophy. *Bone Marrow Transplant*. 1998; 22(11):1119–1122.

More Information on Metachromatic Leukodystrophy

United Leukodystrophy Foundation
2304 Highland Drive
Sycamore, IL 60178
Toll-Free: 800-728-5483
Phone: 815-895-3211
Fax: 815-895-2432
Website: http://www.ulf.org
E-mail: office@ulf.org

Section 60.6

Cerebral X-Linked Adrenoleukodystrophy (ALD)

Definition of Adrenoleukodystrophy

Cerebral X-linked adrenoleukodystrophy (ALD) is an inherited metabolic storage disorder that can cause severe damage to the central nervous system (brain and spinal cord) and the adrenal gland.

A Type of Leukodystrophy

ALD is one of a subgroup of metabolic disorders called the leukodystrophies. The leukodystrophies are caused by a variety of gene mutations (mistakes). Genes carry an inherited code of instructions that tells the body how to make every cell and substance in the body. In the leukodystrophies, the gene mutations lead to damage of the myelin.

Myelin is the fatty substance that forms a sheath around the axons that carry signals to and from nerves in the central nervous system (brain and spinal cord). The myelin sheath is similar to the insulation on a wire. It enables the axons to carry signals very quickly. When the myelin sheath is damaged, the signals slow down or may stop completely.

If the signals from the brain and spinal cord have trouble getting to the rest of the body, a person can have problems controlling the body's movements. If the signals between nerves in the brain are slowed or stopped, a person can have problems with memory, learning, speaking and understanding speech, and other mental functions.

Adrenoleukodystrophy

In people with ALD, the disorder affects the body's ability to break down certain fat molecules known as very long chain fatty acids. Very long chain fatty acids are one of the ten substances that make up myelin. In people with ALD, the body does not break down the very long chain fatty acids, so they build up and damage the myelin. Damage to the myelin causes problems with the function of the nervous system. The very long chain fatty acids also affect the adrenal gland. The adrenal gland makes hormones that help control many body functions.

Childhood Cerebral X-linked ALD

There is a wide variation in how severe ALD is and how it affects people. Signs of ALD can appear in people at different ages and cause symptoms ranging from mild to severe. About 30% to 40% of cases of ALD are the most severe form, childhood cerebral X-linked ALD (which is the form discussed here).

- Childhood ALD appears in boys between two and ten years of age.

- It is called the cerebral form because it damages the brain more severely than other forms of ALD, affecting all mental and body functions.

- The disorder is called X-linked because the mutated gene is on the X chromosome, inherited from the mother. Disorders caused by genes on the X chromosome occur only in males. Females are carriers of the mutated gene but do not get the disorder.

Symptoms and Diagnosis of Cerebral X-Linked ALD

The early symptoms of childhood cerebral X-linked ALD include changes in behavior or learning problems. Without treatment, problems with learning, speaking and understanding speech, hearing, seeing, swallowing, walking, and other movement can get worse quickly. These symptoms are all caused by damage to the central nervous system. If the damage is not stopped, a boy with the disorder will become unable to control his body or respond to life around him, usually within six months to two years. Cerebral ALD leads to death within months to several years.

Diagnosis

For boys showing the symptoms described, a brain scan using magnetic resonance imaging (MRI) shows an abnormal pattern typical of ALD. In boys showing symptoms, the brain MRI is often the first step toward diagnosis.

Doctors can then diagnose ALD using a blood test to check for high levels of very long chain fatty acids. All males in a family affected by

ALD should be carefully screened for ALD. A blood test can diagnose ALD even in boys who do not show symptoms and whose brain MRI is normal. Tests for the gene mutation that causes ALD can also be done. Families affected by ALD may want to talk with a genetic counselor about family planning and the chances of having children with ALD.

Treatment Options for Childhood Cerebral X-Linked ALD

For boys with childhood cerebral X-linked ALD, treatment options may include:

- bone marrow or cord blood transplant (also called a BMT)— the only known treatment that can stop the progression of the disease;

- hormone replacement therapy to make up for problems with the adrenal gland function;

- Lorenzo oil—only if a boy does not yet show signs of the cerebral form of ALD;

- other, newer treatments in clinical trials.

Transplant for Cerebral X-Linked ALD

For boys with cerebral X-linked ALD, a bone marrow or cord blood transplant early in the course of the disease can stop the progression of the disease. Though it has serious risks and is not an option for all patients, a transplant can be life-saving and prevent severe disability for some boys with cerebral X-linked ALD. A transplant is not considered a treatment option for other, less severe forms of ALD because it is not clear transplant offers a benefit in these cases.

One of the earliest transplants for X-linked cerebral ALD was reported in 1990. In this case, a boy received a transplant soon after he began showing signs of nervous system damage. He maintained normal mental function (such as memory and the ability to learn) after the transplant.[1] Since that time, doctors have continued to learn about when and how transplant can help boys with X-linked ALD.

It is a good idea to ask your doctor for help interpreting these data and any other survival outcomes data you find. Your doctor can provide context for these data and discuss your specific situation with you.

Timing of Transplant

Studies show that timing of the transplant is very important. Boys who show early signs of cerebral ALD in MRI scans but have few outward symptoms have a good chance of doing well after transplant. Mild damage may sometimes even be reversed. However, the amount of damage the disorder has already done (amount of myelin already lost) makes a big difference to the outcome of the transplant. Boys who already show major symptoms face higher risks after transplant. Severe damage cannot be reversed, so these boys may have a lower quality of life even if transplant succeeds.

One study reported results for 94 boys with cerebral X-linked ALD who received a transplant between 1982 and 1999.[2]

- For all boys in the study, the likelihood of surviving at least five years after transplant was 56%.

- For the 42 boys who had a related donor, the 5-year likelihood of survival was 64%.

- For the 52 boys who had an unrelated donor, the 5-year likelihood of survival was 53%.

The amount of damage the disease had done before the transplant greatly affected outcomes. The amount of damage was measured with brain MRIs and assessment of the boys' vision, hearing, speech, walking, and other skills.

- For boys who showed the least amount of damage before transplant, the 5-year likelihood of survival was 92%.

- For all other boys (who showed more damage before transplant), the 5-year likelihood of survival was 45%.

- Boys with less damage before transplant were more likely to have stable or improved central nervous system function (such as abilities to learn and to control movement) after transplant. Boys with more damage were likely to continue to get worse.

National Marrow Donor Program (NMDP) Outcomes for Unrelated Donor Transplants

Between 1987 and 2003, 50 boys with ALD received an unrelated donor transplant facilitated by the NMDP. The 5-year likelihood of survival for these boys was 36%.

Long-Term Quality of Life

Another study focused on long-term outcomes by looking at the status of twelve boys five to ten years after their transplants.[3] The study found that problems caused by ALD, such as problems with vision, controlling movement, and reasoning, were improved or became stable in most boys. However, for some boys some problems got worse before becoming stable. All boys continued to receive hormone replacement therapy for problems with the adrenal gland. All boys were able to learn: Eight were in mainstream school classes, including one in college, while four were receiving special help or tutoring.

Hormone Replacement Therapy

Boys with ALD may have a life-long need for treatment with hormone replacement therapy. ALD can alter the adrenal glands so that they do not make enough hormones for the body. This can be life-threatening and requires treatment with hormones.

Lorenzo Oil and Newer Treatments

Another treatment that has been studied is taking Lorenzo oil and eating a low-fat diet. Lorenzo oil is made from olive and rapeseed oils. For some boys who do not yet have the cerebral form of ALD, Lorenzo oil may reduce or delay severe symptoms. Lorenzo oil appears more likely to help boys who have no symptoms of nervous system damage and are younger. However, the benefit of Lorenzo oil remains uncertain and it is not a cure. Even boys who appear to benefit are likely to develop the adult form of ALD. Though the adult form is milder than childhood ALD, it is still a serious disease. Studies have shown that Lorenzo oil does not help boys who already show symptoms.

Newer Treatments

Researchers are trying to develop other treatments for boys with cerebral ALD. Some other treatment options may be available in clinical trials.

Making Treatment Decisions

If your son has cerebral X-linked ALD, it is important for him to see a doctor who is an expert in treating ALD. If your child's doctor has not treated other patients with ALD, ask him or her to refer you to an expert for consultation. Since ALD can get worse quickly, it is important to see an expert as soon as possible. If transplant is a treatment option for your child, talk with your doctor about the risks, limits and possible benefits of transplant.

In a family with a history of ALD, some boys can be diagnosed with ALD when there are no signs of central nervous system damage. The cerebral form of ALD is the only one for which a transplant is a treatment option, because it is not clear whether transplant offers a benefit in other forms of ALD. However, doctors have no way to predict which boys with ALD will develop the cerebral form. If your child is diagnosed with ALD before symptoms appear, it is important for him to be watched carefully for signs the ALD is affecting the central nervous system. Your doctor will schedule regular brain MRIs to watch for these signs.

If your child does develop cerebral ALD, getting a transplant early—before the disease progresses and symptoms become severe—can make a difference to outcomes. Your doctor can take steps to be prepared. He or she can check whether your child has any possible donors in your family. Your doctor can also search the National Marrow Donor Program Registry for potential unrelated volunteer donors or cord blood units. That way, if your child develops cerebral ALD and needs a transplant, the first steps of the donor search will be done and your child may be able to move to transplant more quickly.

References

1. Aubourg P, Blanche S, Jambaqué I, et al. Reversal of early neurologic and neuroradiologic manifestations of X-linked adrenoleukodystrophy by bone marrow transplantation. *N Engl J Med*. 1990; 322(26):1860–1866.

2. Peters C, Charnas LR, Tan Y, et al. Cerebral X-linked adrenoleukodystrophy: the international hematopoietic cell transplantation experience from 1982 to 1999. *Blood*. 2004; 104(3):881–888.

3. Shapiro E, Krivit W, Lockman L, et al. Long-term effect of bone-marrow transplantation for childhood-onset cerebral X-linked adrenoleukodystrophy. *Lancet*. 2000; 356(9231):713–718.

For More Information on Cerebral X-Linked ALD

United Leukodystrophy Foundation
2304 Highland Drive
Sycamore, IL 60178

Toll-Free: 800-728-5483
Phone: 815-895-3211
Fax: 815-895-2432
Website: http://www.ulf.org
E-mail: office@ulf.org

Chapter 61

McCune-Albright Syndrome

The McCune-Albright syndrome is named for the two physicians who described it over 50 years ago. They reported a group of children, most of them girls, with an unusual pattern of associated abnormalities: bone disease with fractures, asymmetry and deformity of the legs, arms and skull; endocrine disease including early puberty with menstrual bleeding, development of breasts and pubic hair and an increased rate of growth; and skin changes with areas of increased pigment distributed in an asymmetric and irregular pattern. Today, we use the term McCune-Albright syndrome to describe patients who have some or all of these bone, endocrine, and skin abnormalities. In the years since it was first identified, however, we have studied many additional patients and have learned that the condition has a broad spectrum of severity. Sometimes, children are diagnosed in early infancy with obvious bone disease and markedly increased endocrine secretions from several glands; a very few of these severely affected children have died. At the opposite end of the spectrum, many children are entirely healthy and have a normal life expectancy. They have little or no outward evidence of bone or endocrine involvement, may enter puberty close to normal age and have no unusual skin pigment at all. Because of this marked variability among some patients, the various components of this complicated syndrome are treated separately in the following sections.

Endocrine Abnormalities

Precocious Puberty

When the signs of puberty (development of breasts, testes, pubic and underarm hair, body odor, menstrual bleeding, and increased growth rate) appear before the age of eight years in a girl and nine and a half years in a boy, it is termed precocious puberty. In the most common form of precocious puberty, there is early activation of the regions in the brain which control the maturation of the gonads (ovaries in a girl, and testes in a boy). One brain center, the hypothalamus, secretes a substance called gonadotropin-releasing-hormone, or GnRH. This acts, in turn, on another part of the brain, the pituitary gland, to cause increased secretion of hormones called gonadotropins (luteinizing hormone [LH] and follicle-stimulating hormone [FSH]) that travel through the bloodstream, and act on the ovaries or testes to stimulate secretion of estrogen or testosterone. Endocrinologists find out whether a child with precocious puberty has early activation of the hypothalamus and pituitary (gonadotropin-dependent precocious puberty) by measuring the levels of LH and FSH in the blood after an injection of a synthetic preparation of GnRH.

After studying many girls with McCune-Albright syndrome, however, we have learned that most do not appear to have early activation of the hypothalamus and pituitary because their levels of LH and FSH are usually low, or similar to those of prepubertal children. The precocious puberty in McCune-Albright girls is caused by estrogens which are secreted into the bloodstream by ovarian cysts which enlarge, and then decrease in size over periods of weeks to days. The cysts can be visualized and measured by ultrasonography, in which sound waves are used to outline the dimensions of the ovaries. The cysts may become quite big, occasionally over 50 cubic centimeters (cc) in volume (about the size of a golf ball). Frequently, menstrual bleeding and breast enlargement accompany the growth of a cyst. In fact, menstrual bleeding under two years of age has been the first symptom of McCune-Albright syndrome in 85% of patients. Although ovarian cysts and irregular menstrual bleeding may continue into adolescence and adulthood, many adult women with McCune-Albright syndrome are fertile and can bear normal children.

The precocious puberty in McCune-Albright syndrome has been difficult to treat. After surgical removal of the cyst or of the entire affected ovary, cysts usually recur in the remaining ovary. A progesterone-like hormone called Provera can be given to suppress the menstrual bleeding, but does not appear to slow the rapid rates of growth and bone development, and may have unwanted effects on adrenal functioning. The biosynthetic forms of GnRH (Deslorelin, Histrelin, and Lupron) which suppress LH and FSH, and are used to treat the common, gonadotropin-dependent form of precocious puberty are not effective in most girls with McCune-Albright syndrome. An investigational form of treatment using oral medications which block estrogen synthesis,(testolactone and fadrozole) is now being tested in girls with McCune-Albright syndrome and has been beneficial in many patients.

Thyroid Function

Almost 50% of patients with McCune-Albright syndrome have thyroid gland abnormalities; these include generalized enlargement called goiter, and irregular masses such as nodules and cysts. Some patients have subtle structural changes detected only by ultrasonography. Pituitary thyroid-stimulating-hormone (TSH) levels are low in these patients, and thyroid hormone levels may be normal or elevated. Therapy with drugs which block thyroid hormone synthesis (Propylthiouracil or Methimazole) can be given if thyroid hormone levels are excessively high.

Growth Hormone

Excessive secretion of pituitary growth hormone has been seen in a few patients with McCune-Albright syndrome. Most of these have been diagnosed as young adults, when they developed the coarsening of facial features, enlargement of hands and feet, and arthritis characteristic of the condition termed acromegaly. Therapy has included surgical removal of the area of the pituitary which is secreting the hormone, and the use of new, synthetic analogs of the hormone somatostatin, which suppress growth hormone secretion.

Other Endocrine Abnormalities

Rarely, adrenal enlargement and excessive secretion of the adrenal hormone cortisol is seen in McCune-Albright syndrome. This may cause obesity of the face and trunk, weight gain, skin fragility, and cessation of growth in childhood. These symptoms are called Cushing syndrome. Treatment is removal of the affected adrenal glands, or use of drugs which block cortisol synthesis.

Some children with McCune-Albright syndrome have very low levels of phosphorus in the blood due to excessive losses of phosphate in the urine. This may cause bone weakening and the condition called rickets. It may be treated with oral phosphates and supplemental vitamin D.

Bone Disease: Polyostotic Fibrous Dysplasia

The term polyostotic fibrous dysplasia means "abnormal fibrous tissue growth in many bones". In affected areas, normal bone is replaced by irregular masses of fibroblast cells. When this occurs in weight-bearing bones, such as the femur (upper leg bone), limping, deformity, and fractures may result. In many children, the arms and/or legs are of unequal length, even in the absence of actual fracture. Regions of fibrous dysplasia are also very common in the bones that form the skull and upper jaw. If these areas begin to expand, skull and facial asymmetry may result. Polyostotic fibrous dysplasia can often be seen in a plain x-ray picture of the skeleton. A more sensitive method of finding lesions is a bone scan, in which a small amount of radioactivity (an isotope of technetium) is injected into a vein, taken up by the abnormal tissues, and detected by a scanner.

The severity of bone disease in McCune-Albright syndrome is quite variable. Some children may be minimally affected, with no asymmetry, deformity, or fracture, and lesions detected only by bone scan. In a few children, lesions are only found in the base of the skull. By repeating bone scans at intervals of one to two years, we have seen that in some children the bone disease may become more extensive over time. Unfortunately, severe bone disease can have permanent effects upon physical appearance and mobility.

There is no known hormonal or medical treatment that has been proven to be effective in controlling progressive polyostotic fibrous dysplasia. Surgical procedures to correct fracture and deformity include grafting, pinning, and casting. Skull and jaw changes are often corrected surgically with great improvement in appearance.

Skin Abnormalities

The irregular, flat areas of increased skin pigment in McCune-Albright syndrome are called cafe-au-lait spots because, in children with light complexions, they are the color of coffee with milk. In dark-skinned individuals, these spots may be difficult to see. Most children have the pigment from birth, and it almost never becomes more extensive. The pattern of the pigment distribution is unique, often starting or ending abruptly at the midline on the abdomen in front or at the spine in back. Some children have no cafe-au-lait pigment at all; in a few, it is confined to small areas, such as the nape of the neck or crease of the buttocks.

There are seldom any medical problems associated with the areas of cafe-au-lait pigment. Some adolescent children may want to use makeup to obscure areas of dark pigment on the face.

Recent Research

So far, we have not found a cure for the bone and endocrine disease in McCune-Albright syndrome. It cannot yet be diagnosed before birth, and we cannot accurately predict how severe the disease may become in an affected child. There are no reported cases of any parent being affected, and the children of women with McCune-Albright syndrome are normal. All races appear to be affected equally. Thus, we are not yet certain of the genetic origin of the defect. It is believed, however, that it may be the result of a mutation occurring early in the development of the embryo.

Recently, researchers have discovered abnormal mutations in deoxyribonucleic acid (DNA) obtained from the affected ovaries, adrenals, and liver of several patients with the McCune-Albright syndrome. The DNA contained the genetic code for one component, called a G protein, of a signaling system which is present in many cells, and which is known to be involved in endocrine cell growth and secretion. The presence of this mutation could result in uncontrolled cell function or hormone secretion. This research is continuing, and it may soon enable us to plan better methods of treatment for patients with the McCune-Albright syndrome.

Additional Information

The MAGIC Foundation
6645 W. North Ave.
Oak Park, IL 60302
Toll-Free: 800-362-4423
Phone: 708-383-0808
Fax: 708-383-0899
Website: http://www.magicfoundation.org

Chapter 62

Metabolic Diseases of the Muscle

What Are Metabolic Diseases of Muscle?

Metabolic diseases of muscle were first recognized in the second half of the 20th century. Each of these disorders is caused by a different genetic defect that impairs the body's metabolism, the collection of chemical changes that occur within cells during normal functioning.

Specifically, the metabolic diseases of muscle interfere with chemical reactions involved in drawing energy from food. Normally, fuel molecules derived from food must be broken down further inside each cell before they can be used by the cells' mitochondria to make the energy molecule adenosine triphosphate (ATP).

The mitochondria inside each cell could be called the cell's engines. The metabolic muscle diseases are caused by problems in the way certain fuel molecules are processed before they enter the mitochondria, or by the inability to get fuel molecules into mitochondria.

Muscles require a lot of energy in the form of ATP to work properly. When energy levels become too low, muscle weakness and exercise intolerance with muscle pain or cramps may occur.

Reprinted from "Facts about Metabolic Diseases of Muscle," with permission of the Muscular Dystrophy Association, www.mda.org. © 2003 The Muscular Dystrophy Association. For additional information, call the Muscular Dystrophy Association National Headquarters toll-free at 800-FIGHT-MD (800-344-4863). To find an MDA office in your area, look in your local telephone book, or search by zip code on the MDA website.

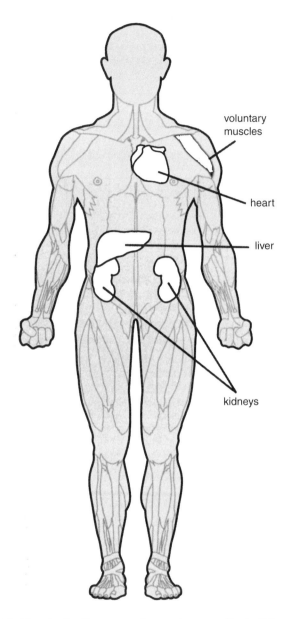

Figure 62.1. *Metabolic diseases of muscle can affect all the body's voluntary muscles, such as those in the arms, legs, and trunk. Some can also involve increased risk of heart or liver diseases, and the effects can damage the kidneys.*

In a few metabolic muscle disorders, symptoms are not caused so much by a lack of energy, but rather by unused fuel molecules that build up inside muscle cells. This buildup may damage the cells, leading to chronic weakness.

Metabolic muscle diseases that have their onset in infancy tend to be the most severe, and some forms are fatal. Those that begin in childhood or adulthood tend to be less severe, and changes in diet and lifestyle can help most people with the milder forms adjust.

There are 10 metabolic diseases of muscle (myopathies) in MDA's program. Each one gets its name from the substance that is lacking:

- acid maltase deficiency (Pompe disease)
- carnitine deficiency
- carnitine palmityl transferase deficiency
- debrancher enzyme deficiency (Cori or Forbes disease)
- lactate dehydrogenase deficiency
- myoadenylate deaminase deficiency
- phosphofructokinase deficiency (Tarui disease)
- phosphoglycerate kinase deficiency
- phosphoglycerate mutase deficiency
- phosphorylase deficiency (McArdle disease)

What Causes Metabolic Diseases?

Nine of the diseases in this chapter are caused by defects in the enzymes that control chemical reactions used to break down food. Enzyme defects are caused by flaws in the genes that govern production of the enzymes.

The 10th disease, carnitine deficiency, is caused by lack of a small, naturally occurring molecule that is not an enzyme but is involved in metabolism.

Enzymes are special types of proteins that act like little machines on a microscopic assembly line, each performing a different function to break down food molecules into fuel. When one of the enzymes in the line is defective, the process goes more slowly or shuts down entirely.

Our bodies can use carbohydrates (starches and sugars), fats, and protein for fuel. Defects in the cells' carbohydrate and fat-processing pathways usually lead to weakness in the voluntary muscles, but may also affect the heart, kidneys, or liver. Although defects in protein-processing pathways can occur as well, these usually lead to different kinds of disorders that affect other organs.

A gene is a "recipe" or set of instructions for making a protein, such as an enzyme. A defect in the gene may cause the protein to be made incorrectly or not at all, leading to a deficiency in the amount of that enzyme. Genes are passed from parents to children. Therefore, gene defects can be inherited.

The metabolic muscle diseases are not contagious, and they are not caused by certain kinds of exercise or lack of exercise. However, exercise or fasting (not eating regularly) may bring on episodes of muscle weakness in a person who has the disease because of a genetic flaw.

What Happens to Someone with a Metabolic Disease?

Exercise Intolerance

The main symptom of most of the metabolic myopathies is difficulty performing some types of exercise, a situation known as exercise intolerance, in which the person becomes tired very easily.

The degree of exercise intolerance in the metabolic myopathies varies greatly between disorders and even from one individual to the next within a disorder. For instance, some people may run into trouble only when jogging, while others may have trouble after mild exertion such as walking across a parking lot or even blow-drying their hair. Each person must learn his activity limitations.

In general, people with defects in their carbohydrate-processing pathways tend to become very tired at the beginning of exercise but may experience a renewed feeling of energy after 10 or 15 minutes. On the other hand, those with carnitine palmityl transferase deficiency (CPT) may experience fatigue only after prolonged exercise.

A person with exercise intolerance may also experience painful muscle cramps and/or injury-induced pain during or after exercising.

The exercise-induced cramps (actually sharp contractions that may seem to temporarily lock the muscles) are especially noted in many of the disorders of carbohydrate metabolism and, rarely, in myoadenylate deaminase deficiency. The injury-induced pain is caused by acute muscle breakdown, a process called rhabdomyolysis, which may occur in any metabolic muscle disorder and is particularly noted in CPT.

Episodes of rhabdomyolysis usually occur when a person with a metabolic myopathy "overdoes it" (sometimes unknowingly). These episodes, often described as "severe muscle pain," may occur during exercise or

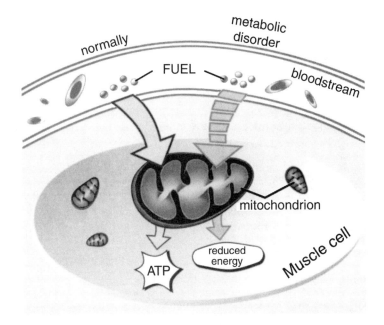

Figure 62.2. In normal metabolism, food provides fuel that is processed inside the cells, producing energy (ATP) for muscle contraction and other cellular functions. In metabolic myopathies, missing enzymes prevent mitochondria from properly processing fuel, and no energy is produced for muscle function.

several hours afterward. In those with carbohydrate-processing disorders, rhabdomyolysis may be triggered by aerobic exercise (such as running or jumping) or isometric exercise (like pushing or pulling heavy objects, squatting, or standing on tiptoes). In people with CPT, rhabdomyolysis is usually brought on by prolonged, moderate exercise, especially if an affected person exercises without eating. In CPT, rhabdomyolysis may also be triggered by illness, cold, fasting, stress, or menstruation.

Because rhabdomyolysis is painful and can cause extensive kidney damage, many people with metabolic muscle diseases try to avoid triggering these episodes by modifying their physical activities or diet. Your MDA clinic director can help you work out a lifestyle plan to optimize your health and abilities.

Muscle Weakness

In acid maltase deficiency, carnitine deficiency, and debrancher enzyme deficiency, progressive muscle weakness, rather than exercise intolerance, is the primary symptom. Over time, people with acid maltase deficiency or debrancher enzyme deficiency may eventually need a wheelchair to get around and, as respiratory muscles weaken, may require ventilatory assistance to provide extra oxygen at night. All three of these disorders may be associated with heart problems.

It is important to realize that, although the metabolic muscle diseases characterized by exercise intolerance are not generally prone to muscle weakness, some chronic or permanent weakness can develop in response to repeated episodes of rhabdomyolysis and to the normal loss of strength that occurs with aging. The degree of muscle weakness that develops in these disorders is extremely variable and may depend on such factors as genetic background and the number of episodes of rhabdomyolysis experienced. The diseases involving exercise intolerance do not usually progress to the degree that a wheelchair or any other mechanical assistance is needed.

Special Issues in Metabolic Disorders

Myoglobinuria: Myoglobinuria refers to rust-colored urine caused by the presence of myoglobin (a muscle protein). When overexertion triggers acute muscle breakdown (rhabdomyolysis), muscle proteins like creatine kinase and myoglobin are released into the blood and ultimately appear in the urine. Myoglobinuria can cause severe kidney damage if untreated. Incidences of myoglobinuria should be dealt with as emergencies and may require intravenous fluids to avoid renal failure.

Emergencies: The metabolic muscle diseases are so rare that emergency room staffs are frequently unfamiliar with them. As a result, they may not treat episodes properly (with fluids and pain medications) or may give the patient food or anesthesia that could trigger further problems.

People with these disorders may want to consider carrying a treatment protocol listing their doctor's phone number, the patient's current medications and dietary requirements, and guidelines for handling emergency situations. A MedicAlert bracelet can also be worn.

Anesthesia: People with metabolic muscle disorders may be at higher risk for a potentially fatal reaction to certain common general anesthetics (typically combinations of halothane and succinylcholine). This reaction, called malignant hyperthermia, can be avoided in planned surgeries by using lower-risk anesthetics. However, it is a good idea to wear a MedicAlert bracelet stating this susceptibility in case of an emergency.

Cardiac care: People with debrancher enzyme deficiency, carnitine deficiency, and acid maltase deficiency may develop significant heart problems. In the case of primary carnitine deficiency, the only symptom may be heart failure; however, this disorder responds well to carnitine supplementation. If you are at risk for cardiac problems, a cardiologist who is familiar with your disorder should monitor your heart function.

Respiratory care: Acid maltase deficiency and debrancher enzyme deficiency tend to weaken the respiratory muscles, those that operate the lungs, meaning that a person with one of these disorders may require supplemental oxygen at some point. If you are at risk for respiratory problems, your breathing should be monitored regularly by a specialist. Also, be conscious of symptoms such as unusual shortness of breath on exertion or morning headaches that may indicate that your breathing is compromised.

How Are the Metabolic Diseases of Muscle Treated?

For many people with metabolic muscle diseases, the only treatment needed is to understand what activities and situations tend to trigger attacks of rhabdomyolysis. A small percentage of adults with metabolic disorders may experience painful muscle cramps that have no obvious triggers; painkillers and meditation techniques may be effective under these circumstances.

In addition, some people with metabolic disorders have benefited from dietary changes. There is evidence that those with carbohydrate-processing problems may be helped by a high-protein diet, while those with difficulty processing fats may do well on a diet high in carbohydrates and low in fat. Carnitine supplements are usually given for carnitine deficiency and can be very effective in reversing heart failure in this disorder.

Please consult your doctor before undertaking any special diets. Your MDA clinic director can help you design a specific plan suited for your metabolic disorder and your individual needs.

There is also emerging evidence that people with some carbohydrate-processing disorders, such as McArdle disease, may benefit from light exercise. Researchers believe that people who are physically fit are better able to use alternative fuel sources to make energy. Because

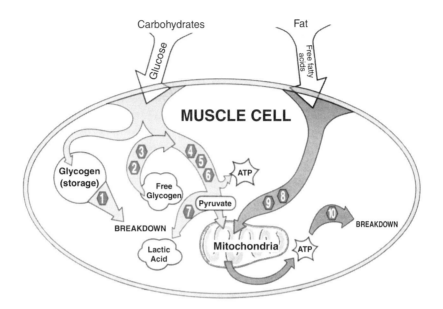

Figure 62.3. *Fueling the Muscles: Roadblocks Lead to Disorders. Where the Problems Are in Each Disease. Skeletal muscles normally depend on energy from carbohydrates and fats. These fuels can be stored in the muscle (glycogen) or imported directly from the bloodstream (glucose and fatty acids). When a genetic defect, interferes with the processing of specific fuels, energy shortages can occur and toxic byproducts may build up. Some people may be able to bypass their defects by adjusting diet or exercise to draw energy more efficiently from unaffected pathways.*

1. Acid maltase deficiency
2. Muscle phosphorylase deficiency
3. Debrancher enzyme deficiency
4. Phosphofructokinase deficiency
5. Phosphoglycerate kinase deficiency
6. Phosphoglycerate mutase deficiency
7. Lactate dehydrogenase deficiency
8. Carnitine palmityl transferase deficiency
9. Carnitine deficiency
10. Myoadenylate deaminase deficiency

overexertion can trigger muscle breakdown, you should only undertake an exercise program under the supervision of a doctor who is familiar with your disorder.

It is unclear whether regular exercise is beneficial in the fat-metabolizing disorders, such as carnitine palmityl transferase deficiency. Note that because of their rarity, the characteristics of several of these diseases are not known well.

Carbohydrate-Processing Disorders

These disorders affect the breakdown of glycogen or glucose (complex and simple carbohydrates) and are also called glycogenosis disorders.

Acid Maltase Deficiency

Also called: Glycogenosis type 2, Pompe disease (infantile form), or lysosomal storage disease.

Onset: Infancy to adulthood.

Inheritance: Autosomal recessive.

Symptoms: Causes slowly progressive weakness, especially of the respiratory muscles and those of the hips, upper legs, shoulders, and upper arms. Enlargement of the tongue occurs in the infantile form, but rarely in the older forms. Cardiac involvement may occur in the childhood form, but is less common in adults. The childhood and adult-onset forms are less severe than the infantile form, but may require use of mechanical ventilation for breathing support as the disease progresses.

The infantile form of Pompe disease often leads to death by age two. An infant with this condition usually requires mechanical ventilation and a feeding tube to help with nourishment. If your infant's condition has been diagnosed as Pompe disease, your MDA clinic director will keep you abreast of ongoing clinical trials for the disease and work with you to make the best decisions for care.

Debrancher Enzyme Deficiency

Also called: Cori disease, Forbes disease, or glycogenosis type 3.

Onset: Childhood to adulthood.

Inheritance: Autosomal recessive.

Symptoms: Principally affects the liver, causing swelling of the liver, slowing of growth, low blood sugar levels, and sometimes, seizures. In children, these symptoms often improve around puberty. Muscle weakness may develop later in life, and is most pronounced in the muscles of the forearms, hands, lower legs, and feet. Weakness is often accompanied by loss of muscle bulk. The heart can be affected as well, and heart function should be monitored closely.

Phosphorylase Deficiency

Also called: Myophosphorylase deficiency, McArdle disease, or glycogenosis type 5.

Onset: Childhood to adulthood.

Inheritance: Autosomal recessive.

Symptoms: Causes exercise intolerance, cramps, muscle pain, and weakness shortly after the beginning of exercise. A person with this disorder may tolerate light-to-moderate exercise such as walking on level ground, but strenuous exercise will usually bring on symptoms quickly. Resting may lead to a "second wind," in which activity is then better tolerated. Isometric exercises that require strength, such as lifting heavy objects, squatting, or standing on tiptoe, also may cause muscle damage.

The symptoms of McArdle disease vary in severity among people and even within the same person from day to day. Symptoms usually do not persist between attacks, although fixed weakness later in life is possible.

Phosphofructokinase Deficiency

Also called: Glycogenosis type 7, or Tarui disease.

Onset: Childhood to adulthood.

Inheritance: Autosomal recessive.

Symptoms: Causes exercise intolerance, with pain, cramps. and occasionally, myoglobinuria. Symptoms are very similar to those of phosphorylase deficiency, but people with this disorder are less likely to experience the "second wind" phenomenon.

A carbohydrate meal typically worsens exercise capacity in this condition by lowering blood levels of fats, which are the major muscle energy fuels for those with the disorder. A partial deficiency of phosphofructokinase in the red blood cells results in the breakdown of those cells and an increase in blood levels of bilirubin, though the person usually experiences no symptoms.

Phosphoglycerate Kinase Deficiency

Also called: Glycogenosis type 9.

Onset: Infancy to early adulthood.

Inheritance: X-linked recessive.

Symptoms: May cause anemia, enlargement of the spleen, mental retardation, and epilepsy. More rarely, weakness, exercise intolerance, muscle cramps, and episodes of myoglobinuria also occur.

Phosphoglycerate Mutase Deficiency

Also called: Glycogenosis type 10.

Onset: Childhood to early adulthood.

Inheritance: Autosomal recessive.

Symptoms: Causes exercise intolerance, cramps, muscle pain, and sometimes, myoglobinuria. Permanent weakness is rare.

Lactate Dehydrogenase Deficiency

Also called: Glycogenosis type 11.

Onset: Early adulthood.

Inheritance: Autosomal recessive.

Symptoms: Causes exercise intolerance and episodes of myoglobinuria. A skin rash is common, probably because skin cells need lactate dehydrogenase.

Fat-Processing Disorders

These disorders affect the breakdown of glycogen or glucose (complex and simple carbohydrates) and are also called glycogenosis disorders.

Carnitine Deficiency

Onset: Childhood.

Inheritance: Autosomal recessive.

Symptoms: This slowly progressive disorder causes cardiac disease and muscle weakness in the hips, shoulders, and upper arms, and legs. The neck and jaw muscles may also be weak. Carnitine deficiency may occur secondary to other metabolic diseases (secondary carnitine deficiency) or in response to a genetic mutation (gene defect) in the protein responsible for bringing carnitine into the cell (primary carnitine deficiency).

Primary carnitine deficiency can often be treated successfully with carnitine supplements.

Carnitine Palmityl Transferase Deficiency

Onset: Childhood to early adulthood.

Inheritance: Autosomal recessive.

Symptoms: Symptoms are usually brought on by prolonged and intense exercise, especially in combination with fasting, but may not appear for several hours after activity stops. Short periods of exercise usually do not provoke symptoms. Symptoms can also be brought on by illness, cold, stress, or menstruation. This disorder causes muscle pain, stiffness. and tenderness, while weakness is less common. Breakdown of muscle tissue during an attack can cause myoglobinuria.

Disorder Affecting ATP Recycling

Myoadenylate Deaminase Deficiency

Onset: Adulthood.

Inheritance: Autosomal recessive.

Symptoms: Interferes with the recycling of the major energy molecule of the cell (called ATP). It may cause exercise intolerance, cramps, and muscle pain, although, in many cases, people with deficiencies in this enzyme may experience no symptoms.

How Are the Metabolic Diseases of Muscle Diagnosed?

It is important to get an accurate diagnosis of a specific metabolic myopathy so the affected person can modify diet and exercise and monitor potentially serious disease effects. Because these diseases are rare, many people with metabolic disorders of muscle have spent some time trying to find out what caused their muscle weakness, myoglobinuria, or other symptoms. The diagnostic process usually begins with a careful medical history, a physical exam, and a neurological exam to test reflexes, strength, and the distribution of weakness.

Several specialized tests are used to confirm a suspected diagnosis of metabolic disease:

- Blood tests can be used to detect the presence of certain chemicals in the blood that may indicate some metabolic diseases.

- An exercise test is used to monitor a person's response to intense or moderate exercise. Blood samples are taken during exercise for testing.

- Electromyography (EMG) uses small needle electrodes to measure the electrical currents in a muscle as it contracts. While an EMG cannot definitively diagnose metabolic disease, it can be used to rule out a number of other types of neuromuscular disease that cause similar patterns of weakness.

- A muscle biopsy requires the removal of a small piece of muscle tissue for microscopic analysis. The procedure is done either surgically, with an incision to expose the target muscle, or with a needle. A skin biopsy is also sometimes performed.

- Other tests that may be needed include an electrocardiogram to test heart function, and brain imaging studies such as computed tomography (CT) or magnetic resonance imaging (MRI) scans.

- Genetic tests, using a blood sample, can analyze the person's genes for particular defects that cause metabolic disease, but these tests often are not necessary for diagnosis or for determining treatment.

Chapter 63

Metabolic Neuropathies

A metabolic neuropathy is a disease of the nerves that is caused by a disruption of the chemical processes in the body. In some cases, nerve damage is caused by the inability to properly use energy in the body. In other cases, dangerous substances (toxins) build up in the body and damage nerves. Some metabolic disorders are passed down through families (inherited), while others are developed due to various diseases.

Causes, Incidence, and Risk Factors

Diabetes is one of the most common causes of metabolic neuropathies. Those who have poorly controlled blood sugar are at the highest risk. People who have damage to the kidneys or eyes from diabetes are also more likely to have nerve damage from diabetes.

Other common metabolic causes of neuropathies include:

- thyroid disease

- hypoglycemia (low blood sugar)

- nutritional deficiencies, including vitamin B_{12}, vitamin B_6, vitamin E, and vitamin B_1 deficiency

- alcoholism

- sepsis (severe systemic infection)
- kidney failure
- porphyria

Symptoms

The symptoms are due to the inability of nerves to send proper signals to and from your brain:

- numbness (inability to feel things properly)
- pain—burning, pins and needles, or shooting pains
- loss of coordination
- clumsy gait
- weakness

Usually, these symptoms start in the toes and feet and progress up the legs, eventually affecting the hands and arms.

Signs and Tests

Your doctor will test your strength, coordination, and sensation. Abnormal reflexes, weakness, or sensation can indicate that you have a neuropathy.

Blood tests are often used to detect most metabolic neuropathies. In some cases, an electrical test of the nerves called electromyogram (EMG) can show how severely the nerves are affected and can indicate if a metabolic disorder is suspected.

Treatment

For most metabolic neuropathies, the best treatment is to correct the underlying metabolic problem. Vitamin deficiencies are treated with an appropriate diet. Abnormal blood sugar or thyroid function may require specific medications to correct the problem.

In some cases, pain is treated with medications that reduce abnormal pain signals from the nerves. Specific lotions, creams, or medicated patches can provide relief in some cases.

Weakness is often treated with physical therapy. Affected patients may need to learn how to use a cane of walker if balance is affected. Special braces on the ankles may be needed to walk better.

Expectations (Prognosis)

The outlook mainly depends on the underlying metabolic cause. In some cases, the problem can easily be fixed. In other cases, the underlying metabolic problem cannot be adequately controlled and nerves may continue to deteriorate.

Complications

- pain
- weakness
- trouble walking
- numbness
- injury to feet

Prevention

Maintaining a healthy lifestyle can reduce the risk of neuropathy. Avoid excess use of alcohol and eat a balanced diet. Regular doctor visits can detect many metabolic disorders before neuropathy develops.

If you already have a metabolic problem, regular doctor visits can help control the problem and reduce the chance of further nerve damage.

Patients who already have metabolic neuropathy can reduce the risk of some complications. A podiatrist can teach patients about inspecting their feet for signs of injury and infection. Proper fitting shoes can lessen the chance of skin breakdown in sensitive areas of the feet.

Chapter 64

Metabolic Syndrome

What is the metabolic syndrome?

The metabolic syndrome is characterized by a group of metabolic risk factors in one person. They include:

- abdominal obesity (excessive fat tissue in and around the abdomen)

- atherogenic dyslipidemia (blood fat disorders—high triglycerides, low high density lipoprotein (HDL) cholesterol and high low density lipoprotein (LDL) cholesterol—that foster plaque buildups in artery walls)

- elevated blood pressure

- insulin resistance or glucose intolerance (the body can't properly use insulin or blood sugar)

- prothrombotic state (for example, high fibrinogen or plasminogen activator inhibitor-1 in the blood)

- proinflammatory state (for example, elevated C-reactive protein in the blood)

Text in this chapter is from "Metabolic Syndrome," and "Metabolic Syndrome Statistics," reproduced with permission from www.americanheart.org. © 2006 American Heart Association, Inc.

People with the metabolic syndrome are at increased risk of coronary heart disease and other diseases related to plaque buildups in artery walls (for example, stroke and peripheral vascular disease) and type 2 diabetes. The metabolic syndrome has become increasingly common in the United States. It's estimated that over 50 million Americans have it.

The dominant underlying risk factors for this syndrome appear to be abdominal obesity and insulin resistance. Insulin resistance is a generalized metabolic disorder, in which the body can't use insulin efficiently. This is why the metabolic syndrome is also called the insulin resistance syndrome.

Other conditions associated with the syndrome include physical inactivity, aging, hormonal imbalance, and genetic predisposition.

Some people are genetically predisposed to insulin resistance. Acquired factors, such as excess body fat and physical inactivity, can elicit insulin resistance and the metabolic syndrome in these people. Most people with insulin resistance have abdominal obesity. The biologic mechanisms at the molecular level between insulin resistance and metabolic risk factors aren't fully understood and appear to be complex.

How is the metabolic syndrome diagnosed?

There are no well-accepted criteria for diagnosing the metabolic syndrome. The criteria proposed by the National Cholesterol Education Program (NCEP) Adult Treatment Panel III (ATP III), with minor modifications, are currently recommended and widely used.

The American Heart Association and the National Heart, Lung, and Blood Institute (NHLBI) recommend that the metabolic syndrome be identified as the presence of three or more of these components:

- Elevated waist circumference:
  - Men—equal to or greater than 40 inches (102 cm)
  - Women—equal to or greater than 35 inches (88 cm)
- Elevated triglycerides: equal to or greater than 150 mg/dL
- Reduced HDL (good) cholesterol:
  - Men—less than 40 mg/dL
  - Women—less than 50 mg/dL
- Elevated blood pressure: equal to or greater than 130/85 mm Hg
- Elevated fasting glucose: equal to or greater than 100 mg/dL

AHA Recommendation for Managing the Metabolic Syndrome

The primary goal of clinical management of the metabolic syndrome is to reduce the risk for cardiovascular disease and type 2 diabetes. Then, the first-line therapy is to reduce the major risk factors for cardiovascular disease: stop smoking, and reduce LDL cholesterol, blood pressure, and glucose levels to the recommended levels.

For managing both long- and short-term risk, lifestyle therapies are the first-line interventions to reduce the metabolic risk factors. These lifestyle interventions include:

- weight loss to achieve a desirable weight (body mass index [BMI] less than 25 kg/m^2);

- increased physical activity, with a goal of at least 30 minutes of moderate-intensity activity on most days of the week;

- healthy eating habits that include reduced intake of saturated fat, trans fat, and cholesterol.

Metabolic Syndrome—Statistics

The Third Report of the National Cholesterol Education Program Expert Panel on Detection, Evaluation, and Treatment of High Blood Cholesterol in Adults (ATP III, NHLBI) defines the metabolic syndrome as three or more of the following abnormalities:

- waist circumference greater than 102 cm (40 inches) in men and 88 cm (35 inches) in women;

- serum triglyceride level of 150 mg/dL or higher;

- high-density lipoprotein (HDL) cholesterol level less than 40 mg/dL in men and 50 mg/dL in women;

- blood pressure of 130/85 mm Hg or higher;

- fasting glucose level of 110 mg/dL or higher.

People with the metabolic syndrome are at increased risk for developing diabetes and cardiovascular disease (CVD) as well as increased mortality from CVD and all causes. Limited information is available about the prevalence of the metabolic syndrome in the United States.

- An estimated 47 million U.S. residents have the metabolic syndrome. (National Health and Nutrition Examination Survey

(NHANES) III [1988–94], Centers for Disease Control and Prevention/National Center for Health Statistics (CDC/NCHS); *Journal of the American Medical Association (JAMA).* 2002;287: 356–359)

- The age-adjusted prevalence of the metabolic syndrome for adults is 23.7 percent.

  - The prevalence ranges from 6.7 percent among people ages 20–29, to 43.5 percent for ages 60–69, and 42.0 percent for those age 70 and older.

  - The age-adjusted prevalence is similar for men (24.0 percent) and women (23.4 percent).

  - Mexican Americans have the highest age-adjusted prevalence of the metabolic syndrome (31.9 percent). The lowest prevalence is among whites (23.8 percent), African Americans (21.6 percent) and people reporting an "other" race or ethnicity (20.3 percent).

  - Among African Americans, women had about a 57 percent higher prevalence than men. Among Mexican Americans, women had a 26 percent higher prevalence than men did.

Source: (NHANES III [1988–94], CDC/NCHS; *JAMA.* 2002;287:356–359)

- The prevalences of people with the metabolic syndrome are:
  - Among whites, 24.3 percent for men and 22.9 percent for women.
  - Among blacks, 13.9 percent for men and 20.9 percent for women.
  - Among Mexican Americans, 20.8 percent for men and 27.2 percent for women.

Source: (NHANES III [1988–94], CDC/NCHS; *Arch Intern Med.* 2003;163, Feb. 24)

Additional Information

American Heart Association
National Center
7272 Greenville Ave.
Dallas, TX 75231
Toll-Free: 800-AHA-USA-1 (242-8721)
Website: http://www.americanheart.org

Chapter 65

Multiple Endocrine Neoplasia Type 1 (MEN1)

Multiple endocrine neoplasia type 1 (MEN1) is an inherited disorder that affects the endocrine glands. It is sometimes called multiple endocrine adenomatosis or Wermer syndrome, after one of the first doctors to recognize it. MEN1 is quite rare, occurring in about three to twenty persons out of 100,000. It affects both sexes equally and shows no geographical, racial, or ethnic preferences.

Endocrine glands are different from other organs in the body because they release hormones into the bloodstream. Hormones are powerful chemicals that travel through the blood, controlling and instructing the functions of various organs. Normally, the hormones released by endocrine glands are carefully balanced to meet the body's needs.

In patients with MEN1, sometimes multiple endocrine glands, such as the parathyroid, the pancreas, and the pituitary, become overactive at the same time. Most people who develop overactivity of only one endocrine gland do not have MEN1.

The Parathyroid Glands

The parathyroids are the endocrine glands earliest and most often affected by MEN1. The human body normally has four parathyroid glands, which are located close to the thyroid gland in the front of the neck. The parathyroids release into the bloodstream a chemical

National Institute of Diabetes and Digestive and Kidney Diseases (NIDDK), NIH Publication No. 06-3048, March 2006.

called parathyroid hormone, which helps maintain a normal supply of calcium in the blood, bones, and urine.

In MEN1, all four parathyroid glands tend to be overactive. They release too much parathyroid hormone, leading to excess calcium in the blood. High blood calcium, known as hypercalcemia, can exist for many years before it is found by accident or by family screening. Unrecognized hypercalcemia can cause excess calcium to spill into the urine, leading to kidney stones or kidney damage.

Nearly everyone who inherits a susceptibility to MEN1 (a "cancer") will develop overactive parathyroid glands (hyperparathyroidism) by age 50, but the disorder can often be detected before age 20. Hyperparathyroidism may cause no problems for many years, or it may cause problems such as tiredness, weakness, muscle or bone pain, constipation, indigestion, kidney stones, or thinning of bones.

Treatment of Hyperparathyroidism

It is sometimes difficult to decide whether hyperparathyroidism in MEN1 is severe enough to need treatment, especially in a person who has no symptoms. The usual treatment is an operation to remove the three largest parathyroid glands and all but a small part of the fourth. After parathyroid surgery, regular testing of blood calcium should continue, since the small piece of remaining parathyroid tissue can grow larger and cause recurrent hyperparathyroidism. People whose parathyroid glands have been completely removed by surgery must take daily supplements of calcium and vitamin D to prevent hypocalcemia (low blood calcium).

The Pancreas Gland

The pancreas gland, located behind the stomach, releases digestive juices into the intestines and releases key hormones into the bloodstream. Some hormones produced in the islet cells of the pancreas and their effects are:

- insulin—lowers blood sugar;
- glucagon—raises blood sugar;
- somatostatin—inhibits many cells;
- gastrin—secretes acid needed for digestion.

Excess gastrin comes from one or more tumors in the pancreas and small intestine. Gastrin normally circulates in the blood, causing the stomach to secrete enough acid needed for digestion. If exposed to too much gastrin, the stomach releases excess acid, leading to the formation of severe ulcers in the stomach and small intestine. Too much gastrin can also cause serious diarrhea.

About one in three patients with MEN1 has gastrin-releasing tumors, called gastrinomas. (The illness associated with these tumors is sometimes called Zollinger-Ellison syndrome.) The ulcers caused by gastrinomas are much more dangerous than typical stomach or intestinal ulcers; left untreated, they can cause rupture of the stomach or intestine and even death.

Treatment of Gastrinomas

The gastrinomas associated with MEN1 are difficult to cure by surgery, because it is difficult to find the multiple small gastrinomas in the pancreas and small intestine. In the past, the standard treatment for gastrinomas was the surgical removal of the entire stomach to prevent acid production. The mainstay of treatment is now very powerful medicines that block stomach acid release, called acid pump inhibitors. Taken by mouth, these have proven effective in controlling the complications from high gastrin in most cases of Zollinger-Ellison syndrome.

The Pituitary Gland

The pituitary is a small gland inside the head, behind the bridge of the nose. Though small, it produces many important hormones that regulate basic body functions. The major pituitary hormones and their effects are:

- prolactin—controls formation of breast milk, influences fertility, and influences bone strength;

- growth hormone—regulates body growth, especially during adolescence;

- adrenocorticotropin (ACTH)—stimulates the adrenal glands to produce cortisol;

- thyrotropin (TSH)—stimulates the thyroid gland to produce thyroid hormones;

- luteinizing hormone (LH)—stimulates the ovaries or testes to produce sex hormones that determine many features of maleness or femaleness; and

- follicle stimulating hormone (FSH)—regulates fertility in men through sperm production and in women through ovulation.

The pituitary gland becomes overactive in about one of four persons with MEN1. This overactivity can usually be traced to a very small, benign tumor in the gland that releases too much prolactin, called a prolactinoma. High prolactin can cause excessive production of breast milk, or it can interfere with fertility in women or with sex drive and fertility in men.

Treatment of Prolactinomas

Some prolactinomas are small, and treatment may not be needed. If treatment is needed, a very effective type of medicine known as a dopamine agonist can lower the production of prolactin and shrink the prolactinoma. Occasionally, prolactinomas do not respond well to this medication. In such cases, surgery, radiation, or both may be needed.

Rare Complications of MEN1

Occasionally, a person who has MEN1 develops an islet tumor of the pancreas which secretes high levels of pancreatic hormones other than gastrin. Insulinomas, for example, produce too much insulin, causing serious low blood sugar, or hypoglycemia. Pancreatic tumors that secrete too much glucagon or somatostatin can cause diabetes, and too much vasoactive intestinal peptide can cause watery diarrhea.

Other rare complications arise from pituitary tumors that release high amounts of ACTH, which in turn stimulates the adrenal glands to produce excess cortisol. Pituitary tumors that produce growth hormone cause excessive bone growth or disfigurement.

Another rare complication is an endocrine tumor inside the chest or in the stomach, known as a carcinoid. In a person with MEN1 a carcinoid tumor rarely secretes a hormone. In general, surgery is the mainstay of treatment for all of these rare types of tumors, except for gastric carcinoids which usually require no treatment.

Are the tumors associated with MEN1 cancerous?

The overactive endocrine glands associated with MEN1 may contain benign tumors, but usually they do not have any signs of cancer. Benign tumors can disrupt normal function by releasing hormones or by crowding nearby tissue. For example, a prolactinoma may become quite large in someone with MEN1. As it grows, the tumor can press against and damage the normal part of the pituitary gland or the nerves that carry vision from the eyes. Sometimes impaired vision is the first sign of a pituitary tumor in MEN1.

Another type of benign tumor often seen in people with MEN1 is a plum-sized, fatty tumor called a lipoma, which grows under the skin. Lipomas cause no health problems and can be removed by simple cosmetic surgery if desired. These tumors are also fairly common in the general population.

Benign tumors do not spread to or invade other parts of the body. Cancer cells, by contrast, break away from the primary tumor and spread, or metastasize, to other parts of the body through the bloodstream or lymphatic system.

The pancreatic islet cell tumors associated with MEN1 tend to be numerous and small, but most are benign and do not release active hormones into the blood.

Eventually, about half of MEN1 cases will develop a cancerous pancreatic tumor or a cancerous carcinoid tumor.

Treatment of Pancreatic Endocrine Cancer in MEN1

Since the type of pancreatic endocrine cancer associated with MEN1 can be difficult to recognize, difficult to treat, and very slow to progress, doctors have different views about the value of surgery in managing these tumors.

One approach is to "watch and wait," using medical, or nonsurgical treatments. According to this school of thought, pancreatic surgery has serious complications, so it should not be attempted unless it will cure a tumor that is secreting too much hormone.

Another school advocates early surgery, perhaps when a tumor grows to a certain size, to prevent or remove pancreatic endocrine cancer in MEN1 (even if it does not over secrete a hormone) before it spreads and becomes dangerous. There is no clear evidence; however, that aggressive surgery to prevent pancreatic endocrine cancer from spreading actually leads to longer survival for patients with MEN1. This is partly because these complex operations can have their own side effects.

Doctors agree that excessive release of certain hormones (such as gastrin) from pancreatic endocrine cancer in MEN1 needs to be treated, and medications are often effective in blocking the effects of these hormones. Some tumors, such as insulin-producing tumors of the pancreas, are usually benign and single and are curable by pancreatic surgery. Such surgery needs to be considered carefully in each patient's case.

Is MEN1 the same in everyone?

Although MEN1 tends to follow certain patterns, it can affect a person's health in many different ways. Not only do the features of MEN1 vary among members of the same family, but some families with MEN1 tend to have a higher rate of prolactin-secreting pituitary tumors and a much lower frequency of gastrin-secreting tumors.

In addition, the age at which MEN1 can begin to cause endocrine gland over-function can differ strikingly from one family member to another. One person may have only mild hyperparathyroidism beginning at age 50, while a relative may develop complications from tumors of the parathyroid, pancreas, and pituitary by age 20.

Sometimes a patient with MEN1 knows of no other case of MEN1 among relatives. The commonest explanation is that knowledge about the family is incomplete; less often, the patient carries a new MEN1 gene mutation.

Can MEN1 be cured?

There is no cure for MEN1 itself, but most of the health problems caused by MEN1 can be recognized at an early stage and controlled or treated before they become serious problems.

If you have been diagnosed with MEN1, it is important to get periodic checkups because MEN1 can affect different glands, and even after treatment, residual tissue can grow back. Careful monitoring enables your doctor to adjust your treatment as needed and to check for any new disturbances caused by MEN1. Most MEN1 cases will have a long and productive life.

How is MEN1 detected?

Each of us has millions of genes in each of our cells, which determine how our cells and bodies function. In people with MEN1, there is a mutation, or mistake, in one gene of every cell. A carrier is a person who has the MEN1 gene mutation. The MEN1 gene mutation is transmitted directly to a child from a parent carrying the gene mutation.

The MEN1 gene was recently identified. As of 2001, a small number of centers around the world began to offer MEN1 gene testing on a research or commercial basis. The likelihood of finding a mutation in an MEN1 family has varied from 60 percent to 95 percent depending on methods. When a mutation is found, further testing in other relatives can become much easier. Many relatives can be tested once and be found without the known MEN1 mutation in their family, and then they can be freed from uncertainty and from any further testing ever for MEN1. When a mutation is not found in a family or isolated case, it does not prove that no MEN1 mutation is present. Depending on the clinical and laboratory information, it may still be very likely that a mutation is present but undetected.

When the MEN1 mutation test is normal in an effected relative or when the test is not available, screening of close relatives of persons with MEN1, who are at high risk, generally involves testing for hyperparathyroidism, the most common and usually the earliest sign of MEN1.

What is the role for genetic counseling with MEN1 gene testing?

Genetic counseling, which should accompany the gene testing, can assist family members address how the test results affect them individually and as a family. In genetic counseling, there can be a review and discussion of issues about the psychosocial benefits and risks of the genetic testing results. Genetic testing results can affect self-image, self-esteem, and individual and family identity. In genetic counseling, issues related to how and with whom genetic test results will be shared, and their possible effect on important matters such as health and life insurance coverage can be reviewed and discussed. The times for these discussions can be when a family member is deciding whether or not to go ahead with the gene testing and again later when the gene testing results are available. The person, who provides the genetic counseling to the family member(s), may be a professional from the disciplines of genetics, nursing, or medicine.

Who should consider MEN1 screening by gene testing?

Screening may be offered to persons with MEN1 or with features resembling them. Affected relatives of persons with MEN1 can be tested. Asymptomatic offspring, brothers, or sisters of a person with MEN1, were born with a 50 percent chance of having inherited the gene; they too can be offered gene testing. While gene testing for any genetic disease can be definitive at any age, it is usually not offered to children below age 18 unless the test outcome would have an important effect on their medical treatment. Since treatable tumors occasionally begin by age five in MEN1, gene testing and tumor surveillance can begin at age five.

Who should consider MEN1 screening by laboratory tests?

MEN1 screening by gene testing will be the most definitive test, when it is available. However, it is not yet widely available, and when no gene mutation is found in a MEN1 family, then it may be necessary to rely upon laboratory tests for diagnosis. Hyperparathyroidism, most often the first sign of MEN1, can usually be detected by blood tests between the ages of five and fifty. Periodic tumor testing should begin between ages five to ten and be repeated every year. There is no age at which periodic testing should stop, since (lacking a specific deoxyribonucleic [DNA] test) doctors cannot rule out the chance that a person has inherited the MEN1 gene mutation. However, a person with normal tumor testing beyond age 50 is very unlikely to have inherited the MEN1 gene mutation.

Why screen for MEN1 tumors?

MEN1 is not an infectious or contagious disease, nor is it caused by environmental factors. Because MEN1 is a genetic disorder inherited from one parent, and its transmission pattern is well understood, family members at 50–50 risk for the disorder can be easily identified.

Streamlined tumor testing can be used to identify an MEN1 carrier. After a carrier is identified, more detailed tumor surveys are generally recommended. Tumor testing can detect the problems caused by MEN1 tumors many years before their later complications develop. Finding these tumors early enables your doctor to begin preventive treatment, reducing the chances that MEN1 will cause problems later.

Should a person who has MEN1 avoid having children?

A person who has MEN1 or who has a MEN1 gene mutation may have a hard time deciding whether to have a child. No one can make this decision for anyone else, but some of the important facts can be summarized as follows:

- A man or a woman with MEN1 has a 50–50 risk with each pregnancy of having a child with MEN1.

- MEN1 tends to fit a broad pattern within a given family, but the severity of the disorder varies widely from one family member to another. In particular, a parent's experience with MEN1 cannot be used to predict the eventual severity of MEN1 in a child.

- The tumors that result from MEN1 do not usually develop until adulthood. Treatment may require regular monitoring and considerable expense, but the disease usually does not prevent an active, productive adulthood.

- Prolactin-releasing tumors in a man or woman with MEN1 may inhibit fertility and make it difficult to conceive. Also, hyperparathyroidism in a woman during pregnancy may raise the risks of complications for mother and child.

Genetic counseling can help individuals and couples through the decision-making process with family planning. Genetic counselors and other professionals will provide information to help with the decision-making process, but they will not tell individuals or couples what decision to make or how to make it.

Research in MEN1

The National Institute of Diabetes and Digestive and Kidney Diseases (NIDDK) conducts and supports a variety of research in endocrine disorders, including MEN1. NIDDK and other National Institutes of Health (NIH) researchers isolated the MEN1 gene in 1997. Researchers have also shown that the MEN1 gene contributes to common endocrine tumors outside of the setting.

Additional Information

Alliance of Genetic Support Groups
4301 Connecticut Ave., N.W., Suite 404
Washington, DC 20008-2304
Phone: 202-966-5557
Toll-Free: 800-336-GENE (4363), Fax: 202-966-8553
Website: http://www.geneticalliance.org
E-mail: info@geneticalliance.org

Endocrine and Metabolic Diseases Information Service
6 Information Way
Bethesda, MD 20892-3569

Toll-Free: 888-828-0904
Fax: 703-738-4929
Website: http://www.endocrine.niddk.nih.gov
E-mail: endoandmeta@info.niddk.nih.gov

March of Dimes Birth Defects Foundation
1275 Mamaroneck Ave.
White Plains, NY 10605
Toll-Free: 888-663-4637
Phone: 914-428-7100
Fax: 914-997-4763
Website: http://www.marchofdimes.com

Pituitary Network Association
P.O. Box 1958
Thousand Oaks, CA 91358
Phone: 805-499-9973
Fax: 805-480-0633
Website: http://www.pituitary.org
E-mail: pna@pituitary.org

National Institute of Diabetes and Digestive and Kidney Diseases (NIDDK)
National Institutes of Health
Building 31, Room 9A06
31 Center Drive, MSC 2560
Bethesda, MD 20892-2560
NIDDK Information Clearinghouse Toll-Free: 800-891-5390
Phone: 301-496-3583
Website: http://www.niddk.nih.gov
E-mail: dwebmaster@extra.niddk.nih.gov

Part Eight

Additional Help and Information

Chapter 66

Glossary of Terms Related to Endocrine and Metabolic Disorders

adenoma: A noncancerous tumor.

adrenal gland: A small gland that makes steroid hormones, adrenaline, and noradrenaline. These hormones help control heart rate, blood pressure, and other important body functions. There are two adrenal glands, one on top of each kidney. Also called suprarenal gland.

benign: Not cancerous. Benign tumors may grow larger but do not spread to other parts of the body.

blood chemistry study: A procedure in which a sample of blood is examined to measure the amounts of certain substances made in the body. An abnormal amount of a substance can be a sign of disease in the organ or tissue that produces it. [1]

calcium: A mineral found in teeth, bones, and other body tissues.

Unmarked definitions in this chapter are excerpted from PDQ® Cancer Information Summary. National Cancer Institute, Bethesda, MD. Pituitary Tumors (PDQ®): Treatment–Patient. Updated 02/2006. Available at http://cancer.gov. Accessed 02/06/2007. Terms marked [1] are reprinted from PDQ® Cancer Information Summary. National Cancer Institute; Bethesda, MD. Parathyroid Cancer (PDQ®): Treatment–Patient. Updated 10/13/2006. Available at http://cancer .gov. Accessed 02/07/2007. Additional terms marked [2] are reprinted with permission from *Stedman's Medical Dictionary, 27th Edition*, Copyright © 2000, Lippincott Williams & Wilkins. All rights reserved.

cancer: A term for diseases in which abnormal cells divide without control. Cancer cells can invade nearby tissues and can spread through the bloodstream and lymphatic system to other parts of the body. There are several main types of cancer.

catheter: A flexible tube used to deliver fluids into or withdraw fluids from the body. [1]

cell: The individual unit that makes up the tissues of the body. All living things are made up of one or more cells.

central nervous system (CNS): The brain and spinal cord.

chemotherapy: Treatment with drugs that kill cancer cells.

clinical trial: A type of research study that tests how well new medical approaches work in people. These studies test new methods of screening, prevention, diagnosis, or treatment of a disease. Also called a clinical study.

contrast material: A dye or other substance that helps show abnormal areas inside the body. It is given by injection into a vein, by enema, or by mouth. Contrast material may be used with x-rays, CT scans, MRI, or other imaging tests. [1]

craniotomy: An operation in which an opening is made in the skull.

computed tomography (CT) scan: A series of detailed pictures of areas inside the body taken from different angles; the pictures are created by a computer linked to an x-ray machine. Also called computed tomography scan, computerized tomography, computerized axial tomography scan, and CAT scan.

diagnosis: The process of identifying a disease by the signs and symptoms. [1]

diabetes mellitus: Chronic metabolic disorder in which utilization of carbohydrate is impaired and that of lipid and protein enhanced; it is caused by an absolute or relative deficiency of insulin. [2]

disorder: In medicine, a disturbance of normal functioning of the mind or body. Disorders may be caused by genetic factors, disease, or trauma. [1]

drug: Any substance, other than food, that is used to prevent, diagnose, treat or relieve symptoms of a disease or abnormal condition.

Also refers to a substance that alters mood or body function, or that can be habit-forming or addictive, especially a narcotic.

endocrine glands: Glands that have no ducts, their secretions being absorbed directly into the blood. [2]

exocrine glands: Glands that release the substances into a duct or opening to the inside or outside of the body.

external radiation: Radiation therapy that uses a machine to aim high-energy rays at the cancer. Also called external-beam radiation.

functioning tumor: A tumor that is found in endocrine tissue and makes hormones (chemicals that travel in the bloodstream and control the actions of other cells or organs).

gland: An organ that makes one or more substances, such as hormones, digestive juices, sweat, tears, saliva, or milk.

glucocorticoid: A compound that belongs to the family of compounds called corticosteroids (steroids). Glucocorticoids affect metabolism and have anti-inflammatory and immunosuppressive effects. They may be naturally produced (hormones) or synthetic (drugs).

glycogen-storage disease: Any of the glycogen deposition diseases characterized by accumulation of glycogen of normal or abnormal chemical structure in tissue; there may be enlargement of the liver, heart, or striated muscle, including the tongue, with progressive muscular weakness. [2]

goiter: An enlargement of the thyroid gland. [2]

gonad: An organ that produces sex cells; a testis or an ovary. [2]

hormone: A chemical made by glands in the body. Hormones circulate in the bloodstream and control the actions of certain cells or organs. Some hormones can also be made in a laboratory.

hyper: Prefix denoting excessive, above normal; opposite of hypo-. [2]

hypercalcemia: Abnormally high blood calcium. [1]

hyperparathyroidism: A condition in which the parathyroid gland (one of four pea-sized organs found on the thyroid) makes too much parathyroid hormone. [1]

hypo: Prefix denoting deficient, below normal. [2]

imaging: Tests that produce pictures of areas inside the body. [1]

impotence: In medicine, refers to the inability to have an erection of the penis adequate for sexual intercourse. Also called erectile dysfunction.

inborn: Initiated during development in utero. In the specific context of inborn error of metabolism, it connotes a genetic disruption of an enzyme. [2]

inherited: Transmitted through genes that have been passed from parents to their offspring (children). [1]

laboratory test: A medical procedure that involves testing a sample of blood, urine, or other substance from the body. Tests can help determine a diagnosis, plan treatment, check to see if treatment is working, or monitor the disease over time.

lipid: "Fat-soluble," an operational term describing a solubility characteristic, not a chemical substance. [2]

localized: Restricted to the site of origin, without evidence of spread. [1]

lymph node: A rounded mass of lymphatic tissue that is surrounded by a capsule of connective tissue. Lymph nodes filter lymph (lymphatic fluid), and they store lymphocytes (white blood cells). They are located along lymphatic vessels. Also called a lymph gland. [1]

malignant: Cancerous. Malignant tumors can invade and destroy nearby tissue and spread to other parts of the body.

medication: A legal drug that is used to prevent, treat, or relieve symptoms of a disease or abnormal condition. Also called medicine. [1]

menstrual cycle: The monthly cycle of hormonal changes from the beginning of one menstrual period to the beginning of the next one.

metabolic disease: Generic term for disease caused by an abnormal metabolic process. It can be congenital, due to inherited enzyme abnormality, or acquired, due to disease of an endocrine organ or failure of function of a metabolic important organ such as the liver. [2]

metabolism: The sum of the chemical and physical changes occurring in tissue, consisting of anabolism, those reactions that convert small molecules into large, and catabolism, those reactions that convert large molecules into small, including both endogenous large molecules as well as biodegradation of xenobiotics. [2]

metastasectomy: Surgery to remove one or more metastases (tumors formed from cells that have spread from the primary tumor). When all metastases are removed, it is called a complete metastasectomy. [1]

metastasize: To spread from one part of the body to another. When cancer cells metastasize and form secondary tumors, the cells in the metastatic tumor are like those in the original (primary) tumor.

millimeter: A measure of length in the metric system. A millimeter is one thousandth of a meter. There are 25 millimeters in an inch.

magnetic resonance imaging (MRI): A procedure in which radio waves and a powerful magnet linked to a computer are used to create detailed pictures of areas inside the body. These pictures can show the difference between normal and diseased tissue. MRI makes better images of organs and soft tissue than other scanning techniques, such as CT or x-ray. MRI is especially useful for imaging the brain, the spine, the soft tissue of joints, and the inside of bones. Also called magnetic resonance imaging, nuclear magnetic resonance imaging, and NMRI.

multiple endocrine neoplasia type 1 syndrome (MEN1 syndrome): A rare, inherited disorder that affects the endocrine glands and can cause tumors in the parathyroid and pituitary glands and the pancreas. Also called MEN1 syndrome, multiple endocrine adenomatosis, and Wermer syndrome. [1]

nonfunctioning tumor: A tumor that is found in endocrine tissue but that does not make extra hormones (chemicals that travel in the blood and control the actions of other cells or organs).

ovary: One of a pair of female reproductive glands in which the ova, or eggs, are formed. The ovaries are located in the pelvis, one on each side of the uterus.

palliative therapy: Treatment given to relieve the symptoms and reduce the suffering caused by cancer and other life-threatening diseases. Palliative cancer therapies are given together with other cancer treatments, from the time of diagnosis, through treatment, survivorship, recurrent or advanced disease, and at the end of life.

pancreas: A glandular organ located in the abdomen. It makes pancreatic juices, which contain enzymes that aid in digestion, and it produces several hormones, including insulin. The pancreas is surrounded by the stomach, intestines, and other organs. [1]

parathyroid cancer: A rare cancer that forms in tissues of one or more of the parathyroid glands.

parathyroid gland: One of four pea-sized glands found on the thyroid. The parathyroid hormone produced by these glands increases the calcium level in the blood. [1]

parathyroid hormone (PTH): A substance made by the parathyroid gland that helps the body store and use calcium. [1]

pituitary gland: The main endocrine gland. The pituitary is a pea-sized organ in the center of the brain above the back of the nose. It produces hormones that control other glands and many body functions, especially growth.

pituitary tumor: A tumor that forms in the pituitary gland. Most pituitary tumors are benign (not cancer).

prognosis: The likely outcome or course of a disease; the chance of recovery or recurrence. [1]

quality of life: The overall enjoyment of life. Many clinical trials assess the effects of cancer and its treatment on the quality of life. These studies measure aspects of an individual's sense of well-being and ability to carry out various activities.

radiation therapy: The use of high-energy radiation from x-rays, gamma rays, neutrons, and other sources to kill cancer cells and shrink tumors. Radiation may come from a machine outside the body (external-beam radiation therapy), or it may come from radioactive material placed in the body near cancer cells (internal radiation therapy, implant radiation, or brachytherapy). Systemic radiation therapy uses a radioactive substance, such as a radiolabeled monoclonal antibody, that circulates throughout the body. Also called radiotherapy.

radionuclide scanning: A test that produces pictures (scans) of internal parts of the body. The person is given an injection or swallows a small amount of radioactive material; a machine called a scanner then measures the radioactivity in certain organs. [1]

recur: To occur again.

recurrent cancer: Cancer that has returned after a period of time during which the cancer could not be detected. The cancer may come back to the same place as the original (primary) tumor or to another place in the body. Also called recurrence.

regional chemotherapy: Treatment with anticancer drugs directed to a specific area of the body. [1]

resection: A procedure that uses surgery to remove tissue or part or all of an organ. [1]

risk factor: Something that may increase the chance of developing a disease. Some examples of risk factors for cancer include age, a family history of certain cancers, use of tobacco products, certain eating habits, obesity, lack of exercise, exposure to radiation or other cancer-causing agents, and certain genetic changes. [1]

scan: A picture of structures inside the body. Scans often used in diagnosing, staging, and monitoring disease include liver scans, bone scans, and computed tomography (CT) or computerized axial tomography (CAT) scans and magnetic resonance imaging (MRI) scans. In liver scanning and bone scanning, radioactive substances that are injected into the bloodstream collect in these organs. A scanner that detects the radiation is used to create pictures. In CT scanning, an x-ray machine linked to a computer is used to produce detailed pictures of organs inside the body. MRI scans use a large magnet connected to a computer to create pictures of areas inside the body. [1]

side effect: A problem that occurs when treatment affects healthy tissues or organs. Some common side effects of cancer treatment are fatigue, pain, nausea, vomiting, decreased blood cell counts, hair loss, and mouth sores.

sonogram: A computer picture of areas inside the body created by bouncing high-energy sound waves (ultrasound) off internal tissues or organs. Also called an ultrasonogram. [1]

staging: Performing exams and tests to learn the extent of the cancer within the body, especially whether the disease has spread from the original site to other parts of the body. It is important to know the stage of the disease in order to plan the best treatment. [1]

standard therapy: In medicine, treatment that experts agree is appropriate, accepted, and widely used. Health care providers are obligated to provide patients with standard therapy. Also called standard of care or best practice.

stereotactic radiosurgery: A radiation therapy procedure that uses special equipment to position the patient and precisely deliver a large radiation dose to a tumor and not to normal tissue. This procedure does not use surgery. It is used to treat brain tumors and other brain disorders. It is also being studied in the treatment of other types of cancer, such as lung cancer. Also called radiation surgery, radiosurgery, stereotactic external-beam radiation, stereotactic radiation therapy, and stereotaxic radiosurgery.

storage disease: A generic term that includes any accumulation of a specific substance within tissues, generally because of congenital deficiency of an enzyme necessary for further metabolism of the substance; for example, glycogen-storage diseases. [2]

supportive care: Care given to improve the quality of life of patients who have a serious or life-threatening disease. The goal of supportive care is to prevent or treat as early as possible the symptoms of the disease, side effects caused by treatment of the disease, and psychological, social, and spiritual problems related to the disease or its treatment. Also called palliative care, comfort care, and symptom management. [1]

symptom: An indication that a person has a condition or disease. Some examples of symptoms are headache, fever, fatigue, nausea, vomiting, and pain.

therapy: Treatment.

thyroid gland: A gland located beneath the voice box (larynx) that produces thyroid hormone. The thyroid helps regulate growth and metabolism. [1]

thyroid hormone: A hormone that affects heart rate, blood pressure, body temperature, and weight. Thyroid hormone is made by the thyroid gland and can also be made in the laboratory.

tumor: An abnormal mass of tissue that results when cells divide more than they should or do not die when they should. Tumors may be benign (not cancerous), or malignant (cancerous). Also called neoplasm. [1]

tumor debulking: Surgically removing as much of the tumor as possible. [1]

ultrasound: A procedure in which high-energy sound waves (ultrasound) are bounced off internal tissues or organs and make echoes. The echo patterns are shown on the screen of an ultrasound machine, forming a picture of body tissues called a sonogram. Also called ultrasonography. [1]

watchful waiting: Closely monitoring a patient's condition but withholding treatment until symptoms appear or change. Also called observation.

x-ray: A type of high-energy radiation. In low doses, x-rays are used to diagnose diseases by making pictures of the inside of the body. In high doses, x-rays are used to treat cancer.

Chapter 67

Finding Resources for Children with Special Needs

Having a child with special needs can be a challenge. You may feel confused and overwhelmed. Parents have said:

"There is so much to learn and know! Where do I begin?"

"There must be an easier way. Our family can't be the first to go through this."

People Who Can Help

Listed are some people that can help you. Their help may be free. Just ask.

Public health nurses (PHN) are registered nurses at your local health department who can help you with general health questions and services like immunizations.

Family resource coordinators (FRC) are case managers who can help you find services if you are worried about how your child under age three is growing or developing.

People at your child's school, including teachers, school nurses, counselors, principals, or therapists, can help your child at school

This chapter includes "Help Finding Resources for Children with Special Needs," "Care Notebook: A Quick Guide," and "Alphabet Soup Acronym Index," used with permission from Children's Hospital & Regional Medical Center, Seattle, and the Washington State Department of Health, 2006.

with medications, equipment, therapies, and homework. If your child goes to a private school, you can still get help from the public school system.

Children with special health care needs (CSHCN) coordinators are public health nurses who help families of children with ongoing health problems. They can help you find resources and health information.

Other parents can tell you about their experiences. They can give you tips, tell you about helpful providers, and give you hope. You can meet other parents at support groups or the doctor's office. Ask your doctor, local hospital, or school about support groups.

Health care providers, including your child's doctors, nurses, or social workers, can also tell you about services and resources.

Create your child's contact list with the names, phone numbers, e-mail, and other important information of pertinent individuals.

- public health nurse
- special health care needs coordinator
- family resource coordinator
- people at school
- other parents
- health care providers

Create a Care Notebook

What is a care notebook?

A care notebook is an organizing tool for families who have children with special health care needs. Use a care notebook to keep track of important information about your child's health and care. A binder with paper and tabbed sections can be used to make a care notebook instead of purchasing one.

How can a care notebook help me?

In caring for your child with special health needs, you may get information and papers from many sources. A care notebook helps you organize the most important information in a central place. A care notebook makes it easier for you to find and share key information with others who are part of your child's care team.

Use your care notebook to:

- track changes in your child's medicines or treatments;
- list phone numbers for health care providers and community organizations;
- prepare for appointments;
- file information about your child's health history; and
- share new information with your child's primary doctor, public health or school nurse, daycare staff, and others caring for your child.

What are some helpful hints for using my child's care notebook?

- Keep the care notebook where it is easy to find. This helps you and anyone who needs information in your absence.
- Add new information to the care notebook when there is a change in your child's treatment.
- Take the care notebook with you to appointments and hospital visits so that information you need will be close at hand.

How do I set up my child's care notebook?

Follow these steps:

1. Gather information. Gather any health information you already have about your child. This may include reports from recent doctor's visits, immunization records, recent summaries of a hospital stay, this year's school plan, test results, or informational pamphlets.

2. Review the care notebook information available on the internet at http://www.cshcn.org. Choose the pages you like. Print copies of any that you think you will use.

3. Choose what to keep in your care notebook.
   - What information do you look up most often?
   - What information is needed by others caring for your child?

- Store other information in a file drawer or box where you can find it if needed.

4. Put a care notebook together.

   - Each of us has our own way of organizing information. The only key is to make it easy for you to find again.
   - Choose a 3-ring notebook or large accordion envelope.
   - Get tabbed dividers or create your own sections.
   - Pocket dividers are handy for storing reports.
   - Plastic pages are helpful for storing business cards and photographs.

Table 67.1 lists a wide variety of acronyms used by professionals who work with families.

For More Information

Children's Hospital and Regional Medical Center
Center for Children with Special Needs
MS: MPW5-2
1100 Olive Way, Suite 500
Seattle, WA 98101
Phone: 206-987-5735
Website: http://www.cshcn.org

- The pages in the Care Notebook are available on the internet at http://www.cshcn.org/resources/CareNtbk.cfm.

- Families in Washington State may order one Care Notebook or one Care Organizer for a child with special needs at no cost. Call the resource line at 866-987-2500, option 4, (WA State only) and provide your name, mailing address, phone number, and item you would like to order.

- Organizations and health professionals may order one sample copy of the Care Notebook and Care Organizer to use as tools to show parents. Additional copies or quantity orders require payment. Call for details.

- Families not from Washington State may order the Care Notebook or Care Organizer for $20.00 each.

Table 67.1. Alphabet Soup Acronym Index(continued on next page)

Acronym	Organization
ADA	Americans with Disabilities Act
ADD	attention deficit disorder
ADHD	attention deficit hyperactivity disorder
AIDS	acquired immune deficiency syndrome
ARC	The Arc: Advocates for the Rights of Citizens with Developmental Disabilities and their families
ARNP	advanced registered nurse practitioner
BIA	Bureau of Indian Affairs
BD	behaviorally disabled
CD	communication disorders
CDS	communication disorders Specialist
CFR	Code of Federal Regulations
CHDD	Center on Human Development and Disability
CP	cerebral palsy
CPS	child protective services
CSHCN	children with special health care needs
CSO	Community Service Office
DCFS	Division of Children and Family Services
DD	developmentally disabled
DDD	Division of Developmental Disabilities
DDPC	Developmental Disabilities Planning Council
DH	developmentally handicapped
DMH	Division of Mental Health
DOH	Department of Health
DSB	Department of Services for the Blind
DSHS	Department of Social and Health Services
DVR	Division of Vocational Rehabilitation
ECEAP	Early Childhood Education and Assistance Program
ED	emotionally disturbed
EEG	electroencephalogram
EEU	experimental education unit
EFMP	Exceptional Family Member Program (helps military families locate to areas with services)

Table 67.1. (continued) Alphabet Soup Acronym Index

Acronym	Organization
EKG	electrocardiogram
EPSDT	early periodic screening, diagnosis, and treatment
ESD	educational service district
FAPE	free appropriate public education
FRC	family resources coordinator
HHS	Health and Human Services
HI	health impaired or hearing impaired
HMO	health maintenance organization
HO	Healthy Options, DSHS Medicaid Managed Care Program
HOH	hard of hearing
ICC	Interagency Coordinating Council; county ICC and state ICC.
IDEA	Individuals with Disabilities Education Act
IEP	individual education plan
IFSP	individual family service plan
I & R	information and referral
ISP	individual service plan
LD	learning disabled
LDA	Learning Disabilities Association
LEA	local education agency
LICWAC	Local Indian Child Welfare Advocacy Board
LRE	least restrictive environment
MCH	maternal and child health
MD	medical doctor
MDT	multi-disciplinary team
MH	multiply handicapped
MR	mentally retarded
MS	multiple sclerosis
NICU	neonatal intensive care unit
NORD	National Association of Rare Disorders
OCR	Office of Civil Rights
OFM	Office of Financial Management
OI	orthopedically impaired

Table 67.1. (continued) Alphabet Soup Acronym Index

Acronym	Organization
OSEP	Office of Special Education Programs
OSERS	Office of Special Education and Rehabilitation Services
OSPI	Office of Superintendent of Public Instruction
OT	occupational therapy or therapist
OTR	licensed and registered occupational therapist
PHN	public health nurse
PL	public law
PT	physical therapy or therapist
PTA	Parent Teacher Association
RN	registered nurse
RPT	registered physical therapist
SBD	seriously behaviorally disabled
SEA	state education agency
SEAC	Special Education Advisory Council
SEPAC	Special Education Parent and Professional Advisory Council
SLD	specific learning disability
SSA	Social Security Administration
SSI	Social Security Income
STOMP	Specialized Training of Military Parents
SW	social work or worker
TANF	Temporary Assistance to Needy Families
TAPP	Technical Assistance for Parents and Professionals
TASH	The Association for Persons with Severe Handicaps
TBI	traumatic brain injury
TDD	telecommunication device for the deaf
TRICARE	U.S. Department of Defense Health Care System
TTY	telecommunication device for deaf, hearing impaired, and speech impaired persons
VI	visually impaired
WIC	Women, Infants and Children Supplemental Food Program

Chapter 68

Additional Resources for Information about Endocrine and Metabolic Disorders

Government Organizations That Provide Additional Information about Endocrine and Metabolic Disorders

Endocrine and Metabolic Diseases Information Service
6 Information Way
Bethesda, MD 20892-3569
Toll-Free: 888-828-0904
Fax: 703-738-4929
Website: http://www.endocrine.niddk.nih.gov
E-mail: endoandmeta@info.niddk.nih.gov

Genetic and Rare Diseases Information Center
P.O. Box 8126
Gaithersburg, MD 20898-8126
Toll-Free: 888-205-2311
Toll-Free TTY: 888-205-3223
Fax: 240-632-9164
Website: http://rarediseases.info.nih.gov

Resources in this chapter were compiled from "Endocrine and Metabolic Diseases Organizations," National Institute of Diabetes and Digestive and Kidney Diseases (NIDDK), 2003, and other sources deemed reliable; all contact information was verified and updated in March 2007.

National Cancer Institute (NCI)
Cancer Information Service
6116 Executive Blvd.
Room 3036A
Bethesda, MD 20892-8322
Toll-Free: 800-4-CANCER
(422-6237)
Toll-Free TTY: 800-332-8615
Website: http://www.cancer.gov
E-mail:
cancergovstaff@mail.nih.gov

National Diabetes Education Program (NDEP)
1 Diabetes Way
Bethesda, MD 20814-9692
Toll-Free: 800-438-5383
Phone: 301-496-3583
Website: http://
www.ndep.nih.gov
E-mail: ndep@mail.nih.gov

National Diabetes Information Clearinghouse
1 Information Way
Bethesda, MD 20892–3560
Toll-Free: 800-860-8747
Phone: 301-654-3327
Fax: 703-738-4929
Website: http://
diabetes.niddk.nih.gov
E-mail: ndic@info.niddk.nih.gov

National Digestive Diseases Information Clearinghouse
2 Information Way
Bethesda, MD 20892-3570
Toll-Free: 800-891-5389
Fax: 703-738-4929
Website: http://
digestive.niddk.nih.gov
E-mail:
nddic@info.niddk.nih.gov

NICHD Information Resource Center
P.O. Box 3006
Rockville, MD 20847
Toll-Free: 800-370-2943
Fax: 301-984-1473
Website: http://
www.nichd.nih.gov
E-mail: NICHDIRC@mail
.nih.gov

National Institute of Child Health and Human Development (NICHD)
31 Center Drive
Bethesda, MD 20892-2425
Toll Free: 800-370-2943
Toll-Free TTY: 888-320-6942
Fax: 301-984-1473
Website: http://
www.nichd.nih.gov

National Institute of Diabetes and Digestive and Kidney Diseases (NIDDK)
National Institutes of Health
Building 31, Room 9A06
31 Center Drive, MSC 2560
Bethesda, MD 20892-2560
NIDDK Information Clearing-house Toll-Free: 800-891-5390
Phone: 301-496-3583
Website: http://
www.niddk.nih.gov
E-mail: dwebmaster@extra
.niddk.nih.gov

National Institute of Environmental Health Sciences
P.O. Box 12233
Research Triangle Park
NC 27709
Phone: 919-541-3345
TTY: 919-541-0731
Website: http://
www.niehs.nih.gov
E-mail:
webcenter@niehs.nih.gov

National Institute of Neurological Disorders and Stroke (NINDS)
P.O. Box 5801
Bethesda, MD 20824
Toll-Free: 800-352-9424
Phone: 301-496-5751
Fax: 301-468-5981
Website: http://
www.ninds.nih.gov
E-mail: braininfo@ninds.nih.gov

National Kidney and Urologic Diseases Information Clearinghouse (NKUDIC)
3 Information Way
Bethesda, MD 20892-3580
Toll-Free: 800-891-5390
Fax: 703-738-4929
Website: http://
www.kidney.niddk.nih.gov
E-mail:
nkudic@info.niddk.nih.gov

National Library of Medicine (NLM)
8600 Rockville Pike
Bethesda, MD 20894
Toll Free: 888-FIND-NLM
(346-3656)
Phone: 301-594-5983
Fax: 301-402-1384
Website: http://www.nlm.nih.gov
E-mail: custserv@nlm.nih.gov

National Women's Health Information Center (NWHIC)
8270 Willow Oaks Corporate Dr.
Fairfax, VA 22031
Toll-Free: 800-994-9662
Toll-Free TDD: 888-220-5446
Website: http://
www.4woman.gov; or
http://www.womenshealth.gov

Weight-control Information Network (WIN)
1 WIN Way
Bethesda, MD 20892-3665
Toll-Free: 877-946-4627
Phone: 202-828-1025
Fax: 202-828-1028
Website: http://
win.niddk.nih.gov
E-mail: win@info.niddk.nih.gov

Private Organizations That Provide Information about Endocrine and Metabolic Disorders

Alliance of Genetic Support Groups
4301 Connecticut Ave., N.W.,
Suite 404
Washington, DC 20008-2304
Toll-Free: 800-336-GENE (4363)
Phone: 202-966-5557
Fax: 202-966-8553
Website: http://
www.geneticalliance.org
E-mail: info@geneticalliance.org

American Association of Clinical Endocrinologists (AACE)
245 Riverside Ave.
Suite 200
Jacksonville, FL 32202
Phone: 904-353-7878
Fax: 904-353-8185
Website: http://www.aace.com
E-mail: info@aace.com

American Autoimmune Related Diseases Association
National Office
22100 Gratiot Ave.
East Detroit, MI 48021
Phone: 586-776-3900
Website: http://www.aarda.org
E-mail: aarda@aarda.org

American College of Radiology
1891 Preston White Dr.
Reston, VA 20191-4397
Toll-Free: 800-227-5463
Phone: 703-648-8900
Fax: 703-295-6773
Website: http://www.acr.org
E-mail: info@acr.org

American Diabetes Association (ADA)
701 N. Beauregard Street
Alexandria, VA 22311
Toll-Free: 800-DIABETES
(342-2383)
Fax: 703-549-6995
Website: http://www.diabetes.org
E-mail: askada@diabetes.org

American Gastroenterological Association (AGA)
National Office
4930 Del Ray Ave.
Bethesda, MD 20814
Phone: 301-654-2055
Fax: 301-654-5920
Website: http://www.gastro.org
E-mail: info@gastro.org

American Society for Reproductive Medicine (ASRM)
1209 Montgomery Hwy.
Birmingham, AL 35216-2809
Phone: 205-978-5000
Fax: 205-978-5005
Website: http://www.asrm.org
E-mail: asrm@asrm.org

American Thyroid Association
6066 Leesburg Pike, Suite 550
Falls Church, VA 22041
Toll-Free: 800-THYROID
(849-7643)
Phone: 703-998-8890
Fax: 703-998-8893
Website: http://www.thyroid.org
E-mail: thyroid@thyroid.org

Association for Glycogen-Storage Disease
P.O. Box 896
Durant, IA 52747
Phone: 563-785-6038
Website: http://www.agsdus.org

CARES Foundation, Inc.
Congenital Adrenal Hyperplasia Support
2414 Morris Ave.
Suite 110
Union, NJ 07083
Toll-Free: 866-227-3737
Phone: 973-912-3895
Fax: 973-912-8990
Website: http://www.caresfoundation.org
E-mail: info@caresfoundation.org

Children's Gaucher Research Fund
P.O. Box 2123
Granite Bay, CA 95746-2123
Phone: 916-797-3700
Fax: 916-797-3707
Website: http://www.childrensgaucher.org
E-mail: research@childrensgaucher.org

Children's PKU Network (CPN)
3790 Via De la Valle, Suite 120
Del Mar, CA 92014
Phone: 858-509-0767
Fax: 858-509-0768
Website: http://www.pkunetwork.org
E-mail: pkunetwork@aol.com

CLIMB (Children Living with Inherited Metabolic Diseases)
Climb Building
176 Nantwich Road
Crewe CW2 6BG
United Kingdom
Phone: +44-87-0-7700-325
Fax: +44-87-0-7700-327
Website: http://
www.CLIMB.org.uk
E-mail: infosvcs@climb.org.uk

Creutzfeldt-Jakob Disease Foundation Inc.
P.O. Box 5312
Akron, OH 44334
Toll-Free: 800-659-1991
Phone: 330-665-5590
Website: http://
www.cjdfoundation.org
E-mail: help@cjdfoundation.org

Cushing's Support and Research Foundation, Inc.
65 East India Row, Suite 22B
Boston, MA 02110
Phone/Fax: 617-723-3674
Website: http://www.CSRF.net
E-mail: cushinfo@csrf.net

Cystic Fibrosis Foundation
6931 Arlington Road
Bethesda, MD 20814
Toll-Free: 800-FIGHT-CF
(344-4823)
Phone: 301-951-4422
Website: http://www.cff.org

Endocrine Society
8401 Connecticut Ave., Suite 900
Chevy Chase, MD 20815
Phone: 301-941-0200
Website: http://
www.endo-society.org

The Genetic Alliance
(formerly the Alliance of Genetic Support Groups)
4301 Connecticut Ave., N.W., Suite 404
Washington, DC 20008
Toll-Free: 800-336-GENE (4363)
Phone: 202-966-5557
Fax: 202-966-8553
Website: http://
www.geneticalliance.org
E-mail: info@geneticalliance.org

Hormone Foundation
8401 Connecticut Ave.
Suite 900
Chevy Chase, MD 20815
Toll-Free: 800-HORMONE
(467-6663)
Fax: 301-941-0259
Website: http://
www.hormone.org
E-mail: hormone@endo-society.org

Human Growth Foundation (HGF)
997 Glen Cove Ave., Suite 5
Glen Head, NY 11545
Toll-Free: 800-451-6434
Fax: 516-671-4055
Website: http://
www.hgfound.org.
E-mail: hgf1@hgfound.org

InterNational Council on Infertility Information Dissemination, Inc. (INCIID)
P.O. Box 6836
Arlington, VA 22206
Phone: 703-379-9178
Fax: 703-379-1593
Website: http://www.inciid.org
E-mail: alert@inciid.org

Juvenile Diabetes Research Foundation (JDRF)
120 Wall Street
New York, NY 10005-4001
Toll-Free: 800-533-CURE (2873)
Fax: 212-785-9595
Website: http://www.jdrf.org
E-mail: info@jdrf.org

The MAGIC Foundation
6645 W. North Ave.
Oak Park, IL 60302
Toll-Free: 800-362-4423
Phone: 708-383-0808
Fax: 708-383-0899
Website: http://
www.magicfoundation.org

March of Dimes Birth Defects Foundation
1275 Mamaroneck Avenue
White Plains, NY 10605
Toll-Free: 888-MODIMES
(663-4637)
Phone: 914-428-7100
Fax: 914-428-8203
Website: http://
www.marchofdimes.com
E-mail:
askus@marchofdimes.com

MUMS: National Parent to Parent Network
150 Custer Court
Green Bay, WI 54301-1243
Toll-Free: 877-336-5333 (Parents only please)
Phone: 920-336-5333
Fax: 920-339-0995
Website: http://www.netnet.net/mums
E-mail: mums@netnet.net

Muscular Dystrophy Association
3300 E. Sunrise Dr.
Tucson, AZ 85718
Toll-Free: 800-344-4863
Phone: 520-529-2000
Fax: 520-529-5300
Website: http://www.mdausa.org
E-mail: mda@mdausa.org

National Adrenal Diseases Foundation (NADF)
505 Northern Blvd.
Great Neck, NY 11021
Phone: 516-487-4992
Fax: 516-829-5710
Website: http://www.nadf.us
E-mail: nadfmail@aol.com

National Gaucher Foundation
2227 Idlewood Rd., Suite 12
Tucker, GA 30084
Toll-Free: 800-504-3189
Fax: 770-934-2911
Website: http://
www.gaucherdisease.org
E-mail:
rhonda@gaucherdisease.org

National Organization for Rare Disorders (NORD)
P.O. Box 1968
Danbury, CT 06813-1968
Toll-Free: 800-999-NORD (6673)
Phone: 203-744-0100
Fax: 203-798-2291
Website: http://
www.rarediseases.org
E-mail:
orphan@rarediseases.org

National Osteoporosis Foundation
1232 22nd Street, N.W.
Washington, DC 20037
Phone: 202-223-2226
Website: http://www.nof.org
E-mail: webmaster@nof.org

National Tay-Sachs and Allied Diseases Association
2001 Beacon Street, Suite 204
Brighton, MA 02135
Toll-Free: 800-906-8723
Phone: 617-277-4463
Fax: 616-277-0134
Website: http://www.ntsad.org
E-mail: info@ntsad.org

National Urea Cycle Disorders Foundation
4841 Hill Street
La Canada, CA 91011
Toll-Free: 800-38-NUCDF
(68233)
Fax: 818-248-9770
Website: http://www.nucdf.org
E-mail: info@nucdf.org

Pituitary Network Association
P.O. Box 1958
Thousand Oaks, CA 91358
Phone: 805-499-9973
Fax: 805-480-0633
Website: http://
www.pituitary.org
E-mail: pna@pituitary.org

Radiological Society of North America
820 Jorie Blvd.
Oak Brook, IL 60523-2251
Toll-Free: 800-381-6660
Phone: 630-571-2670
Fax: 630-571-7837
Website: http://www.rsna.org
E-mail: webmaster@rsna.org

Thyroid Foundation of America
One Longfellow Place
Suite 1518
Boston, MA 02114
Toll-Free: 800-832-8321
Fax: 617-534-1515
Website: http://www.tsh.org
E-mail: info@allthyroid.org

United Leukodystrophy Foundation
2304 Highland Drive
Sycamore, IL 60178
Toll-Free: 800-728-5483
Phone: 815-895-3211
Fax: 815-895-2432
Website: http://www.ulf.org
E-mail: office@ulf.org

Index

Index

Page numbers followed by 'n' indicate a footnote. Page numbers in *italics* indicate a table or illustration.

K

Kansas, newborn screening
tests *106, 108, 110*
Kentucky, newborn screening
tests *106, 108, 110*
ketoconazole 302
Krabbe disease
described 470–71
overview 487–92

L

laboratory tests
defined 548
described 64
see also tests
lactase deficiency *428*
lactate dehydrogenase deficiency,
described 521
lansoprazole 388
"Laparoscopic Adrenal Gland
Removal" (SAGES) 311n
leptin, food intake 45–47
levothyroxine 213
LH *see* luteinizing hormone
limit dextrinosis *see* Forbes disease
lipid disorders, described 54
lipidoses *see* lipid storage diseases
lipids
defined 548
described 464
"Lipid Storage Diseases Fact Sheet"
(NINDS) 464n
lipid storage diseases, overview
464–73
lipoprotein lipase deficiency *429*
Lippincott Williams and Wilkins,
dictionary publication 545n
liver, digestive system 15, 17
liver phosphorylase deficiency
see Hers disease
localized, defined 548
Lorenzo oil 502
Louisiana, newborn screening
tests *106, 108, 110*
low blood sugar *see* hypoglycemia

luteinizing hormone (LH)
described 535
reproductive system 413
lymph nodes, defined 548
lysinuric protein intolerance *428, 429*
lysosomal storage disease *see* Pompe
disease

M

macroadenomas, described 184
The MAGIC Foundation
contact information 509, 569
publications
adult growth hormone
deficiency 139n
growth hormone therapy 147n
McCune-Albright syndrome 505n
magnetic resonance imaging (MRI)
Creutzfeldt-Jakob disease 157
Cushing disease 168
defined 549
described 70–71, 551
pancreas function 322
pancreatic cancer 369–70
pituitary disorders 191
pituitary tumors 186
thyroid nodule 227
Maine, newborn screening
tests *106, 108, 110*
malignant, defined 548
malignant tumors, described 366
maple syrup urine disease (MSUD)
newborn screening 103–4
overview 440–41
statistics *432*
"Maple Syrup Urine Disease"
(Washington State Department
of Health Newborn Screening
Program) 440n
March of Dimes Birth Defects
Foundation, contact information
473, 542, 569
Maryland, newborn screening
tests *106, 108, 110*
Massachusetts, newborn screening
tests *106, 108, 110*
master gland *see* pituitary gland

Health Reference Series

COMPLETE CATALOG

List price $87 per volume. **School and library price $78 per volume.**

Adolescent Health Sourcebook, 2nd Edition

Basic Consumer Health Information about the Physical, Mental, and Emotional Growth and Development of Adolescents, Including Medical Care, Nutritional and Physical Activity Requirements, Puberty, Sexual Activity, Acne, Tanning, Body Piercing, Common Physical Illnesses and Disorders, Eating Disorders, Attention Deficit Hyperactivity Disorder, Depression, Bullying, Hazing, and Adolescent Injuries Related to Sports, Driving, and Work

Along with Substance Abuse Information about Nicotine, Alcohol, and Drug Use, a Glossary, and Directory of Additional Resources

Edited by Joyce Brennfleck Shannon. 683 pages. 2006. 978-0-7808-0943-7.

"It is written in clear, nontechnical language aimed at general readers. . . . Recommended for public libraries, community colleges, and other agencies serving health care consumers."
— *American Reference Books Annual, 2003*

"Recommended for school and public libraries. Parents and professionals dealing with teens will appreciate the easy-to-follow format and the clearly written text. This could become a 'must have' for every high school teacher." — *E-Streams, Jan '03*

"A good starting point for information related to common medical, mental, and emotional concerns of adolescents." — *School Library Journal, Nov '02*

"This book provides accurate information in an easy to access format. It addresses topics that parents and caregivers might not be aware of and provides practical, useable information."
— *Doody's Health Sciences Book Review Journal, Sep-Oct '02*

"Recommended reference source."
— *Booklist, American Library Association, Sep '02*

AIDS Sourcebook, 3rd Edition

Basic Consumer Health Information about Acquired Immune Deficiency Syndrome (AIDS) and Human Immunodeficiency Virus (HIV) Infection, Including Facts about Transmission, Prevention, Diagnosis, Treatment, Opportunistic Infections, and Other Complications, with a Section for Women and Children, Including Details about Associated Gynecological Concerns, Pregnancy, and Pediatric Care

Along with Updated Statistical Information, Reports on Current Research Initiatives, a Glossary, and Directories of Internet, Hotline, and Other Resources

Edited by Dawn D. Matthews. 664 pages. 2003. 978-0-7808-0631-3.

"The 3rd edition of the *AIDS Sourcebook*, part of Omnigraphics' *Health Reference Series*, is a welcome update. . . . This resource is highly recommended for academic and public libraries."
— *American Reference Books Annual, 2004*

"Excellent sourcebook. This continues to be a highly recommended book. There is no other book that provides as much information as this book provides."
— *AIDS Book Review Journal, Dec-Jan '00*

"Recommended reference source."
— *Booklist, American Library Association, Dec '99*

Alcoholism Sourcebook, 2nd Edition

Basic Consumer Health Information about Alcohol Use, Abuse, and Dependence, Featuring Facts about the Physical, Mental, and Social Health Effects of Alcohol Addiction, Including Alcoholic Liver Disease, Pancreatic Disease, Cardiovascular Disease, Neurological Disorders, and the Effects of Drinking during Pregnancy

Along with Information about Alcohol Treatment, Medications, and Recovery Programs, in Addition to Tips for Reducing the Prevalence of Underage Drinking, Statistics about Alcohol Use, a Glossary of Related Terms, and Directories of Resources for More Help and Information

Edited by Amy L. Sutton. 653 pages. 2006. 978-0-7808-0942-0.

"This title is one of the few reference works on alcoholism for general readers. For some readers this will be a welcome complement to the many self-help books on the market. Recommended for collections serving general readers and consumer health collections."
— *E-Streams, Mar '01*

"This book is an excellent choice for public and academic libraries."
— *American Reference Books Annual, 2001*

"Recommended reference source."
— *Booklist, American Library Association, Dec '00*

"Presents a wealth of information on alcohol use and abuse and its effects on the body and mind, treatment, and prevention." — *SciTech Book News, Dec '00*

"Important new health guide which packs in the latest consumer information about the problems of alcoholism." — *Reviewer's Bookwatch, Nov '00*

SEE ALSO Drug Abuse Sourcebook

Allergies Sourcebook, 3rd Edition

Basic Consumer Health Information about Allergic Disorders, Such as Anaphylaxis, Hives, Eczema, Rhinitis, Sinusitis, and Conjunctivitis, and Their Triggers, Including Pollen, Mold, Dust Mites, Animal Dander, Insects, Chemicals, Food, Food Additives, and Medications;

Along with Advice about the Diagnosis and Treatment of Allergy Symptoms, a Glossary of Related Terms, a Directory of Resources for Help and Information, and Suggestions for Additional Reading

Edited by Amy L. Sutton. 616 pages. 2007. 978-0-7808-0950-5.

"This book brings a great deal of useful material together. . . . This is an excellent addition to public and consumer health library collections."
— *American Reference Books Annual, 2003*

"This second edition would be useful to laypersons with little or advanced knowledge of the subject matter. This book would also serve as a resource for nursing and other health care professions students. It would be useful in public, academic, and hospital libraries with consumer health collections." — *E-Streams, Jul '02*

Alternative Medicine Sourcebook

SEE Complementary & Alternative Medicine Sourcebook

Alzheimer's Disease Sourcebook, 3rd Edition

Basic Consumer Health Information about Alzheimer's Disease, Other Dementias, and Related Disorders, Including Multi-Infarct Dementia, AIDS Dementia Complex, Dementia with Lewy Bodies, Huntington's Disease, Wernicke-Korsakoff Syndrome (Alcohol-Related Dementia), Delirium, and Confusional States

Along with Information for People Newly Diagnosed with Alzheimer's Disease and Caregivers, Reports Detailing Current Research Efforts in Prevention, Diagnosis, and Treatment, Facts about Long-Term Care Issues, and Listings of Sources for Additional Information

Edited by Karen Bellenir. 645 pages. 2003. 978-0-7808-0666-5.

"This very informative and valuable tool will be a great addition to any library serving consumers, students and health care workers."
— *American Reference Books Annual, 2004*

"This is a valuable resource for people affected by dementias such as Alzheimer's. It is easy to navigate and includes important information and resources."
— *Doody's Review Service, Feb '04*

"Recommended reference source."
— *Booklist, American Library Association, Oct '99*

SEE ALSO *Brain Disorders Sourcebook*

Arthritis Sourcebook, 2nd Edition

Basic Consumer Health Information about Osteoarthritis, Rheumatoid Arthritis, Other Rheumatic Disorders, Infectious Forms of Arthritis, and Diseases with Symptoms Linked to Arthritis, Featuring Facts about Diagnosis, Pain Management, and Surgical Therapies

Along with Coping Strategies, Research Updates, a Glossary, and Resources for Additional Help and Information

Edited by Amy L. Sutton. 593 pages. 2004. 978-0-7808-0667-2.

"This easy-to-read volume is recommended for consumer health collections within public or academic libraries." — *E-Streams, May '05*

"As expected, this updated edition continues the excellent reputation of this series in providing sound, usable health information. . . . Highly recommended."
— *American Reference Books Annual, 2005*

"Excellent reference." — *The Bookwatch, Jan '05*

Asthma Sourcebook, 2nd Edition

Basic Consumer Health Information about the Causes, Symptoms, Diagnosis, and Treatment of Asthma in Infants, Children, Teenagers, and Adults, Including Facts about Different Types of Asthma, Common Co-Occurring Conditions, Asthma Management Plans, Triggers, Medications, and Medication Delivery Devices

Along with Asthma Statistics, Research Updates, a Glossary, a Directory of Asthma-Related Resources, and More

Edited by Karen Bellenir. 609 pages. 2006. 978-0-7808-0866-9.

"A worthwhile reference acquisition for public libraries and academic medical libraries whose readers desire a quick introduction to the wide range of asthma information." — *Choice, Association of College & Research Libraries, Jun '01*

"Recommended reference source."
— *Booklist, American Library Association, Feb '01*

"Highly recommended." — *The Bookwatch, Jan '01*

"There is much good information for patients and their families who deal with asthma daily."
— *American Medical Writers Association Journal, Winter '01*

"This informative text is recommended for consumer health collections in public, secondary school, and community college libraries and the libraries of universities with a large undergraduate population."
— *American Reference Books Annual, 2001*

Attention Deficit Disorder Sourcebook

Basic Consumer Health Information about Attention Deficit/Hyperactivity Disorder in Children and Adults,

Including Facts about Causes, Symptoms, Diagnostic Criteria, and Treatment Options Such as Medications, Behavior Therapy, Coaching, and Homeopathy

Along with Reports on Current Research Initiatives, Legal Issues, and Government Regulations, and Featuring a Glossary of Related Terms, Internet Resources, and a List of Additional Reading Material

Edited by Dawn D. Matthews. 470 pages. 2002. 978-0-7808-0624-5.

"Recommended reference source."
—Booklist, American Library Association, Jan '03

"This book is recommended for all school libraries and the reference or consumer health sections of public libraries." —American Reference Books Annual, 2003

Back & Neck Sourcebook, 2nd Edition

Basic Consumer Health Information about Spinal Pain, Spinal Cord Injuries, and Related Disorders, Such as Degenerative Disk Disease, Osteoarthritis, Scoliosis, Sciatica, Spina Bifida, and Spinal Stenosis, and Featuring Facts about Maintaining Spinal Health, Self-Care, Pain Management, Rehabilitative Care, Chiropractic Care, Spinal Surgeries, and Complementary Therapies

Along with Suggestions for Preventing Back and Neck Pain, a Glossary of Related Terms, and a Directory of Resources

Edited by Amy L. Sutton. 633 pages. 2004. 978-0-7808-0738-9.

"Recommended . . . an easy to use, comprehensive medical reference book." —E-Streams, Sep '05

"The strength of this work is its basic, easy-to-read format. Recommended." —Reference and User Services Quarterly, American Library Association, Winter '97

Blood & Circulatory Disorders Sourcebook, 2nd Edition

Basic Consumer Health Information about the Blood and Circulatory System and Related Disorders, Such as Anemia and Other Hemoglobin Diseases, Cancer of the Blood and Associated Bone Marrow Disorders, Clotting and Bleeding Problems, and Conditions That Affect the Veins, Blood Vessels, and Arteries, Including Facts about the Donation and Transplantation of Bone Marrow, Stem Cells, and Blood and Tips for Keeping the Blood and Circulatory System Healthy

Along with a Glossary of Related Terms and Resources for Additional Help and Information

Edited by Amy L. Sutton. 659 pages. 2005. 978-0-7808-0746-4.

"Highly recommended pick for basic consumer health reference holdings at all levels."
—The Bookwatch, Aug '05

"Recommended reference source."
—Booklist, American Library Association, Feb '99

"An important reference sourcebook written in simple language for everyday, non-technical users. "
—Reviewer's Bookwatch, Jan '99

Brain Disorders Sourcebook, 2nd Edition

Basic Consumer Health Information about Acquired and Traumatic Brain Injuries, Infections of the Brain, Epilepsy and Seizure Disorders, Cerebral Palsy, and Degenerative Neurological Disorders, Including Amyotrophic Lateral Sclerosis (ALS), Dementias, Multiple Sclerosis, and More

Along with Information on the Brain's Structure and Function, Treatment and Rehabilitation Options, Reports on Current Research Initiatives, a Glossary of Terms Related to Brain Disorders and Injuries, and a Directory of Sources for Further Help and Information

Edited by Sandra J. Judd. 625 pages. 2005. 978-0-7808-0744-0.

"Highly recommended pick for basic consumer health reference holdings at all levels."
—The Bookwatch, Aug '05

"Belongs on the shelves of any library with a consumer health collection." —E-Streams, Mar '00

"Recommended reference source."
—Booklist, American Library Association, Oct '99

SEE ALSO Alzheimer's Disease Sourcebook

Breast Cancer Sourcebook, 2nd Edition

Basic Consumer Health Information about Breast Cancer, Including Facts about Risk Factors, Prevention, Screening and Diagnostic Methods, Treatment Options, Complementary and Alternative Therapies, Post-Treatment Concerns, Clinical Trials, Special Risk Populations, and New Developments in Breast Cancer Research

Along with Breast Cancer Statistics, a Glossary of Related Terms, and a Directory of Resources for Additional Help and Information

Edited by Sandra J. Judd. 595 pages. 2004. 978-0-7808-0668-9.

"This book will be an excellent addition to public, community college, medical, and academic libraries."
—American Reference Books Annual, 2006

"It would be a useful reference book in a library or on loan to women in a support group."
—Cancer Forum, Mar '03

"Recommended reference source."
—Booklist, American Library Association, Jan '02

"This reference source is highly recommended. It is quite informative, comprehensive and detailed in nature, and yet it offers practical advice in easy-to-read language. It could be thought of as the 'bible' of breast cancer for the consumer." — *E-Streams, Jan '02*

"From the pros and cons of different screening methods and results to treatment options, *Breast Cancer Sourcebook* provides the latest information on the subject." — *Library Bookwatch, Dec '01*

"This thoroughgoing, very readable reference covers all aspects of breast health and cancer. . . . Readers will find much to consider here. Recommended for all public and patient health collections." — *Library Journal, Sep '01*

SEE ALSO *Cancer Sourcebook for Women, Women's Health Concerns Sourcebook*

■

Breastfeeding Sourcebook

Basic Consumer Health Information about the Benefits of Breastmilk, Preparing to Breastfeed, Breastfeeding as a Baby Grows, Nutrition, and More, Including Information on Special Situations and Concerns Such as Mastitis, Illness, Medications, Allergies, Multiple Births, Prematurity, Special Needs, and Adoption

Along with a Glossary and Resources for Additional Help and Information

Edited by Jenni Lynn Colson. 388 pages. 2002. 978-0-7808-0332-9.

"Particularly useful is the information about professional lactation services and chapters on breastfeeding when returning to work. . . . *Breastfeeding Sourcebook* will be useful for public libraries, consumer health libraries, and technical schools offering nurse assistant training, especially in areas where Internet access is problematic." — *American Reference Books Annual, 2003*

SEE ALSO *Pregnancy & Birth Sourcebook*

■

Burns Sourcebook

Basic Consumer Health Information about Various Types of Burns and Scalds, Including Flame, Heat, Cold, Electrical, Chemical, and Sun Burns

Along with Information on Short-Term and Long-Term Treatments, Tissue Reconstruction, Plastic Surgery, Prevention Suggestions, and First Aid

Edited by Allan R. Cook. 604 pages. 1999. 978-0-7808-0204-9.

"This is an exceptional addition to the series and is highly recommended for all consumer health collections, hospital libraries, and academic medical centers." — *E-Streams, Mar '00*

"This key reference guide is an invaluable addition to all health care and public libraries in confronting this ongoing health issue." — *American Reference Books Annual, 2000*

"Recommended reference source." —*Booklist, American Library Association, Dec '99*

SEE ALSO *Dermatological Disorders Sourcebook*

Cancer Sourcebook, 5th Edition

Basic Consumer Health Information about Major Forms and Stages of Cancer, Featuring Facts about Head and Neck Cancers, Lung Cancers, Gastrointestinal Cancers, Genitourinary Cancers, Lymphomas, Blood Cell Cancers, Endocrine Cancers, Skin Cancers, Bone Cancers, Metastatic Cancers, and More

Along with Facts about Cancer Treatments, Cancer Risks and Prevention, a Glossary of Related Terms, Statistical Data, and a Directory of Resources for Additional Information

Edited by Karen Bellenir. 1,133 pages. 2007. 978-0-7808-0947-5.

"With cancer being the second leading cause of death for Americans, a prodigious work such as this one, which locates centrally so much cancer-related information, is clearly an asset to this nation's citizens and others." — *Journal of the National Medical Association, 2004*

"This title is recommended for health sciences and public libraries with consumer health collections." — *E-Streams, Feb '01*

". . . can be effectively used by cancer patients and their families who are looking for answers in a language they can understand. Public and hospital libraries should have it on their shelves." — *American Reference Books Annual, 2001*

"Recommended reference source." —*Booklist, American Library Association, Dec '00*

SEE ALSO *Breast Cancer Sourcebook, Cancer Sourcebook for Women, Pediatric Cancer Sourcebook, Prostate Cancer Sourcebook*

■

Cancer Sourcebook for Women, 3rd Edition

Basic Consumer Health Information about Leading Causes of Cancer in Women, Featuring Facts about Gynecologic Cancers and Related Concerns, Such as Breast Cancer, Cervical Cancer, Endometrial Cancer, Uterine Sarcoma, Vaginal Cancer, Vulvar Cancer, and Common Non-Cancerous Gynecologic Conditions, in Addition to Facts about Lung Cancer, Colorectal Cancer, and Thyroid Cancer in Women

Along with Information about Cancer Risk Factors, Screening and Prevention, Treatment Options, and Tips on Coping with Life after Cancer Treatment, a Glossary of Cancer Terms, and a Directory of Resources for Additional Help and Information

Edited by Amy L. Sutton. 715 pages. 2006. 978-0-7808-0867-6.

"An excellent addition to collections in public, consumer health, and women's health libraries." — *American Reference Books Annual, 2003*

"Overall, the information is excellent, and complex topics are clearly explained. As a reference book for the consumer it is a valuable resource to assist them to make informed decisions about cancer and its treatments." — *Cancer Forum, Nov '02*

"Highly recommended for academic and medical reference collections." — *Library Bookwatch, Sep '02*

"This is a highly recommended book for any public or consumer library, being reader friendly and containing accurate and helpful information."
— *E-Streams, Aug '02*

"Recommended reference source."
—*Booklist, American Library Association, Jul '02*

SEE ALSO *Breast Cancer Sourcebook, Women's Health Concerns Sourcebook*

Cancer Survivorship Sourcebook

Basic Consumer Health Information about the Physical, Educational, Emotional, Social, and Financial Needs of Cancer Patients from Diagnosis, through Cancer Treatment, and Beyond, Including Facts about Researching Specific Types of Cancer and Learning about Clinical Trials and Treatment Options, and Featuring Tips for Coping with the Side Effects of Cancer Treatments and Adjusting to Life after Cancer Treatment Concludes

Along with Suggestions for Caregivers, Friends, and Family Members of Cancer Patients, a Glossary of Cancer Care Terms, and Directories of Related Resources

Edited by Karen Bellenir. 6561 pages. 2007. 978-0-7808-0985-7.

Cardiovascular Diseases & Disorders Sourcebook, 3rd Edition

Basic Consumer Health Information about Heart and Vascular Diseases and Disorders, Such as Angina, Heart Attacks, Arrhythmias, Cardiomyopathy, Valve Disease, Atherosclerosis, and Aneurysms, with Information about Managing Cardiovascular Risk Factors and Maintaining Heart Health, Medications and Procedures Used to Treat Cardiovascular Disorders, and Concerns of Special Significance to Women

Along with Reports on Current Research Initiatives, a Glossary of Related Medical Terms, and a Directory of Sources for Further Help and Information

Edited by Sandra J. Judd. 713 pages. 2005. 978-0-7808-0739-6.

"This updated sourcebook is still the best first stop for comprehensive introductory information on cardiovascular diseases."
— *American Reference Books Annual, 2006*

"Recommended for public libraries and libraries supporting health care professionals."
— *E-Streams, Sep '05*

"This should be a standard health library reference."
—*The Bookwatch, Jun '05*

"Recommended reference source."
—*Booklist, American Library Association, Dec '00*

". . . comprehensive format provides an extensive overview on this subject."
— *Choice, Association of College & Research Libraries*

Caregiving Sourcebook

Basic Consumer Health Information for Caregivers, Including a Profile of Caregivers, Caregiving Responsibilities and Concerns, Tips for Specific Conditions, Care Environments, and the Effects of Caregiving

Along with Facts about Legal Issues, Financial Information, and Future Planning, a Glossary, and a Listing of Additional Resources

Edited by Joyce Brennfleck Shannon. 600 pages. 2001. 978-0-7808-0331-2.

"Essential for most collections."
— *Library Journal, Apr 1, 2002*

"An ideal addition to the reference collection of any public library. Health sciences information professionals may also want to acquire the *Caregiving Sourcebook* for their hospital or academic library for use as a ready reference tool by health care workers interested in aging and caregiving."
—*E-Streams, Jan '02*

"Recommended reference source."
—*Booklist, American Library Association, Oct '01*

Child Abuse Sourcebook

Basic Consumer Health Information about the Physical, Sexual, and Emotional Abuse of Children, with Additional Facts about Neglect, Munchausen Syndrome by Proxy (MSBP), Shaken Baby Syndrome, and Controversial Issues Related to Child Abuse, Such as Withholding Medical Care, Corporal Punishment, and Child Maltreatment in Youth Sports, and Featuring Facts about Child Protective Services, Foster Care, Adoption, Parenting Challenges, and Other Abuse Prevention Efforts

Along with a Glossary of Related Terms and Resources for Additional Help and Information

Edited by Dawn D. Matthews. 620 pages. 2004. 978-0-7808-0705-1.

"A valuable and highly recommended resource for school, academic and public libraries whether used on its own or as a starting point for more in-depth research."
— *E-Streams, Apr '05*

"Every week the news brings cases of child abuse or neglect, so it is useful to have a source that supplies so much helpful information. . . . Recommended. Public and academic libraries, and child welfare offices."
— *Choice, Association of College & Research Libraries, Mar '05*

"Packed with insights on all kinds of issues, from foster care and adoption to parenting and abuse prevention."
—*The Bookwatch, Nov '04*

SEE ALSO: *Domestic Violence Sourcebook*

Childhood Diseases & Disorders Sourcebook

Basic Consumer Health Information about Medical Problems Often Encountered in Pre-Adolescent Children, Including Respiratory Tract Ailments, Ear Infections, Sore Throats, Disorders of the Skin and Scalp, Digestive and Genitourinary Diseases, Infectious Diseases, Inflammatory Disorders, Chronic Physical and Developmental Disorders, Allergies, and More

Along with Information about Diagnostic Tests, Common Childhood Surgeries, and Frequently Used Medications, with a Glossary of Important Terms and Resource Directory

Edited by Chad T. Kimball. 662 pages. 2003. 978-0-7808-0458-6.

"This is an excellent book for new parents and should be included in all health care and public libraries."
—American Reference Books Annual, 2004

SEE ALSO: *Healthy Children Sourcebook*

Colds, Flu & Other Common Ailments Sourcebook

Basic Consumer Health Information about Common Ailments and Injuries, Including Colds, Coughs, the Flu, Sinus Problems, Headaches, Fever, Nausea and Vomiting, Menstrual Cramps, Diarrhea, Constipation, Hemorrhoids, Back Pain, Dandruff, Dry and Itchy Skin, Cuts, Scrapes, Sprains, Bruises, and More

Along with Information about Prevention, Self-Care, Choosing a Doctor, Over-the-Counter Medications, Folk Remedies, and Alternative Therapies, and Including a Glossary of Important Terms and a Directory of Resources for Further Help and Information

Edited by Chad T. Kimball. 638 pages. 2001. 978-0-7808-0435-7.

"A good starting point for research on common illnesses. It will be a useful addition to public and consumer health library collections."
— American Reference Books Annual, 2002

"Will prove valuable to any library seeking to maintain a current, comprehensive reference collection of health resources. . . . Excellent reference."
— The Bookwatch, Aug '01

"Recommended reference source."
— Booklist, American Library Association, Jul '01

Communication Disorders Sourcebook

Basic Information about Deafness and Hearing Loss, Speech and Language Disorders, Voice Disorders, Balance and Vestibular Disorders, and Disorders of Smell, Taste, and Touch

Edited by Linda M. Ross. 533 pages. 1996. 978-0-7808-0077-9.

"This is skillfully edited and is a welcome resource for the layperson. It should be found in every public and medical library." *— Booklist Health Sciences Supplement, American Library Association, Oct '97*

Complementary & Alternative Medicine Sourcebook, 3rd Edition

Basic Consumer Health Information about Complementary and Alternative Medical Therapies, Including Acupuncture, Ayurveda, Traditional Chinese Medicine, Herbal Medicine, Homeopathy, Naturopathy, Biofeedback, Hypnotherapy, Yoga, Art Therapy, Aromatherapy, Clinical Nutrition, Vitamin and Mineral Supplements, Chiropractic, Massage, Reflexology, Crystal Therapy, Therapeutic Touch, and More

Along with Facts about Alternative and Complementary Treatments for Specific Conditions Such as Cancer, Diabetes, Osteoarthritis, Chronic Pain, Menopause, Gastrointestinal Disorders, Headaches, and Mental Illness, a Glossary, and a Resource List for Additional Help and Information

Edited by Sandra J. Judd. 657 pages. 2006. 978-0-7808-0864-5.

"Recommended for public, high school, and academic libraries that have consumer health collections. Hospital libraries that also serve the public will find this to be a useful resource." *— E-Streams, Feb '03*

"Recommended reference source."
—Booklist, American Library Association, Jan '03

"An important alternate health reference."
— MBR Bookwatch, Oct '02

"A great addition to the reference collection of every type of library." *— American Reference Books Annual, 2000*

Congenital Disorders Sourcebook, 2nd Edition

Basic Consumer Health Information about Nonhereditary Birth Defects and Disorders Related to Prematurity, Gestational Injuries, Congenital Infections, and Birth Complications, Including Heart Defects, Hydrocephalus, Spina Bifida, Cleft Lip and Palate, Cerebral Palsy, and More

Along with Facts about the Prevention of Birth Defects, Fetal Surgery and Other Treatment Options, Research Initiatives, a Glossary of Related Terms, and Resources for Additional Information and Support

Edited by Sandra J. Judd. 647 pages. 2006. 978-0-7808-0945-1.

"Recommended reference source."
— Booklist, American Library Association, Oct '97

SEE ALSO *Pregnancy & Birth Sourcebook*

Contagious Diseases Sourcebook

Basic Consumer Health Information about Infectious Diseases Spread by Person-to-Person Contact through

Direct Touch, Airborne Transmission, Sexual Contact, or Contact with Blood or Other Body Fluids, Including Hepatitis, Herpes, Influenza, Lice, Measles, Mumps, Pinworm, Ringworm, Severe Acute Respiratory Syndrome (SARS), Streptococcal Infections, Tuberculosis, and Others

Along with Facts about Disease Transmission, Antimicrobial Resistance, and Vaccines, with a Glossary and Directories of Resources for More Information

Edited by Karen Bellenir. 643 pages. 2004. 978-0-7808-0736-5.

"This easy-to-read volume is recommended for consumer health collections within public or academic libraries." — E-Streams, May '05

"This informative book is highly recommended for public libraries, consumer health collections, and secondary schools and undergraduate libraries."
— American Reference Books Annual, 2005

"Excellent reference." — The Bookwatch, Jan '05

■

Death & Dying Sourcebook, 2nd Edition

Basic Consumer Health Information about End-of-Life Care and Related Perspectives and Ethical Issues, Including End-of-Life Symptoms and Treatments, Pain Management, Quality-of-Life Concerns, the Use of Life Support, Patients' Rights and Privacy Issues, Advance Directives, Physician-Assisted Suicide, Caregiving, Organ and Tissue Donation, Autopsies, Funeral Arrangements, and Grief

Along with Statistical Data, Information about the Leading Causes of Death, a Glossary, and Directories of Support Groups and Other Resources

Edited by Joyce Brennfleck Shannon. 653 pages. 2006. 978-0-7808-0871-3.

"Public libraries, medical libraries, and academic libraries will all find this sourcebook a useful addition to their collections."
— American Reference Books Annual, 2001

"An extremely useful resource for those concerned with death and dying in the United States."
— Respiratory Care, Nov '00

"Recommended reference source."
—Booklist, American Library Association, Aug '00

"This book is a definite must for all those involved in end-of-life care." — Doody's Review Service, 2000

■

Dental Care & Oral Health Sourcebook, 2nd Edition

Basic Consumer Health Information about Dental Care, Including Oral Hygiene, Dental Visits, Pain Management, Cavities, Crowns, Bridges, Dental Implants, and Fillings, and Other Oral Health Concerns, Such as Gum Disease, Bad Breath, Dry Mouth, Genetic and Developmental Abnormalities, Oral Cancers, Orthodontics, and Temporomandibular Disorders

Along with Updates on Current Research in Oral Health, a Glossary, a Directory of Dental and Oral Health Organizations, and Resources for People with Dental and Oral Health Disorders

Edited by Amy L. Sutton. 609 pages. 2003. 978-0-7808-0634-4.

"This book could serve as a turning point in the battle to educate consumers in issues concerning oral health."
— American Reference Books Annual, 2004

"Unique source which will fill a gap in dental sources for patients and the lay public. A valuable reference tool even in a library with thousands of books on dentistry. Comprehensive, clear, inexpensive, and easy to read and use. It fills an enormous gap in the health care literature." — Reference & User Services Quarterly, American Library Association, Summer '98

"Recommended reference source."
— Booklist, American Library Association, Dec '97

■

Depression Sourcebook

Basic Consumer Health Information about Unipolar Depression, Bipolar Disorder, Postpartum Depression, Seasonal Affective Disorder, and Other Types of Depression in Children, Adolescents, Women, Men, the Elderly, and Other Selected Populations

Along with Facts about Causes, Risk Factors, Diagnostic Criteria, Treatment Options, Coping Strategies, Suicide Prevention, a Glossary, and a Directory of Sources for Additional Help and Information

Edited by Karen Bellenir. 602 pages. 2002. 978-0-7808-0611-5.

"Depression Sourcebook is of a very high standard. Its purpose, which is to serve as a reference source to the lay reader, is very well served."
— Journal of the National Medical Association, 2004

"Invaluable reference for public and school library collections alike." — Library Bookwatch, Apr '03

"Recommended for purchase."
— American Reference Books Annual, 2003

■

Dermatological Disorders Sourcebook, 2nd Edition

Basic Consumer Health Information about Conditions and Disorders Affecting the Skin, Hair, and Nails, Such as Acne, Rosacea, Rashes, Dermatitis, Pigmentation Disorders, Birthmarks, Skin Cancer, Skin Injuries, Psoriasis, Scleroderma, and Hair Loss, Including Facts about Medications and Treatments for Dermatological Disorders and Tips for Maintaining Healthy Skin, Hair, and Nails

Along with Information about How Aging Affects the Skin, a Glossary of Related Terms, and a Directory of Resources for Additional Help and Information

Edited by Amy L. Sutton. 645 pages. 2005. 978-0-7808-0795-2.

"*. . . comprehensive, easily read reference book.*"
—*Doody's Health Sciences Book Reviews, Oct '97*

SEE ALSO Burns Sourcebook

Diabetes Sourcebook, 3rd Edition

Basic Consumer Health Information about Type 1 Diabetes (Insulin-Dependent or Juvenile-Onset Diabetes), Type 2 Diabetes (Noninsulin-Dependent or Adult-Onset Diabetes), Gestational Diabetes, Impaired Glucose Tolerance (IGT), and Related Complications, Such as Amputation, Eye Disease, Gum Disease, Nerve Damage, and End-Stage Renal Disease, Including Facts about Insulin, Oral Diabetes Medications, Blood Sugar Testing, and the Role of Exercise and Nutrition in the Control of Diabetes

Along with a Glossary and Resources for Further Help and Information

Edited by Dawn D. Matthews. 622 pages. 2003. 978-0-7808-0629-0.

"**This edition is even more helpful than earlier versions. . . . It is a truly valuable tool for anyone seeking readable and authoritative information on diabetes.**"
— *American Reference Books Annual, 2004*

"**An invaluable reference.**" — *Library Journal, May '00*

Selected as one of the 250 "Best Health Sciences Books of 1999." — *Doody's Rating Service, Mar-Apr '00*

"**Provides useful information for the general public.**"
— *Healthlines, University of Michigan Health Management Research Center, Sep/Oct '99*

"*. . . provides reliable mainstream medical information . . . belongs on the shelves of any library with a consumer health collection.*" — *E-Streams, Sep '99*

"**Recommended reference source.**"
— *Booklist, American Library Association, Feb '99*

Diet & Nutrition Sourcebook, 3rd Edition

Basic Consumer Health Information about Dietary Guidelines and the Food Guidance System, Recommended Daily Nutrient Intakes, Serving Proportions, Weight Control, Vitamins and Supplements, Nutrition Issues for Different Life Stages and Lifestyles, and the Needs of People with Specific Medical Concerns, Including Cancer, Celiac Disease, Diabetes, Eating Disorders, Food Allergies, and Cardiovascular Disease

Along with Facts about Federal Nutrition Support Programs, a Glossary of Nutrition and Dietary Terms, and Directories of Additional Resources for More Information about Nutrition

Edited by Joyce Brennfleck Shannon. 633 pages. 2006. 978-0-7808-0800-3.

"**This book is an excellent source of basic diet and nutrition information.**" — *Booklist Health Sciences Supplement, American Library Association, Dec '00*

"**This reference document should be in any public library, but it would be a very good guide for beginning students in the health sciences. If the other books in this publisher's series are as good as this, they should all be in the health sciences collections.**"
— *American Reference Books Annual, 2000*

"**This book is an excellent general nutrition reference for consumers who desire to take an active role in their health care for prevention. Consumers of all ages who select this book can feel confident they are receiving current and accurate information.**" — *Journal of Nutrition for the Elderly, Vol. 19, No. 4, 2000*

SEE ALSO Digestive Diseases & Disorders Sourcebook, Eating Disorders Sourcebook, Gastrointestinal Diseases & Disorders Sourcebook, Vegetarian Sourcebook

---

Digestive Diseases & Disorders Sourcebook

Basic Consumer Health Information about Diseases and Disorders that Impact the Upper and Lower Digestive System, Including Celiac Disease, Crohn's Disease, Cyclic Vomiting Syndrome, Diarrhea, Diverticulosis and Diverticulitis, Gallstones, Heartburn, Hemorrhoids, Hernias, Indigestion (Dyspepsia), Irritable Bowel Syndrome, Lactose Intolerance, Ulcers, and More

Along with Information about Medications and Other Treatments, Tips for Maintaining a Healthy Digestive Tract, a Glossary, and Directory of Digestive Diseases Organizations

Edited by Karen Bellenir. 335 pages. 2000. 978-0-7808-0327-5.

"**This title would be an excellent addition to all public or patient-research libraries.**"
— *American Reference Books Annual, 2001*

"**This title is recommended for public, hospital, and health sciences libraries with consumer health collections.**" — *E-Streams, Jul-Aug '00*

"**Recommended reference source.**"
— *Booklist, American Library Association, May '00*

SEE ALSO Eating Disorders Sourcebook, Gastrointestinal Diseases & Disorders Sourcebook

---

Disabilities Sourcebook

Basic Consumer Health Information about Physical and Psychiatric Disabilities, Including Descriptions of Major Causes of Disability, Assistive and Adaptive Aids, Workplace Issues, and Accessibility Concerns

Along with Information about the Americans with Disabilities Act, a Glossary, and Resources for Additional Help and Information

Edited by Dawn D. Matthews. 616 pages. 2000. 978-0-7808-0389-3.

"**It is a must for libraries with a consumer health section.**" — *American Reference Books Annual, 2002*

"A much needed addition to the Omnigraphics *Health Reference Series*. A current reference work to provide people with disabilities, their families, caregivers or those who work with them, a broad range of information in one volume, has not been available until now. . . . It is recommended for all public and academic library reference collections." —*E-Streams, May '01*

"An excellent source book in easy-to-read format covering many current topics; highly recommended for all libraries." —*Choice, Association of College & Research Libraries, Jan '01*

"Recommended reference source."
—*Booklist, American Library Association, Jul '00*

■

Domestic Violence Sourcebook, 2nd Edition

Basic Consumer Health Information about the Causes and Consequences of Abusive Relationships, Including Physical Violence, Sexual Assault, Battery, Stalking, and Emotional Abuse, and Facts about the Effects of Violence on Women, Men, Young Adults, and the Elderly, with Reports about Domestic Violence in Selected Populations, and Featuring Facts about Medical Care, Victim Assistance and Protection, Prevention Strategies, Mental Health Services, and Legal Issues

Along with a Glossary of Related Terms and Resources for Additional Help and Information

Edited by Dawn D. Matthews. 628 pages. 2004. 978-0-7808-0669-6.

"Educators, clergy, medical professionals, police, and victims and their families will benefit from this realistic and easy-to-understand resource."
—*American Reference Books Annual, 2005*

"Recommended for all collections supporting consumer health information. It should also be considered for any collection needing general, readable information on domestic violence." —*E-Streams, Jan '05*

"This sourcebook complements other books in its field, providing a one-stop resource . . . Recommended."
—*Choice, Association of College & Research Libraries, Jan '05*

"Interested lay persons should find the book extremely beneficial. . . . A copy of *Domestic Violence and Child Abuse Sourcebook* should be in every public library in the United States."
—*Social Science & Medicine, No. 56, 2003*

"This is important information. The Web has many resources but this sourcebook fills an important societal need. I am not aware of any other resources of this type." —*Doody's Review Service, Sep '01*

"Recommended reference source."
—*Booklist, American Library Association, Apr '01*

"Important pick for college-level health reference libraries." —*The Bookwatch, Mar '01*

"Because this problem is so widespread and because this book includes a lot of issues within one volume, this work is recommended for all public libraries."
—*American Reference Books Annual, 2001*

SEE ALSO Child Abuse Sourcebook

■

Drug Abuse Sourcebook, 2nd Edition

Basic Consumer Health Information about Illicit Substances of Abuse and the Misuse of Prescription and Over-the-Counter Medications, Including Depressants, Hallucinogens, Inhalants, Marijuana, Stimulants, and Anabolic Steroids

Along with Facts about Related Health Risks, Treatment Programs, Prevention Programs, a Glossary of Abuse and Addiction Terms, a Glossary of Drug-Related Street Terms, and a Directory of Resources for More Information

Edited by Catherine Ginther. 607 pages. 2004. 978-0-7808-0740-2.

"Commendable for organizing useful, normally scattered government and association-produced data into a logical sequence."
—*American Reference Books Annual, 2006*

"This easy-to-read volume is recommended for consumer health collections within public or academic libraries." —*E-Streams, Sep '05*

"An excellent library reference."
—*The Bookwatch, May '05*

"Containing a wealth of information, this book will be useful to the college student just beginning to explore the topic of substance abuse. This resource belongs in libraries that serve a lower-division undergraduate or community college clientele as well as the general public." —*Choice, Association of College & Research Libraries, Jun '01*

"Recommended reference source."
—*Booklist, American Library Association, Feb '01*

SEE ALSO Alcoholism Sourcebook

■

Ear, Nose & Throat Disorders Sourcebook, 2nd Edition

Basic Consumer Health Information about Disorders of the Ears, Hearing Loss, Vestibular Disorders, Nasal and Sinus Problems, Throat and Vocal Cord Disorders, and Otolaryngologic Cancers, Including Facts about Ear Infections and Injuries, Genetic and Congenital Deafness, Sensorineural Hearing Disorders, Tinnitus, Vertigo, Ménière Disease, Rhinitis, Sinusitis, Snoring, Sore Throats, Hoarseness, and More

Along with Reports on Current Research Initiatives, a Glossary of Related Medical Terms, and a Directory of Sources for Further Help and Information

Edited by Sandra J. Judd. 659 pages. 2006. 978-0-7808-0872-0.

"Overall, this sourcebook is helpful for the consumer seeking information on ENT issues. It is recommended for public libraries."
—*American Reference Books Annual, 1999*

"Recommended reference source."
—*Booklist, American Library Association, Dec '98*

■

Eating Disorders Sourcebook, 2nd Edition

Basic Consumer Health Information about Anorexia Nervosa, Bulimia Nervosa, Binge Eating, Compulsive Exercise, Female Athlete Triad, and Other Eating Disorders, Including Facts about Body Image and Other Cultural and Age-Related Risk Factors, Prevention Efforts, Adverse Health Effects, Treatment Options, and the Recovery Process

Along with Guidelines for Healthy Weight Control, a Glossary, and Directories of Additional Resources

Edited by Joyce Brennfleck Shannon. 585 pages. 2007. 978-0-7808-0948-2.

"Recommended for health science libraries that are open to the public, as well as hospital libraries. This book is a good resource for the consumer who is concerned about eating disorders." — *E-Streams, Mar '02*

"This volume is another convenient collection of excerpted articles. Recommended for school and public library patrons; lower-division undergraduates; and two-year technical program students."
—*Choice, Association of College & Research Libraries, Jan '02*

"Recommended reference source."
— *Booklist, American Library Association, Oct '01*

SEE ALSO *Diet & Nutrition Sourcebook, Digestive Diseases & Disorders Sourcebook, Gastrointestinal Diseases & Disorders Sourcebook*

■

Emergency Medical Services Sourcebook

Basic Consumer Health Information about Preventing, Preparing for, and Managing Emergency Situations, When and Who to Call for Help, What to Expect in the Emergency Room, the Emergency Medical Team, Patient Issues, and Current Topics in Emergency Medicine

Along with Statistical Data, a Glossary, and Sources of Additional Help and Information

Edited by Jenni Lynn Colson. 494 pages. 2002. 978-0-7808-0420-3.

"Handy and convenient for home, public, school, and college libraries. Recommended."
— *Choice, Association of College & Research Libraries, Apr '03*

"This reference can provide the consumer with answers to most questions about emergency care in the United States, or it will direct them to a resource where the answer can be found."
— *American Reference Books Annual, 2003*

"Recommended reference source."
— *Booklist, American Library Association, Feb '03*

■

Endocrine & Metabolic Disorders Sourcebook

Basic Information for the Layperson about Pancreatic and Insulin-Related Disorders Such as Pancreatitis, Diabetes, and Hypoglycemia; Adrenal Gland Disorders Such as Cushing's Syndrome, Addison's Disease, and Congenital Adrenal Hyperplasia; Pituitary Gland Disorders Such as Growth Hormone Deficiency, Acromegaly, and Pituitary Tumors; Thyroid Disorders Such as Hypothyroidism, Graves' Disease, Hashimoto's Disease, and Goiter; Hyperparathyroidism; and Other Diseases and Syndromes of Hormone Imbalance or Metabolic Dysfunction

Along with Reports on Current Research Initiatives

Edited by Linda M. Shin. 574 pages. 1998. 978-0-7808-0207-0.

"Omnigraphics has produced another needed resource for health information consumers."
—*American Reference Books Annual, 2000*

"Recommended reference source."
— *Booklist, American Library Association, Dec '98*

■

Environmental Health Sourcebook, 2nd Edition

Basic Consumer Health Information about the Environment and Its Effect on Human Health, Including the Effects of Air Pollution, Water Pollution, Hazardous Chemicals, Food Hazards, Radiation Hazards, Biological Agents, Household Hazards, Such as Radon, Asbestos, Carbon Monoxide, and Mold, and Information about Associated Diseases and Disorders, Including Cancer, Allergies, Respiratory Problems, and Skin Disorders

Along with Information about Environmental Concerns for Specific Populations, a Glossary of Related Terms, and Resources for Further Help and Information

Edited by Dawn D. Matthews. 673 pages. 2003. 978-0-7808-0632-0.

"This recently updated edition continues the level of quality and the reputation of the numerous other volumes in Omnigraphics' *Health Reference Series.*"
— *American Reference Books Annual, 2004*

"An excellent updated edition."
— *The Bookwatch, Oct '03*

"Recommended reference source."
— *Booklist, American Library Association, Sep '98*

"This book will be a useful addition to anyone's library." — *Choice Health Sciences Supplement, Association of College & Research Libraries, May '98*

". . . a good survey of numerous environmentally induced physical disorders . . . a useful addition to anyone's library."
— *Doody's Health Sciences Book Reviews, Jan '98*

Ethnic Diseases Sourcebook

Basic Consumer Health Information for Ethnic and Racial Minority Groups in the United States, Including General Health Indicators and Behaviors, Ethnic Diseases, Genetic Testing, the Impact of Chronic Diseases, Women's Health, Mental Health Issues, and Preventive Health Care Services

Along with a Glossary and a Listing of Additional Resources

Edited by Joyce Brennfleck Shannon. 664 pages. 2001. 978-0-7808-0336-7.

"Recommended for health sciences libraries where public health programs are a priority."
— *E-Streams, Jan '02*

"Not many books have been written on this topic to date, and the *Ethnic Diseases Sourcebook* is a strong addition to the list. It will be an important introductory resource for health consumers, students, health care personnel, and social scientists. It is recommended for public, academic, and large hospital libraries."
— *American Reference Books Annual, 2002*

"Recommended reference source."
— *Booklist, American Library Association, Oct '01*

"Will prove valuable to any library seeking to maintain a current, comprehensive reference collection of health resources.... An excellent source of health information about genetic disorders which affect particular ethnic and racial minorities in the U.S."
— *The Bookwatch, Aug '01*

■

Eye Care Sourcebook, 2nd Edition

Basic Consumer Health Information about Eye Care and Eye Disorders, Including Facts about the Diagnosis, Prevention, and Treatment of Common Refractive Problems Such as Myopia, Hyperopia, Astigmatism, and Presbyopia, and Eye Diseases, Including Glaucoma, Cataract, Age-Related Macular Degeneration, and Diabetic Retinopathy

Along with a Section on Vision Correction and Refractive Surgeries, Including LASIK and LASEK, a Glossary, and Directories of Resources for Additional Help and Information

Edited by Amy L. Sutton. 543 pages. 2003. 978-0-7808-0635-1.

"... a solid reference tool for eye care and a valuable addition to a collection."
— *American Reference Books Annual, 2004*

■

Family Planning Sourcebook

Basic Consumer Health Information about Planning for Pregnancy and Contraception, Including Traditional Methods, Barrier Methods, Hormonal Methods, Permanent Methods, Future Methods, Emergency Contraception, and Birth Control Choices for Women at Each Stage of Life

Along with Statistics, a Glossary, and Sources of Additional Information

Edited by Amy Marcaccio Keyzer. 520 pages. 2001. 978-0-7808-0379-4.

"Recommended for public, health, and undergraduate libraries as part of the circulating collection."
— *E-Streams, Mar '02*

"Information is presented in an unbiased, readable manner, and the sourcebook will certainly be a necessary addition to those public and high school libraries where Internet access is restricted or otherwise problematic." — *American Reference Books Annual, 2002*

"Recommended reference source."
— *Booklist, American Library Association, Oct '01*

"Will prove valuable to any library seeking to maintain a current, comprehensive reference collection of health resources.... Excellent reference."
— *The Bookwatch, Aug '01*

SEE ALSO Pregnancy & Birth Sourcebook

■

Fitness & Exercise Sourcebook, 3rd Edition

Basic Consumer Health Information about the Physical and Mental Benefits of Fitness, Including Cardiorespiratory Endurance, Muscular Strength, Muscular Endurance, and Flexibility, with Facts about Sports Nutrition and Exercise-Related Injuries and Tips about Physical Activity and Exercises for People of All Ages and for People with Health Concerns

Along with Advice on Selecting and Using Exercise Equipment, Maintaining Exercise Motivation, a Glossary of Related Terms, and a Directory of Resources for More Help and Information

Edited by Amy L. Sutton. 663 pages. 2007. 978-0-7808-0946-8.

"This work is recommended for all general reference collections."
— *American Reference Books Annual, 2002*

"Highly recommended for public, consumer, and school grades fourth through college." — *E-Streams, Nov '01*

"Recommended reference source."
— *Booklist, American Library Association, Oct '01*

"The information appears quite comprehensive and is considered reliable.... This second edition is a welcomed addition to the series."
— *Doody's Review Service, Sep '01*

■

Food Safety Sourcebook

Basic Consumer Health Information about the Safe Handling of Meat, Poultry, Seafood, Eggs, Fruit Juices, and Other Food Items, and Facts about Pesticides, Drinking Water, Food Safety Overseas, and the Onset, Duration, and Symptoms of Foodborne Illnesses, Including Types of Pathogenic Bacteria, Parasitic Protozoa, Worms, Viruses, and Natural Toxins

Along with the Role of the Consumer, the Food Handler, and the Government in Food Safety; a Glossary, and Resources for Additional Help and Information

Edited by Dawn D. Matthews. 339 pages. 1999. 978-0-7808-0326-8.

"This book is recommended for public libraries and universities with home economic and food science programs." — *E-Streams, Nov '00*

"Recommended reference source."
— *Booklist, American Library Association, May '00*

"This book takes the complex issues of food safety and foodborne pathogens and presents them in an easily understood manner. [It does] an excellent job of covering a large and often confusing topic."
— *American Reference Books Annual, 2000*

■

Forensic Medicine Sourcebook

Basic Consumer Information for the Layperson about Forensic Medicine, Including Crime Scene Investigation, Evidence Collection and Analysis, Expert Testimony, Computer-Aided Criminal Identification, Digital Imaging in the Courtroom, DNA Profiling, Accident Reconstruction, Autopsies, Ballistics, Drugs and Explosives Detection, Latent Fingerprints, Product Tampering, and Questioned Document Examination

Along with Statistical Data, a Glossary of Forensics Terminology, and Listings of Sources for Further Help and Information

Edited by Annemarie S. Muth. 574 pages. 1999. 978-0-7808-0232-2.

"Given the expected widespread interest in its content and its easy to read style, this book is recommended for most public and all college and university libraries."
— *E-Streams, Feb '01*

"Recommended for public libraries."
— *Reference & User Services Quarterly, American Library Association, Spring 2000*

"Recommended reference source."
— *Booklist, American Library Association, Feb '00*

"A wealth of information, useful statistics, references are up-to-date and extremely complete. This wonderful collection of data will help students who are interested in a career in any type of forensic field. It is a great resource for attorneys who need information about types of expert witnesses needed in a particular case. It also offers useful information for fiction and nonfiction writers whose work involves a crime. A fascinating compilation. All levels."
— *Choice, Association of College & Research Libraries, Jan '00*

"There are several items that make this book attractive to consumers who are seeking certain forensic data. . . . This is a useful current source for those seeking general forensic medical answers."
— *American Reference Books Annual, 2000*

Gastrointestinal Diseases & Disorders Sourcebook, 2nd Edition

Basic Consumer Health Information about the Upper and Lower Gastrointestinal (GI) Tract, Including the Esophagus, Stomach, Intestines, Rectum, Liver, and Pancreas, with Facts about Gastroesophageal Reflux Disease, Gastritis, Hernias, Ulcers, Celiac Disease, Diverticulitis, Irritable Bowel Syndrome, Hemorrhoids, Gastrointestinal Cancers, and Other Diseases and Disorders Related to the Digestive Process

Along with Information about Commonly Used Diagnostic and Surgical Procedures, Statistics, Reports on Current Research Initiatives and Clinical Trials, a Glossary, and Resources for Additional Help and Information

Edited by Sandra J. Judd. 681 pages. 2006. 978-0-7808-0798-3.

". . . very readable form. The successful editorial work that brought this material together into a useful and understandable reference makes accessible to all readers information that can help them more effectively understand and obtain help for digestive tract problems."
— *Choice, Association of College & Research Libraries, Feb '97*

SEE ALSO *Diet & Nutrition Sourcebook, Digestive Diseases & Disorders Sourcebook, Eating Disorders Sourcebook*

■

Genetic Disorders Sourcebook, 3rd Edition

Basic Consumer Health Information about Hereditary Diseases and Disorders, Including Facts about the Human Genome, Genetic Inheritance Patterns, Disorders Associated with Specific Genes, Such as Sickle Cell Disease, Hemophilia, and Cystic Fibrosis, Chromosome Disorders, Such as Down Syndrome, Fragile X Syndrome, and Turner Syndrome, and Complex Diseases and Disorders Resulting from the Interaction of Environmental and Genetic Factors, Such as Allergies, Cancer, and Obesity

Along with Facts about Genetic Testing, Suggestions for Parents of Children with Special Needs, Reports on Current Research Initiatives, a Glossary of Genetic Terminology, and Resources for Additional Help and Information

Edited by Karen Bellenir. 777 pages. 2004. 978-0-7808-0742-6.

"This text is recommended for any library with an interest in providing consumer health resources."
— *E-Streams, Aug '05*

"This is a valuable resource for anyone wishing to have an understandable description of any of the topics or disorders included. The editor succeeds in making complex genetic issues understandable."
— *Doody's Book Review Service, May '05*

"A good acquisition for public libraries."
— *American Reference Books Annual, 2005*

Head Trauma Sourcebook

Basic Information for the Layperson about Open-Head and Closed-Head Injuries, Treatment Advances, Recovery, and Rehabilitation

Along with Reports on Current Research Initiatives

Edited by Karen Bellenir. 414 pages. 1997. 978-0-7808-0208-7.

Headache Sourcebook

Basic Consumer Health Information about Migraine, Tension, Cluster, Rebound and Other Types of Headaches, with Facts about the Cause and Prevention of Headaches, the Effects of Stress and the Environment, Headaches during Pregnancy and Menopause, and Childhood Headaches

Along with a Glossary and Other Resources for Additional Help and Information

Edited by Dawn D. Matthews. 362 pages. 2002. 978-0-7808-0337-4.

Healthy Aging Sourcebook

Basic Consumer Health Information about Maintaining Health through the Aging Process, Including Advice on Nutrition, Exercise, and Sleep, Help in Making Decisions about Midlife Issues and Retirement, and Guidance Concerning Practical and Informed Choices in Health Consumerism

Along with Data Concerning the Theories of Aging, Different Experiences in Aging by Minority Groups, and Facts about Aging Now and Aging in the Future; and Featuring a Glossary, a Guide to Consumer Help, Additional Suggested Reading, and Practical Resource Directory

Edited by Jenifer Swanson. 536 pages. 1999. 978-0-7808-0390-9.

SEE ALSO *Physical & Mental Issues in Aging Sourcebook*

Healthy Children Sourcebook

Basic Consumer Health Information about the Physical and Mental Development of Children between the Ages of 3 and 12, Including Routine Health Care, Preventative Health Services, Safety and First Aid, Healthy Sleep, Dental Care, Nutrition, and Fitness, and Featuring Parenting Tips on Such Topics as Bedwetting, Choosing Day Care, Monitoring TV and Other Media, and Establishing a Foundation for Substance Abuse Prevention

Along with a Glossary of Commonly Used Pediatric Terms and Resources for Additional Help and Information

Edited by Chad T. Kimball. 647 pages. 2003. 978-0-7808-0247-6.

SEE ALSO *Childhood Diseases & Disorders Sourcebook*

Healthy Heart Sourcebook for Women

Basic Consumer Health Information about Cardiac Issues Specific to Women, Including Facts about Major Risk Factors and Prevention, Treatment and Control Strategies, and Important Dietary Issues

Along with a Special Section Regarding the Pros and Cons of Hormone Replacement Therapy and Its Impact on Heart Health, and Additional Help, Including Recipes, a Glossary, and a Directory of Resources

Edited by Dawn D. Matthews. 336 pages. 2000. 978-0-7808-0329-9.

SEE ALSO *Cardiovascular Diseases & Disorders Sourcebook, Women's Health Concerns Sourcebook*

Hepatitis Sourcebook

Basic Consumer Health Information about Hepatitis A, Hepatitis B, Hepatitis C, and Other Forms of Hepatitis, Including Autoimmune Hepatitis, Alcoholic Hepatitis, Nonalcoholic Steatohepatitis, and Toxic Hepatitis, with

Facts about Risk Factors, Screening Methods, Diagnostic Tests, and Treatment Options

Along with Information on Liver Health, Tips for People Living with Chronic Hepatitis, Reports on Current Research Initiatives, a Glossary of Terms Related to Hepatitis, and a Directory of Sources for Further Help and Information

Edited by Sandra J. Judd. 597 pages. 2005. 978-0-7808-0749-5.

"Highly recommended."
— *American Reference Books Annual, 2006*

▪

Household Safety Sourcebook

Basic Consumer Health Information about Household Safety, Including Information about Poisons, Chemicals, Fire, and Water Hazards in the Home

Along with Advice about the Safe Use of Home Maintenance Equipment, Choosing Toys and Nursery Furniture, Holiday and Recreation Safety, a Glossary, and Resources for Further Help and Information

Edited by Dawn D. Matthews. 606 pages. 2002. 978-0-7808-0338-1.

"This work will be useful in public libraries with large consumer health and wellness departments."
— *American Reference Books Annual, 2003*

"As a sourcebook on household safety this book meets its mark. It is encyclopedic in scope and covers a wide range of safety issues that are commonly seen in the home." — *E-Streams, Jul '02*

▪

Hypertension Sourcebook

Basic Consumer Health Information about the Causes, Diagnosis, and Treatment of High Blood Pressure, with Facts about Consequences, Complications, and Co-Occurring Disorders, Such as Coronary Heart Disease, Diabetes, Stroke, Kidney Disease, and Hypertensive Retinopathy, and Issues in Blood Pressure Control, Including Dietary Choices, Stress Management, and Medications

Along with Reports on Current Research Initiatives and Clinical Trials, a Glossary, and Resources for Additional Help and Information

Edited by Dawn D. Matthews and Karen Bellenir. 613 pages. 2004. 978-0-7808-0674-0.

"Academic, public, and medical libraries will want to add the *Hypertension Sourcebook* to their collections."
— *E-Streams, Aug '05*

"The strength of this source is the wide range of information given about hypertension."
— *American Reference Books Annual, 2005*

▪

Immune System Disorders Sourcebook, 2nd Edition

Basic Consumer Health Information about Disorders of the Immune System, Including Immune System Function and Response, Diagnosis of Immune Disorders, Information about Inherited Immune Disease, Acquired Immune Disease, and Autoimmune Diseases, Including Primary Immune Deficiency, Acquired Immunodeficiency Syndrome (AIDS), Lupus, Multiple Sclerosis, Type 1 Diabetes, Rheumatoid Arthritis, and Graves' Disease

Along with Treatments, Tips for Coping with Immune Disorders, a Glossary, and a Directory of Additional Resources.

Edited by Joyce Brennfleck Shannon. 671 pages. 2005. 978-0-7808-0748-8.

"Highly recommended for academic and public libraries." — *American Reference Books Annual, 2006*

"The updated second edition is a 'must' for any consumer health library seeking a solid resource covering the treatments, symptoms, and options for immune disorder sufferers. . . . An excellent guide."
— *MBR Bookwatch, Jan '06*

▪

Infant & Toddler Health Sourcebook

Basic Consumer Health Information about the Physical and Mental Development of Newborns, Infants, and Toddlers, Including Neonatal Concerns, Nutrition Recommendations, Immunization Schedules, Common Pediatric Disorders, Assessments and Milestones, Safety Tips, and Advice for Parents and Other Caregivers

Along with a Glossary of Terms and Resource Listings for Additional Help

Edited by Jenifer Swanson. 585 pages. 2000. 978-0-7808-0246-9.

"As a reference for the general public, this would be useful in any library." — *E-Streams, May '01*

"Recommended reference source."
— *Booklist, American Library Association, Feb '01*

"This is a good source for general use."
— *American Reference Books Annual, 2001*

▪

Infectious Diseases Sourcebook

Basic Consumer Health Information about Non-Contagious Bacterial, Viral, Prion, Fungal, and Parasitic Diseases Spread by Food and Water, Insects and Animals, or Environmental Contact, Including Botulism, E. Coli, Encephalitis, Legionnaires' Disease, Lyme Disease, Malaria, Plague, Rabies, Salmonella, Tetanus, and Others, and Facts about Newly Emerging Diseases, Such as Hantavirus, Mad Cow Disease, Monkeypox, and West Nile Virus

Along with Information about Preventing Disease Transmission, the Threat of Bioterrorism, and Current Research Initiatives, with a Glossary and Directory of Resources for More Information

Edited by Karen Bellenir. 634 pages. 2004. 978-0-7808-0675-7.

"This reference continues the excellent tradition of the *Health Reference Series* in consolidating a wealth of information on a selected topic into a format that is easy to use and accessible to the general public."
— *American Reference Books Annual, 2005*

"Recommended for public and academic libraries."
— *E-Streams, Jan '05*

Injury & Trauma Sourcebook

Basic Consumer Health Information about the Impact of Injury, the Diagnosis and Treatment of Common and Traumatic Injuries, Emergency Care, and Specific Injuries Related to Home, Community, Workplace, Transportation, and Recreation

Along with Guidelines for Injury Prevention, a Glossary, and a Directory of Additional Resources

Edited by Joyce Brennfleck Shannon. 696 pages. 2002. 978-0-7808-0421-0.

"This publication is the most comprehensive work of its kind about injury and trauma."
— *American Reference Books Annual, 2003*

"This sourcebook provides concise, easily readable, basic health information about injuries. . . . This book is well organized and an easy to use reference resource suitable for hospital, health sciences and public libraries with consumer health collections."
— *E-Streams, Nov '02*

"Practitioners should be aware of guides such as this in order to facilitate their use by patients and their families."
— *Doody's Health Sciences Book Review Journal, Sep-Oct '02*

"Recommended reference source."
— *Booklist, American Library Association, Sep '02*

"Highly recommended for academic and medical reference collections."
— *Library Bookwatch, Sep '02*

Kidney & Urinary Tract Diseases & Disorders Sourcebook

SEE Urinary Tract & Kidney Diseases & Disorders Sourcebook

Learning Disabilities Sourcebook, 2nd Edition

Basic Consumer Health Information about Learning Disabilities, Including Dyslexia, Developmental Speech and Language Disabilities, Non-Verbal Learning Disorders, Developmental Arithmetic Disorder, Developmental Writing Disorder, and Other Conditions That Impede Learning Such as Attention Deficit/Hyperactivity Disorder, Brain Injury, Hearing Impairment, Klinefelter Syndrome, Dyspraxia, and Tourette's Syndrome

Along with Facts about Educational Issues and Assistive Technology, Coping Strategies, a Glossary of Related Terms, and Resources for Further Help and Information

Edited by Dawn D. Matthews. 621 pages. 2003. 978-0-7808-0626-9.

"The second edition of Learning Disabilities Sourcebook far surpasses the earlier edition in that it is more focused on information that will be useful as a consumer health resource."
— *American Reference Books Annual, 2004*

"Teachers as well as consumers will find this an essential guide to understanding various syndromes and their latest treatments. [An] invaluable reference for public and school library collections alike."
— *Library Bookwatch, Apr '03*

Named "Outstanding Reference Book of 1999."
— *New York Public Library, Feb '00*

"An excellent candidate for inclusion in a public library reference section. It's a great source of information. Teachers will also find the book useful. Definitely worth reading."
— *Journal of Adolescent & Adult Literacy, Feb 2000*

"Readable . . . provides a solid base of information regarding successful techniques used with individuals who have learning disabilities, as well as practical suggestions for educators and family members. Clear language, concise descriptions, and pertinent information for contacting multiple resources add to the strength of this book as a useful tool."
— *Choice, Association of College & Research Libraries, Feb '99*

"Recommended reference source."
— *Booklist, American Library Association, Sep '98*

"A useful resource for libraries and for those who don't have the time to identify and locate the individual publications."
— *Disability Resources Monthly, Sep '98*

Leukemia Sourcebook

Basic Consumer Health Information about Adult and Childhood Leukemias, Including Acute Lymphocytic Leukemia (ALL), Chronic Lymphocytic Leukemia (CLL), Acute Myelogenous Leukemia (AML), Chronic Myelogenous Leukemia (CML), and Hairy Cell Leukemia, and Treatments Such as Chemotherapy, Radiation Therapy, Peripheral Blood Stem Cell and Marrow Transplantation, and Immunotherapy

Along with Tips for Life During and After Treatment, a Glossary, and Directories of Additional Resources

Edited by Joyce Brennfleck Shannon. 587 pages. 2003. 978-0-7808-0627-6.

"Unlike other medical books for the layperson, . . . the language does not talk down to the reader. . . . This volume is highly recommended for all libraries."
— *American Reference Books Annual, 2004*

". . . a fine title which ranges from diagnosis to alternative treatments, staging, and tips for life during and after diagnosis."
— *The Bookwatch, Dec '03*

Liver Disorders Sourcebook

Basic Consumer Health Information about the Liver and How It Works; Liver Diseases, Including Cancer, Cirrhosis, Hepatitis, and Toxic and Drug Related Diseases; Tips for Maintaining a Healthy Liver; Laboratory Tests, Radiology Tests, and Facts about Liver Transplantation

Along with a Section on Support Groups, a Glossary, and Resource Listings

Edited by Joyce Brennfleck Shannon. 591 pages. 2000. 978-0-7808-0383-1.

"A valuable resource."
—American Reference Books Annual, 2001

"This title is recommended for health sciences and public libraries with consumer health collections."
—E-Streams, Oct '00

"Recommended reference source."
—Booklist, American Library Association, Jun '00

Lung Disorders Sourcebook

Basic Consumer Health Information about Emphysema, Pneumonia, Tuberculosis, Asthma, Cystic Fibrosis, and Other Lung Disorders, Including Facts about Diagnostic Procedures, Treatment Strategies, Disease Prevention Efforts, and Such Risk Factors as Smoking, Air Pollution, and Exposure to Asbestos, Radon, and Other Agents

Along with a Glossary and Resources for Additional Help and Information

Edited by Dawn D. Matthews. 678 pages. 2002. 978-0-7808-0339-8.

"This title is a great addition for public and school libraries because it provides concise health information on the lungs."
—American Reference Books Annual, 2003

"Highly recommended for academic and medical reference collections." *—Library Bookwatch, Sep '02*

SEE ALSO *Respiratory Diseases & Disorders Sourcebook*

Medical Tests Sourcebook, 2nd Edition

Basic Consumer Health Information about Medical Tests, Including Age-Specific Health Tests, Important Health Screenings and Exams, Home-Use Tests, Blood and Specimen Tests, Electrical Tests, Scope Tests, Genetic Testing, and Imaging Tests, Such as X-Rays, Ultrasound, Computed Tomography, Magnetic Resonance Imaging, Angiography, and Nuclear Medicine

Along with a Glossary and Directory of Additional Resources

Edited by Joyce Brennfleck Shannon. 654 pages. 2004. 978-0-7808-0670-2.

"Recommended for hospital and health sciences

libraries with consumer health collections."
—E-Streams, Mar '00

"This is an overall excellent reference with a wealth of general knowledge that may aid those who are reluctant to get vital tests performed."
—Today's Librarian, Jan '00

"A valuable reference guide."
—American Reference Books Annual, 2000

Men's Health Concerns Sourcebook, 2nd Edition

Basic Consumer Health Information about the Medical and Mental Concerns of Men, Including Theories about the Shorter Male Lifespan, the Leading Causes of Death and Disability, Physical Concerns of Special Significance to Men, Reproductive and Sexual Concerns, Sexually Transmitted Diseases, Men's Mental and Emotional Health, and Lifestyle Choices That Affect Wellness, Such as Nutrition, Fitness, and Substance Use

Along with a Glossary of Related Terms and a Directory of Organizational Resources in Men's Health

Edited by Robert Aquinas McNally. 644 pages. 2004. 978-0-7808-0671-9.

"A very accessible reference for non-specialist general readers and consumers." *—The Bookwatch, Jun '04*

"This comprehensive resource and the series are highly recommended."
—American Reference Books Annual, 2000

"Recommended reference source."
—Booklist, American Library Association, Dec '98

Mental Health Disorders Sourcebook, 3rd Edition

Basic Consumer Health Information about Mental and Emotional Health and Mental Illness, Including Facts about Depression, Bipolar Disorder, and Other Mood Disorders, Phobias, Post-Traumatic Stress Disorder (PTSD), Obsessive-Compulsive Disorder, and Other Anxiety Disorders, Impulse Control Disorders, Eating Disorders, Personality Disorders, and Psychotic Disorders, Including Schizophrenia and Dissociative Disorders

Along with Statistical Information, a Special Section Concerning Mental Health Issues in Children and Adolescents, a Glossary, and Directories of Resources for Additional Help and Information

Edited by Karen Bellenir. 661 pages. 2005. 978-0-7808-0747-1.

"Recommended for public libraries and academic libraries with an undergraduate program in psychology."
—American Reference Books Annual, 2006

"Recommended reference source."
—Booklist, American Library Association, Jun '00

Mental Retardation Sourcebook

Basic Consumer Health Information about Mental Retardation and Its Causes, Including Down Syndrome, Fetal Alcohol Syndrome, Fragile X Syndrome, Genetic Conditions, Injury, and Environmental Sources

Along with Preventive Strategies, Parenting Issues, Educational Implications, Health Care Needs, Employment and Economic Matters, Legal Issues, a Glossary, and a Resource Listing for Additional Help and Information

Edited by Joyce Brennfleck Shannon. 642 pages. 2000. 978-0-7808-0377-0.

"Public libraries will find the book useful for reference and as a beginning research point for students, parents, and caregivers."
— *American Reference Books Annual, 2001*

"The strength of this work is that it compiles many basic fact sheets and addresses for further information in one volume. It is intended and suitable for the general public. This sourcebook is relevant to any collection providing health information to the general public."
— *E-Streams, Nov '00*

"From preventing retardation to parenting and family challenges, this covers health, social and legal issues and will prove an invaluable overview."
— *Reviewer's Bookwatch, Jul '00*

Movement Disorders Sourcebook

Basic Consumer Health Information about Neurological Movement Disorders, Including Essential Tremor, Parkinson's Disease, Dystonia, Cerebral Palsy, Huntington's Disease, Myasthenia Gravis, Multiple Sclerosis, and Other Early-Onset and Adult-Onset Movement Disorders, Their Symptoms and Causes, Diagnostic Tests, and Treatments

Along with Mobility and Assistive Technology Information, a Glossary, and a Directory of Additional Resources

Edited by Joyce Brennfleck Shannon. 655 pages. 2003. 978-0-7808-0628-3.

". . . a good resource for consumers and recommended for public, community college and undergraduate libraries." — *American Reference Books Annual, 2004*

Muscular Dystrophy Sourcebook

Basic Consumer Health Information about Congenital, Childhood-Onset, and Adult-Onset Forms of Muscular Dystrophy, Such as Duchenne, Becker, Emery-Dreifuss, Distal, Limb-Girdle, Facioscapulohumeral (FSHD), Myotonic, and Ophthalmoplegic Muscular Dystrophies, Including Facts about Diagnostic Tests, Medical and Physical Therapies, Management of Co-Occurring Conditions, and Parenting Guidelines

Along with Practical Tips for Home Care, a Glossary, and Directories of Additional Resources

Edited by Joyce Brennfleck Shannon. 577 pages. 2004. 978-0-7808-0676-4.

"This book is highly recommended for public and academic libraries as well as health care offices that support the information needs of patients and their families."
— *E-Streams, Apr '05*

"Excellent reference." — *The Bookwatch, Jan '05*

Obesity Sourcebook

Basic Consumer Health Information about Diseases and Other Problems Associated with Obesity, and Including Facts about Risk Factors, Prevention Issues, and Management Approaches

Along with Statistical and Demographic Data, Information about Special Populations, Research Updates, a Glossary, and Source Listings for Further Help and Information

Edited by Wilma Caldwell and Chad T. Kimball. 376 pages. 2001. 978-0-7808-0333-6.

"The book synthesizes the reliable medical literature on obesity into one easy-to-read and useful resource for the general public."
— *American Reference Books Annual, 2002*

"This is a very useful resource book for the lay public."
— *Doody's Review Service, Nov '01*

"Well suited for the health reference collection of a public library or an academic health science library that serves the general population." — *E-Streams, Sep '01*

"Recommended reference source."
— *Booklist, American Library Association, Apr '01*

"Recommended pick both for specialty health library collections and any general consumer health reference collection." — *The Bookwatch, Apr '01*

Oral Health Sourcebook

SEE Dental Care & Oral Health Sourcebook

Osteoporosis Sourcebook

Basic Consumer Health Information about Primary and Secondary Osteoporosis and Juvenile Osteoporosis and Related Conditions, Including Fibrous Dysplasia, Gaucher Disease, Hyperthyroidism, Hypophosphatasia, Myeloma, Osteopetrosis, Osteogenesis Imperfecta, and Paget's Disease

Along with Information about Risk Factors, Treatments, Traditional and Non-Traditional Pain Management, a Glossary of Related Terms, and a Directory of Resources

Edited by Allan R. Cook. 584 pages. 2001. 978-0-7808-0239-1.

"This would be a book to be kept in a staff or patient library. The targeted audience is the layperson, but the therapist who needs a quick bit of information on a particular topic will also find the book useful."
— *Physical Therapy, Jan '02*

"This resource is recommended as a great reference source for public, health, and academic libraries, and is another triumph for the editors of Omnigraphics."
—*American Reference Books Annual, 2002*

"Recommended for all public libraries and general health collections, especially those supporting patient education or consumer health programs."
—*E-Streams, Nov '01*

"Will prove valuable to any library seeking to maintain a current, comprehensive reference collection of health resources. . . . From prevention to treatment and associated conditions, this provides an excellent survey."
—*The Bookwatch, Aug '01*

"Recommended reference source."
—*Booklist, American Library Association, Jul '01*

SEE ALSO *Healthy Aging Sourcebook, Physical &* *Mental Issues in Aging Sourcebook, Women's Health Concerns Sourcebook*

Pain Sourcebook, 2nd Edition

Basic Consumer Health Information about Specific Forms of Acute and Chronic Pain, Including Muscle and Skeletal Pain, Nerve Pain, Cancer Pain, and Disorders Characterized by Pain, Such as Fibromyalgia, Shingles, Angina, Arthritis, and Headaches

Along with Information about Pain Medications and Management Techniques, Complementary and Alternative Pain Relief Options, Tips for People Living with Chronic Pain, a Glossary, and a Directory of Sources for Further Information

Edited by Karen Bellenir. 670 pages. 2002. 978-0-7808-0612-2.

"A source of valuable information. . . . This book offers help to nonmedical people who need information about pain and pain management. It is also an excellent reference for those who participate in patient education."
—*Doody's Review Service, Sep '02*

"Highly recommended for academic and medical reference collections." —*Library Bookwatch, Sep '02*

"The text is readable, easily understood, and well indexed. This excellent volume belongs in all patient education libraries, consumer health sections of public libraries, and many personal collections."
—*American Reference Books Annual, 1999*

"The information is basic in terms of scholarship and is appropriate for general readers. Written in journalistic style . . . intended for non-professionals. Quite thorough in its coverage of different pain conditions and summarizes the latest clinical information regarding pain treatment." —*Choice, Association of College and Research Libraries, Jun '98*

"Recommended reference source."
—*Booklist, American Library Association, Mar '98*

Pediatric Cancer Sourcebook

Basic Consumer Health Information about Leukemias, Brain Tumors, Sarcomas, Lymphomas, and Other Cancers in Infants, Children, and Adolescents, Including Descriptions of Cancers, Treatments, and Coping Strategies

Along with Suggestions for Parents, Caregivers, and Concerned Relatives, a Glossary of Cancer Terms, and Resource Listings

Edited by Edward J. Prucha. 587 pages. 1999. 978-0-7808-0245-2.

"An excellent source of information. Recommended for public, hospital, and health science libraries with consumer health collections." —*E-Streams, Jun '00*

"Recommended reference source."
—*Booklist, American Library Association, Feb '00*

"A valuable addition to all libraries specializing in health services and many public libraries."
—*American Reference Books Annual, 2000*

SEE ALSO *Childhood Diseases &* *Disorders Sourcebook, Healthy Children Sourcebook*

Physical & Mental Issues in Aging Sourcebook

Basic Consumer Health Information on Physical and Mental Disorders Associated with the Aging Process, Including Concerns about Cardiovascular Disease, Pulmonary Disease, Oral Health, Digestive Disorders, Musculoskeletal and Skin Disorders, Metabolic Changes, Sexual and Reproductive Issues, and Changes in Vision, Hearing, and Other Senses

Along with Data about Longevity and Causes of Death, Information on Acute and Chronic Pain, Descriptions of Mental Concerns, a Glossary of Terms, and Resource Listings for Additional Help

Edited by Jenifer Swanson. 660 pages. 1999. 978-0-7808-0233-9.

"This is a treasure of health information for the layperson." — *Choice Health Sciences Supplement, Association of College &* *Research Libraries, May '00*

"Recommended for public libraries."
—*American Reference Books Annual, 2000*

"Recommended reference source."
—*Booklist, American Library Association, Oct '99*

SEE ALSO *Healthy Aging Sourcebook*

Podiatry Sourcebook, 2nd Edition

Basic Consumer Health Information about Disorders, Diseases, Deformities, and Injuries that Affect the Foot and Ankle, Including Sprains, Corns, Calluses, Bunions, Plantar Warts, Plantar Fasciitis, Neuromas, Clubfoot, Flat Feet, Achilles Tendonitis, and Much More

Along with Information about Selecting a Foot Care Specialist, Foot Fitness, Shoes and Socks, Diagnostic Tests and Corrective Procedures, Financial Assistance for Corrective Devices, a Glossary of Related Terms, and a *Directory of Resources for Additional Help and Information*

Edited by Ivy L. Alexander. 543 pages. 2007. 978-0-7808-0944-4.

"Recommended reference source."
— *Booklist, American Library Association, Feb '02*

"There is a lot of information presented here on a topic that is usually only covered sparingly in most larger comprehensive medical encyclopedias."
— *American Reference Books Annual, 2002*

■

Pregnancy & Birth Sourcebook, 2nd Edition

Basic Consumer Health Information about Conception and Pregnancy, Including Facts about Fertility, Infertility, Pregnancy Symptoms and Complications, Fetal Growth and Development, Labor, Delivery, and the Postpartum Period, as Well as Information about Maintaining Health and Wellness during Pregnancy and Caring for a Newborn

Along with Information about Public Health Assistance for Low-Income Pregnant Women, a Glossary, and Directories of Agencies and Organizations Providing Help and Support

Edited by Amy L. Sutton. 626 pages. 2004. 978-0-7808-0672-6.

"Will appeal to public and school reference collections strong in medicine and women's health. . . . Deserves a spot on any medical reference shelf."
— *The Bookwatch, Jul '04*

"A well-organized handbook. Recommended."
— *Choice, Association of College & Research Libraries, Apr '98*

"Recommended reference source."
— *Booklist, American Library Association, Mar '98*

"Recommended for public libraries."
— *American Reference Books Annual, 1998*

SEE ALSO *Breastfeeding Sourcebook, Congenital Disorders Sourcebook, Family Planning Sourcebook*

■

Prostate & Urological Disorders Sourcebook

Basic Consumer Health Information about Urogenital and Sexual Disorders in Men, Including Prostate and Other Andrological Cancers, Prostatitis, Benign Prostatic Hyperplasia, Testicular and Penile Trauma, Cryptorchidism, Peyronie Disease, Erectile Dysfunction, and Male Factor Infertility, and Facts about Commonly Used Tests and Procedures, Such as Prostatectomy, Vasectomy, Vasectomy Reversal, Penile Implants, and Semen Analysis

Along with a Glossary of Andrological Terms and a Directory of Resources for Additional Information

Edited by Karen Bellenir. 631 pages. 2005. 978-0-7808-0797-6.

Prostate Cancer Sourcebook

Basic Consumer Health Information about Prostate Cancer, Including Information about the Associated Risk Factors, Detection, Diagnosis, and Treatment of Prostate Cancer

Along with Information on Non-Malignant Prostate Conditions, and Featuring a Section Listing Support and Treatment Centers and a Glossary of Related Terms

Edited by Dawn D. Matthews. 358 pages. 2001. 978-0-7808-0324-4.

"Recommended reference source."
— *Booklist, American Library Association, Jan '02*

"A valuable resource for health care consumers seeking information on the subject. . . . All text is written in a clear, easy-to-understand language that avoids technical jargon. Any library that collects consumer health resources would strengthen their collection with the addition of the *Prostate Cancer Sourcebook*."
— *American Reference Books Annual, 2002*

SEE ALSO *Men's Health Concerns Sourcebook*

■

Reconstructive & Cosmetic Surgery Sourcebook

Basic Consumer Health Information on Cosmetic and Reconstructive Plastic Surgery, Including Statistical Information about Different Surgical Procedures, Things to Consider Prior to Surgery, Plastic Surgery Techniques and Tools, Emotional and Psychological Considerations, and Procedure-Specific Information

Along with a Glossary of Terms and a Listing of Resources for Additional Help and Information

Edited by M. Lisa Weatherford. 374 pages. 2001. 978-0-7808-0214-8.

"An excellent reference that addresses cosmetic and medically necessary reconstructive surgeries. . . . The style of the prose is calm and reassuring, discussing the many positive outcomes now available due to advances in surgical techniques."
— *American Reference Books Annual, 2002*

"Recommended for health science libraries that are open to the public, as well as hospital libraries that are open to the patients. This book is a good resource for the consumer interested in plastic surgery."
— *E-Streams, Dec '01*

"Recommended reference source."
— *Booklist, American Library Association, Jul '01*

■

Rehabilitation Sourcebook

Basic Consumer Health Information about Rehabilitation for People Recovering from Heart Surgery, Spinal Cord Injury, Stroke, Orthopedic Impairments, Amputation, Pulmonary Impairments, Traumatic Injury, and More, Including Physical Therapy, Occupational Therapy, Speech/Language Therapy, Massage Therapy, Dance Therapy, Art Therapy, and Recreational Therapy

Along with Information on Assistive and Adaptive Devices, a Glossary, and Resources for Additional Help and Information

Edited by Dawn D. Matthews. 531 pages. 1999. 978-0-7808-0236-0.

"This is an excellent resource for public library reference and health collections."
— American Reference Books Annual, 2001

"Recommended reference source."
— Booklist, American Library Association, May '00

Respiratory Diseases & Disorders Sourcebook

Basic Information about Respiratory Diseases and Disorders, Including Asthma, Cystic Fibrosis, Pneumonia, the Common Cold, Influenza, and Others, Featuring Facts about the Respiratory System, Statistical and Demographic Data, Treatments, Self-Help Management Suggestions, and Current Research Initiatives

Edited by Allan R. Cook and Peter D. Dresser. 771 pages. 1995. 978-0-7808-0037-3.

"Designed for the layperson and for patients and their families coping with respiratory illness. . . . an extensive array of information on diagnosis, treatment, management, and prevention of respiratory illnesses for the general reader." — Choice, Association of College & Research Libraries, Jun '96

"A highly recommended text for all collections. It is a comforting reminder of the power of knowledge that good books carry between their covers."
— Academic Library Book Review, Spring '96

"A comprehensive collection of authoritative information presented in a nontechnical, humanitarian style for patients, families, and caregivers."
—Association of Operating Room Nurses, Sep/Oct '95

SEE ALSO Lung Disorders Sourcebook

Sexually Transmitted Diseases Sourcebook, 3rd Edition

Basic Consumer Health Information about Chlamydial Infections, Gonorrhea, Hepatitis, Herpes, HIV/AIDS, Human Papillomavirus, Pubic Lice, Scabies, Syphilis, Trichomoniasis, Vaginal Infections, and Other Sexually Transmitted Diseases, Including Facts about Risk Factors, Symptoms, Diagnosis, Treatment, and the Prevention of Sexually Transmitted Infections

Along with Updates on Current Research Initiatives, a Glossary of Related Terms, and Resources for Additional Help and Information

Edited by Amy L. Sutton. 629 pages. 2006. 978-0-7808-0824-9.

"Recommended for consumer health collections in public libraries, and secondary school and community college libraries."
— American Reference Books Annual, 2002

"Every school and public library should have a copy of this comprehensive and user-friendly reference book."
— Choice, Association of College & Research Libraries, Sep '01

"This is a highly recommended book. This is an especially important book for all school and public libraries."
— AIDS Book Review Journal, Jul-Aug '01

"Recommended reference source."
— Booklist, American Library Association, Apr '01

Sleep Disorders Sourcebook, 2nd Edition

Basic Consumer Health Information about Sleep and Sleep Disorders, Including Insomnia, Sleep Apnea, Restless Legs Syndrome, Narcolepsy, Parasomnias, and Other Health Problems That Affect Sleep, Plus Facts about Diagnostic Procedures, Treatment Strategies, Sleep Medications, and Tips for Improving Sleep Quality

Along with a Glossary of Related Terms and Resources for Additional Help and Information

Edited by Amy L. Sutton. 567 pages. 2005. 978-0-7808-0743-3.

"This book will be useful for just about everybody, especially the 40 million Americans with sleep disorders."
— American Reference Books Annual, 2006

"Recommended for public libraries and libraries supporting health care professionals." — E-Streams, Sep '05

". . . key medical library acquisition."
— The Bookwatch, Jun '05

Smoking Concerns Sourcebook

Basic Consumer Health Information about Nicotine Addiction and Smoking Cessation, Featuring Facts about the Health Effects of Tobacco Use, Including Lung and Other Cancers, Heart Disease, Stroke, and Respiratory Disorders, Such as Emphysema and Chronic Bronchitis

Along with Information about Smoking Prevention Programs, Suggestions for Achieving and Maintaining a Smoke-Free Lifestyle, Statistics about Tobacco Use, Reports on Current Research Initiatives, a Glossary of Related Terms, and Directories of Resources for Additional Help and Information

Edited by Karen Bellenir. 621 pages. 2004. 978-0-7808-0323-7.

"Provides everything needed for the student or general reader seeking practical details on the effects of tobacco use." — The Bookwatch, Mar '05

"Public libraries and consumer health care libraries will find this work useful."
— American Reference Books Annual, 2005

Sports Injuries Sourcebook, 3rd Edition

Basic Consumer Health Information about Sprains and Strains, Fractures, Growth Plate Injuries, Overtraining Injuries, and Injuries to the Head, Face, Shoulders, Elbows, Hands, Spinal Column, Knees, Ankles, and Feet, and with Facts about Heat-Related Illness, Steroids and Sport Supplements, Protective Equipment, Diagnostic Procedures, Treatment Options, and Rehabilitation

Along with a Glossary of Related Terms and a Directory of Resources for Additional Help and Information

Edited by Sandra J. Judd. 651 pages. 2007. 978-0-7808-0949-9.

"This is an excellent reference for consumers and it is recommended for public, community college, and undergraduate libraries."
— *American Reference Books Annual, 2003*

"Recommended reference source."
— *Booklist, American Library Association, Feb '03*

■

Stress-Related Disorders Sourcebook

Basic Consumer Health Information about Stress and Stress-Related Disorders, Including Stress Origins and Signals, Environmental Stress at Work and Home, Mental and Emotional Stress Associated with Depression, Post-Traumatic Stress Disorder, Panic Disorder, Suicide, and the Physical Effects of Stress on the Cardiovascular, Immune, and Nervous Systems

Along with Stress Management Techniques, a Glossary, and a Listing of Additional Resources

Edited by Joyce Brennfleck Shannon. 610 pages. 2002. 978-0-7808-0560-6.

"Well written for a general readership, the *Stress-Related Disorders Sourcebook* is a useful addition to the health reference literature."
— *American Reference Books Annual, 2003*

"I am impressed by the amount of information. It offers a thorough overview of the causes and consequences of stress for the layperson. . . . A well-done and thorough reference guide for professionals and nonprofessionals alike."
— *Doody's Review Service, Dec '02*

■

Stroke Sourcebook

Basic Consumer Health Information about Stroke, Including Ischemic, Hemorrhagic, Transient Ischemic Attack (TIA), and Pediatric Stroke, Stroke Triggers and Risks, Diagnostic Tests, Treatments, and Rehabilitation Information

Along with Stroke Prevention Guidelines, Legal and Financial Information, a Glossary, and a Directory of Additional Resources

Edited by Joyce Brennfleck Shannon. 606 pages. 2003. 978-0-7808-0630-6.

"This volume is highly recommended and should be in every medical, hospital, and public library."
— *American Reference Books Annual, 2004*

"Highly recommended for the amount and variety of topics and information covered." — *Choice, Nov '03*

■

Surgery Sourcebook

Basic Consumer Health Information about Inpatient and Outpatient Surgeries, Including Cardiac, Vascular, Orthopedic, Ocular, Reconstructive, Cosmetic, Gynecologic, and Ear, Nose, and Throat Procedures and More

Along with Information about Operating Room Policies and Instruments, Laser Surgery Techniques, Hospital Errors, Statistical Data, a Glossary, and Listings of Sources for Further Help and Information

Edited by Annemarie S. Muth and Karen Bellenir. 596 pages. 2002. 978-0-7808-0380-0.

"Large public libraries and medical libraries would benefit from this material in their reference collections."
— *American Reference Books Annual, 2004*

"Invaluable reference for public and school library collections alike." — *Library Bookwatch, Apr '03*

■

Thyroid Disorders Sourcebook

Basic Consumer Health Information about Disorders of the Thyroid and Parathyroid Glands, Including Hypothyroidism, Hyperthyroidism, Graves Disease, Hashimoto Thyroiditis, Thyroid Cancer, and Parathyroid Disorders, Featuring Facts about Symptoms, Risk Factors, Tests, and Treatments

Along with Information about the Effects of Thyroid Imbalance on Other Body Systems, Environmental Factors That Affect the Thyroid Gland, a Glossary, and a Directory of Additional Resources

Edited by Joyce Brennfleck Shannon. 599 pages. 2005. 978-0-7808-0745-7.

"Recommended for consumer health collections."
— *American Reference Books Annual, 2006*

"Highly recommended pick for basic consumer health reference holdings at all levels."
— *The Bookwatch, Aug '05*

■

Transplantation Sourcebook

Basic Consumer Health Information about Organ and Tissue Transplantation, Including Physical and Financial Preparations, Procedures and Issues Relating to Specific Solid Organ and Tissue Transplants, Rehabilitation, Pediatric Transplant Information, the Future of Transplantation, and Organ and Tissue Donation

Along with a Glossary and Listings of Additional Resources

Edited by Joyce Brennfleck Shannon. 628 pages. 2002. 978-0-7808-0322-0.

"Along with these advances [in transplantation technology] have come a number of daunting questions for potential transplant patients, their families, and their health care providers. This reference text is the best single tool to address many of these questions. . . . It will be a much-needed addition to the reference collections in health care, academic, and large public libraries."
— *American Reference Books Annual, 2003*

"Recommended for libraries with an interest in offering consumer health information." — *E-Streams, Jul '02*

"This is a unique and valuable resource for patients facing transplantation and their families."
— *Doody's Review Service, Jun '02*

▪

Traveler's Health Sourcebook

Basic Consumer Health Information for Travelers, Including Physical and Medical Preparations, Transportation Health and Safety, Essential Information about Food and Water, Sun Exposure, Insect and Snake Bites, Camping and Wilderness Medicine, and Travel with Physical or Medical Disabilities

Along with International Travel Tips, Vaccination Recommendations, Geographical Health Issues, Disease Risks, a Glossary, and a Listing of Additional Resources

Edited by Joyce Brennfleck Shannon. 613 pages. 2000. 978-0-7808-0384-8.

"Recommended reference source."
— *Booklist, American Library Association, Feb '01*

"This book is recommended for any public library, any travel collection, and especially any collection for the physically disabled."
— *American Reference Books Annual, 2001*

SEE ALSO Worldwide Health Sourcebook

▪

Urinary Tract & Kidney Diseases & Disorders Sourcebook, 2nd Edition

Basic Consumer Health Information about the Urinary System, Including the Bladder, Urethra, Ureters, and Kidneys, with Facts about Urinary Tract Infections, Incontinence, Congenital Disorders, Kidney Stones, Cancers of the Urinary Tract and Kidneys, Kidney Failure, Dialysis, and Kidney Transplantation

Along with Statistical and Demographic Information, Reports on Current Research in Kidney and Urologic Health, a Summary of Commonly Used Diagnostic Tests, a Glossary of Related Terms, and a Directory of Resources for Additional Help and Information

Edited by Ivy L. Alexander. 649 pages. 2005. 978-0-7808-0750-1.

"A good choice for a consumer health information library or for a medical library needing information to refer to their patients."
— *American Reference Books Annual, 2006*

Vegetarian Sourcebook

Basic Consumer Health Information about Vegetarian Diets, Lifestyle, and Philosophy, Including Definitions of Vegetarianism and Veganism, Tips about Adopting Vegetarianism, Creating a Vegetarian Pantry, and Meeting Nutritional Needs of Vegetarians, with Facts Regarding Vegetarianism's Effect on Pregnant and Lactating Women, Children, Athletes, and Senior Citizens

Along with a Glossary of Commonly Used Vegetarian Terms and Resources for Additional Help and Information

Edited by Chad T. Kimball. 360 pages. 2002. 978-0-7808-0439-5.

"Organizes into one concise volume the answers to the most common questions concerning vegetarian diets and lifestyles. This title is recommended for public and secondary school libraries." — *E-Streams, Apr '03*

"Invaluable reference for public and school library collections alike." — *Library Bookwatch, Apr '03*

"The articles in this volume are easy to read and come from authoritative sources. The book does not necessarily support the vegetarian diet but instead provides the pros and cons of this important decision. The Vegetarian Sourcebook is recommended for public libraries and consumer health libraries."
— *American Reference Books Annual, 2003*

SEE ALSO Diet & Nutrition Sourcebook

▪

Women's Health Concerns Sourcebook, 2nd Edition

Basic Consumer Health Information about the Medical and Mental Concerns of Women, Including Maintaining Health and Wellness, Gynecological Concerns, Breast Health, Sexuality and Reproductive Issues, Menopause, Cancer in Women, Leading Causes of Death and Disability among Women, Physical Concerns of Special Significance to Women, and Women's Mental and Emotional Health

Along with a Glossary of Related Terms and Directories of Resources for Additional Help and Information

Edited by Amy L. Sutton. 746 pages. 2004. 978-0-7808-0673-3.

"This is a useful reference book, which makes the reader knowledgeable about several issues that concern women's health. It is recommended for public libraries and home library collections." — *E-Streams, May '05*

"A useful addition to public and consumer health library collections."
— *American Reference Books Annual, 2005*

"A highly recommended title."
— *The Bookwatch, May '04*

"Handy compilation. There is an impressive range of diseases, devices, disorders, procedures, and other physical and emotional issues covered . . . well organized, illustrated, and indexed." — *Choice, Association of College & Research Libraries, Jan '98*

SEE ALSO *Breast Cancer Sourcebook, Cancer Sourcebook for Women, Healthy Heart Sourcebook for Women, Osteoporosis Sourcebook*

Workplace Health & Safety Sourcebook

Basic Consumer Health Information about Workplace Health and Safety, Including the Effect of Workplace Hazards on the Lungs, Skin, Heart, Ears, Eyes, Brain, Reproductive Organs, Musculoskeletal System, and Other Organs and Body Parts

Along with Information about Occupational Cancer, Personal Protective Equipment, Toxic and Hazardous Chemicals, Child Labor, Stress, and Workplace Violence

Edited by Chad T. Kimball. 626 pages. 2000. 978-0-7808-0231-5.

"As a reference for the general public, this would be useful in any library." — *E-Streams, Jun '01*

"Provides helpful information for primary care physicians and other caregivers interested in occupational medicine. . . . General readers; professionals."
— *Choice, Association of College & Research Libraries, May '01*

"Recommended reference source."
— *Booklist, American Library Association, Feb '01*

"Highly recommended." — *The Bookwatch, Jan '01*

Worldwide Health Sourcebook

Basic Information about Global Health Issues, Including Malnutrition, Reproductive Health, Disease Dispersion and Prevention, Emerging Diseases, Risky Health Behaviors, and the Leading Causes of Death

Along with Global Health Concerns for Children, Women, and the Elderly, Mental Health Issues, Research and Technology Advancements, and Economic, Environmental, and Political Health Implications, a Glossary, and a Resource Listing for Additional Help and Information

Edited by Joyce Brennfleck Shannon. 614 pages. 2001. 978-0-7808-0330-5.

"Named an Outstanding Academic Title."
— *Choice, Association of College & Research Libraries, Jan '02*

"Yet another handy but also unique compilation in the extensive *Health Reference Series*, this is a useful work because many of the international publications reprinted or excerpted are not readily available. Highly recommended." — *Choice, Association of College & Research Libraries, Nov '01*

"Recommended reference source."
— *Booklist, American Library Association, Oct '01*

SEE ALSO *Traveler's Health Sourcebook*

621

Teen Health Series

Helping Young Adults Understand, Manage, and Avoid Serious Illness

List price $65 per volume. **School and library price $58 per volume.**

Alcohol Information for Teens

Health Tips about Alcohol and Alcoholism

Including Facts about Underage Drinking, Preventing Teen Alcohol Use, Alcohol's Effects on the Brain and the Body, Alcohol Abuse Treatment, Help for Children of Alcoholics, and More

Edited by Joyce Brennfleck Shannon. 370 pages. 2005. 978-0-7808-0741-9.

"Boxed facts and tips add visual interest to the well-researched and clearly written text."
— *Curriculum Connection, Apr '06*

Allergy Information for Teens

Health Tips about Allergic Reactions Such as Anaphylaxis, Respiratory Problems, and Rashes

Including Facts about Identifying and Managing Allergies to Food, Pollen, Mold, Animals, Chemicals, Drugs, and Other Substances

Edited by Karen Bellenir. 410 pages. 2006. 978-0-7808-0799-0.

Asthma Information for Teens

Health Tips about Managing Asthma and Related Concerns

Including Facts about Asthma Causes, Triggers, Symptoms, Diagnosis, and Treatment

Edited by Karen Bellenir. 386 pages. 2005. 978-0-7808-0770-9.

"Highly recommended for medical libraries, public school libraries, and public libraries."
— *American Reference Books Annual, 2006*

"It is so clearly written and well organized that even hesitant readers will be able to find the facts they need, whether for reports or personal information. . . . A succinct but complete resource."
— *School Library Journal, Sep '05*

Body Information for Teens

Health Tips about Maintaining Well-Being for a Lifetime

Including Facts about the Development and Functioning of the Body's Systems, Organs, and Structures and the Health Impact of Lifestyle Choices

Edited by Sandra Augustyn Lawton. 458 pages. 2007. 978-0-7808-0443-2.

Cancer Information for Teens

Health Tips about Cancer Awareness, Prevention, Diagnosis, and Treatment

Including Facts about Frequently Occurring Cancers, Cancer Risk Factors, and Coping Strategies for Teens Fighting Cancer or Dealing with Cancer in Friends or Family Members

Edited by Wilma R. Caldwell. 428 pages. 2004. 978-0-7808-0678-8.

"Recommended for school libraries, or consumer libraries that see a lot of use by teens."
— *E-Streams, May '05*

"A valuable educational tool."
— *American Reference Books Annual, 2005*

"Young adults and their parents alike will find this new addition to the *Teen Health Series* an important reference to cancer in teens."
— *Children's Bookwatch, Feb '05*

Complementary and Alternative Medicine Information for Teens

Health Tips about Non-Traditional and Non-Western Medical Practices

Including Information about Acupuncture, Chiropractic Medicine, Dietary and Herbal Supplements, Hypnosis, Massage Therapy, Prayer and Spirituality, Reflexology, Yoga, and More

Edited by Sandra Augustyn Lawton. 405 pages. 2006. 978-0-7808-0966-6.

Diabetes Information for Teens

Health Tips about Managing Diabetes and Preventing Related Complications

Including Information about Insulin, Glucose Control, Healthy Eating, Physical Activity, and Learning to Live with Diabetes

Edited by Sandra Augustyn Lawton. 410 pages. 2006. 978-0-7808-0811-9.

Diet Information for Teens, 2nd Edition

Health Tips about Diet and Nutrition

Including Facts about Dietary Guidelines, Food Groups, Nutrients, Healthy Meals, Snacks, Weight Control, Medical Concerns Related to Diet, and More

Edited by Karen Bellenir. 432 pages. 2006. 978-0-7808-0820-1.

"Full of helpful insights and facts throughout the book. ... An excellent resource to be placed in public libraries or even in personal collections."
— American Reference Books Annual, 2002

"Recommended for middle and high school libraries and media centers as well as academic libraries that educate future teachers of teenagers. It is also a suitable addition to health science libraries that serve patrons who are interested in teen health promotion and education."
— E-Streams, Oct '01

"This comprehensive book would be beneficial to collections that need information about nutrition, dietary guidelines, meal planning, and weight control. ... This reference is so easy to use that its purchase is recommended."
— The Book Report, Sep-Oct '01

"This book is written in an easy to understand format describing issues that many teens face every day, and then provides thoughtful explanations so that teens can make informed decisions. This is an interesting book that provides important facts and information for today's teens."
— Doody's Health Sciences Book Review Journal, Jul-Aug '01

"A comprehensive compendium of diet and nutrition. The information is presented in a straightforward, plain-spoken manner. This title will be useful to those working on reports on a variety of topics, as well as to general readers concerned about their dietary health."
— School Library Journal, Jun '01

Drug Information for Teens, 2nd Edition

Health Tips about the Physical and Mental Effects of Substance Abuse

Including Information about Marijuana, Inhalants, Club Drugs, Stimulants, Hallucinogens, Opiates, Prescription and Over-the-Counter Drugs, Herbal Products, Tobacco, Alcohol, and More

Edited by Sandra Augustyn Lawton. 468 pages. 2006. 978-0-7808-0862-1.

"A clearly written resource for general readers and researchers alike." *— School Library Journal*

"This book is well-balanced. ... a must for public and school libraries."
— VOYA: Voice of Youth Advocates, Dec '03

"The chapters are quick to make a connection to their teenage reading audience. The prose is straightforward and the book lends itself to spot reading. It should be useful both for practical information and for research, and it is suitable for public and school libraries."
— American Reference Books Annual, 2003

"Recommended reference source."
— Booklist, American Library Association, Feb '03

"This is an excellent resource for teens and their parents. Education about drugs and substances is key to discouraging teen drug abuse and this book provides this much needed information in a way that is interesting and factual." *— Doody's Review Service, Dec '02*

Eating Disorders Information for Teens

Health Tips about Anorexia, Bulimia, Binge Eating, and Other Eating Disorders

Including Information on the Causes, Prevention, and Treatment of Eating Disorders, and Such Other Issues as Maintaining Healthy Eating and Exercise Habits

Edited by Sandra Augustyn Lawton. 337 pages. 2005. 978-0-7808-0783-9.

"An excellent resource for teens and those who work with them."
— VOYA: Voice of Youth Advocates, Apr '06

"A welcome addition to high school and undergraduate libraries." *— American Reference Books Annual, 2006*

"This book covers the topic in a lucid manner but delves deeper into every aspect of an eating disorder. A solid addition for any nonfiction or reference collection." *— School Library Journal, Dec '05*

Fitness Information for Teens

Health Tips about Exercise, Physical Well-Being, and Health Maintenance

Including Facts about Aerobic and Anaerobic Conditioning, Stretching, Body Shape and Body Image, Sports Training, Nutrition, and Activities for Non-Athletes

Edited by Karen Bellenir. 425 pages. 2004. 978-0-7808-0679-5.

"Another excellent offering from Omnigraphics in their *Teen Health Series*. ... This book will be a great addition to any public, junior high, senior high, or secondary school library."
— American Reference Books Annual, 2005

Learning Disabilities Information for Teens

Health Tips about Academic Skills Disorders and Other Disabilities That Affect Learning

Including Information about Common Signs of Learning Disabilities, School Issues, Learning to Live with a Learning Disability, and Other Related Issues

Edited by Sandra Augustyn Lawton. 337 pages. 2005. 978-0-7808-0796-9.

"This book provides a wealth of information for any reader interested in the signs, causes, and consequences

of learning disabilities, as well as related legal rights and educational interventions. . . . Public and academic libraries should want this title for both students and general readers."
— *American Reference Books Annual, 2006*

Mental Health Information for Teens, 2nd Edition
Health Tips about Mental Wellness and Mental Illness
Including Facts about Mental and Emotional Health, Depression and Other Mood Disorders, Anxiety Disorders, Behavior Disorders, Self-Injury, Psychosis, Schizophrenia, and More

Edited by Karen Bellenir. 400 pages. 2006. 978-0-7808-0863-8.

"In both language and approach, this user-friendly entry in the *Teen Health Series* is on target for teens needing information on mental health concerns."
— *Booklist, American Library Association, Jan '02*

"Readers will find the material accessible and informative, with the shaded notes, facts, and embedded glossary insets adding appropriately to the already interesting and succinct presentation."
— *School Library Journal, Jan '02*

"This title is highly recommended for any library that serves adolescents and parents/caregivers of adolescents." — *E-Streams, Jan '02*

"Recommended for high school libraries and young adult collections in public libraries. Both health professionals and teenagers will find this book useful."
— *American Reference Books Annual, 2002*

"This is a nice book written to enlighten the society, primarily teenagers, about common teen mental health issues. It is highly recommended to teachers and parents as well as adolescents."
— *Doody's Review Service, Dec '01*

Pregnancy Information for Teens
Health Tips about Teen Pregnancy and Teen Parenting
Including Facts about Prenatal Care, Pregnancy Complications, Labor and Delivery, Postpartum Care, Pregnancy-Related Lifestyle Concerns, and More

Edited by Robert Aquinas McNally. 425 pages. 2007. 978-0-7808-0984-0.

Sexual Health Information for Teens
Health Tips about Sexual Development, Human Reproduction, and Sexually Transmitted Diseases
*Including Facts about Puberty, Reproductive Health, Chlamydia, Human Papillomavirus, Pelvic Inflam-*matory *Disease, Herpes, AIDS, Contraception, Pregnancy, and More*

Edited by Deborah A. Stanley. 391 pages. 2003. 978-0-7808-0445-6.

"This work should be included in all high school libraries and many larger public libraries. . . . highly recommended."
— *American Reference Books Annual, 2004*

"*Sexual Health* approaches its subject with appropriate seriousness and offers easily accessible advice and information." — *School Library Journal, Feb '04*

Skin Health Information for Teens
Health Tips about Dermatological Concerns and Skin Cancer Risks
Including Facts about Acne, Warts, Hives, and Other Conditions and Lifestyle Choices, Such as Tanning, Tattooing, and Piercing, That Affect the Skin, Nails, Scalp, and Hair

Edited by Robert Aquinas McNally. 429 pages. 2003. 978-0-7808-0446-3.

"This volume, as with others in the series, will be a useful addition to school and public library collections." — *American Reference Books Annual, 2004*

"There is no doubt that this reference tool is valuable."
— *VOYA: Voice of Youth Advocates, Feb '04*

"This volume serves as a one-stop source and should be a necessity for any health collection."
— *Library Media Connection*

Sports Injuries Information for Teens
Health Tips about Sports Injuries and Injury Protection
Including Facts about Specific Injuries, Emergency Treatment, Rehabilitation, Sports Safety, Competition Stress, Fitness, Sports Nutrition, Steroid Risks, and More

Edited by Joyce Brennfleck Shannon. 405 pages. 2003. 978-0-7808-0447-0.

"This work will be useful in the young adult collections of public libraries as well as high school libraries."
— *American Reference Books Annual, 2004*

Suicide Information for Teens
Health Tips about Suicide Causes and Prevention
Including Facts about Depression, Risk Factors, Getting Help, Survivor Support, and More

Edited by Joyce Brennfleck Shannon. 368 pages. 2005. 978-0-7808-0737-2.

Tobacco Information for Teens

Health Tips about the Hazards of Using Cigarettes, Smokeless Tobacco, and Other Nicotine Products

Including Facts about Nicotine Addiction, Immediate and Long-Term Health Effects of Tobacco Use, Related Cancers, Smoking Cessation, Tobacco Use Prevention, and Tobacco Use Statistics

Edited by Karen Bellenir. 440 pages. 2007. 978-0-7808-0976-5.